ISAACS REPORT – CONTENTS

Department of Health

Isaacs Report

The Investigation of Events that followed the death of **Cyril Mark Isaacs**

London: TSO

TSO

Published by TSO (The Stationery Office) and available from:

Online
www.tso.co.uk/bookshop

Mail, Telephone, Fax & E-mail
TSO
PO Box 29, Norwich, NR3 1GN
Telephone orders/General enquiries: 0870 600 5522
Fax orders: 0870 600 5533
E-mail: book.orders@tso.co.uk
Textphone 0870 240 3701

TSO Shops
123 Kingsway, London, WC2B 6PQ
020 7242 6393 Fax 020 7242 6394
68-69 Bull Street, Birmingham B4 6AD
0121 236 9696 Fax 0121 236 9699
9-21 Princess Street, Manchester M60 8AS
0161 834 7201 Fax 0161 833 0634
16 Arthur Street, Belfast BT1 4GD
028 9023 8451 Fax 028 9023 5401
18-19 High Street, Cardiff CF10 1PT
029 2039 5548 Fax 029 2038 4347
71 Lothian Road, Edinburgh EH3 9AZ
0870 606 5566 Fax 0870 606 5588

TSO Accredited Agents
(see Yellow Pages)

and through good booksellers

Published with the permission of the Department of Health on behalf of the Controller of Her Majesty's Stationery Office.

First published 2003

ISBN 0 11 322611 X

Printed in the United Kingdom for The Stationery Office
139946 C70 5/03

FOREWORD

This report was instigated by the events that took place following the untimely death of Mr Cyril Isaacs on 26 February 1987, and the post mortem examination that was carried out the following day at Prestwich Hospital mortuary on the instructions of the Coroner.

The need for an investigation of these events followed the discovery by Mr Isaacs' widow, Mrs Elaine Isaacs, on 5 April 2000 that the brain of her late husband had been retained during the post mortem on the morning of 27 February 1987 and taken later that day to Manchester University for use in research.

The retention of Mr Isaacs' brain and the intended use for research took place without the knowledge of Mr Isaacs' relatives. Had Mr Isaacs' family been aware at the time of the retention of any of Mr Isaacs' organs, this would have been vigorously opposed.

Mrs Isaacs submitted a detailed statement for the Chief Medical Officer's Summit on Organ Retention held on 11 January 2001. On 30 January in a debate in the House of Commons on the issues raised at the Summit, Mr Ivan Lewis MP drew attention to Mrs Isaacs' discovery that Mr Isaacs' brain had been retained without the consent of the family.

Annex 1

Appendix 1

Following the debate in the House of Commons, Mrs Isaacs' son, Dr Austin Isaacs, wrote on 19 March on behalf of himself and Mrs Isaacs to Mr Alan Milburn, the Secretary of State for Health, requesting an investigation into what occurred following the death of Mr Isaacs.

Annex 2

The Chief Medical Officer, at the request of the Secretary of State, held a meeting on 4 May 2001 with Mrs Isaacs, Dr Austin Isaacs, and Mr Ivan Lewis. The meeting, which was also attended by officials of the Home Office and Department of Health, agreed that further investigation was needed to find out what had taken place following Mr Isaacs' death, and why.

On 28 July I was appointed by the Secretary of State for Health, in my capacity as HM Inspector of Anatomy, to undertake the investigation of Mr Isaacs' death and, in particular, the retention and intended use for research of his brain.

Terms of Reference

In October 2001, following consideration of the scope of the investigation, I was given the following Terms of Reference:

"H.M. Inspector of Anatomy has been asked to carry out an independent investigation with the following Terms of Reference:

1. To investigate and document the procedures and circumstances which led to the removal and retention of organs of the late Cyril Mark Isaacs during the autopsy performed at Prestwich Mortuary on 27 February 1987;

2. To investigate what subsequently happened to the organs removed and retained;
3. To review whether similar removals of organs occurred at other public mortuaries after deaths outside hospitals;
4. To examine these events in the light of clinical and ethical policies, relevant legislation, religious beliefs, and the expectations and rights of relatives;
5. To report conclusions and recommendations to the Secretary of State for Health."

While the starting point of my investigation is the death of Mr Isaacs, my Terms of Reference were intentionally widely drawn. This was to require me also to investigate whether the circumstances of Mr Isaacs' death were unique, or whether similar retention of organs for use in research had taken place in other locations after post mortem examinations undertaken on the instructions of Coroners.

Procedure and method of working

While the Terms of Reference of my investigation were not formally announced, copies of these were made available to everyone who I have asked to assist me with this investigation, and to anyone else who enquired about the investigation, its scope and purposes.

Throughout the investigation I was assisted by Mr Jim Connelly of the Department of Health. We undertook all discussions jointly, with the single exception of my first meeting with Mrs Isaacs and Dr Isaacs in August 2000. This meeting took place before Mr Connelly had been appointed.

The first step in this investigation was to collate and read the considerable volume of papers that Mrs Elaine Isaacs had collected about the death of her husband. Thereafter the investigation was structured in four phases, which were sequentially:

i. identification of what happened after Mr Isaacs' death;
ii. investigation of organ retention for research at Manchester University;
iii. documentation of post mortem brain research at other locations;
iv. collation of the beliefs and views on the research use of retained organs from organisations representing religious, research and medical interests.

To prepare for the first phase of the investigation, the papers collected by Mrs Isaacs identified the persons who were directly involved in the police investigation of Mr Isaacs' death, the post mortem examination at Prestwich mortuary and the research team at Manchester University which received Mr Isaacs' brain.

In the first phase of the investigation, everyone identified during my initial review of records, letters and other documents were contacted by letter. An invitation was sent to everyone who could have relevant information to contribute to the investigation. The letters were modified to match each person's involvement in the events of February 1987. All those I wrote to were invited to tell me at a face to face meeting their recollection of events, procedures and practices that were in place at the time of Mr Isaacs' death sixteen years ago.

A similar methodology was used for later phases of the investigation. A summary record was prepared of every meeting or significant telephone conversation. Contemporaneous documents still available were obtained and copies made.

After the initial review of paper work, the pattern of working from then on followed the course of an investigation rather than a formal inquiry.

At this stage it is important to record that although no powers were available to me to compel anyone to respond, **all those who were invited agreed to a meeting and/or provided access to relevant documents that were still in their possession**. A full list of persons and organisations that responded to these requests or contributed to the investigation is at Annex 4. Annex 4

Phase one

During the first phase of the investigation its scope was broadened significantly for the following reasons:

- at a meeting at Manchester University in November 2001 the records of the brains received for research between 1985 and 1997 were provided. These records showed that large numbers of brains had been received from Coroners' post mortems undertaken in several different mortuaries in the Manchester area. As cases from Coroners' post mortems relevant to the investigation had been undertaken in hospital mortuaries as well as public mortuaries, and included some deaths of hospital inpatients, the categories of brain retention to be investigated were reviewed. It was decided that the investigation **would include all deaths where brains had been retained for research except for those where the post mortem examination had been undertaken with the consent of the relatives** following a death in hospital;

- the geographical coverage of the investigation was widened after the records reviewed during the first phase indicated that research or teaching on brains obtained from Coroners' post mortems had taken place in many other locations in England;

- a number of families who suspected that organs had been retained after Coroners' post mortems on their relatives in other locations contacted me.

Phases two and three

In phases two and three of the investigation these many contacts were followed up with visits to the research teams and NHS Trusts in other coronial districts. These visits included discussions with the Coroners and the staff of mortuaries and pathology departments. The visits are listed in Annex 5. Annex 5

To provide an overview of brain retention from Coroners' cases at locations that had not been identified from the above contacts, the Chief Medical Officer provided me with access to the returns received in response to the Survey of Retained Organs and Tissues that he had conducted in 2000. A questionnaire was sent to those NHS Trusts that I had not already visited to discover what policies and consent procedures they had operated in the late 1980s and early 1990s.

Phase four

In the context of my fourth Terms of Reference, contact was made with representatives of religious faiths to explore the acceptability or prohibition on post mortems and organ retention to those of different faiths. It should be noted that objections to these procedures are not confined to those who hold religious beliefs.

Validation of factual matters

To ensure the factual accuracy of this report, references to persons identified in it were shown, in draft, to the person concerned, except for those believed to be still alive, whose present whereabouts I could not discover. Where corrections of fact were required in the light of the comments received, these have been incorporated.

Structure of the report

The report is structured so that each chapter describes a different aspect of post mortems or organ retention. **I must emphasise that the Summary, Main Conclusions and Unanswered Questions sections of the report should not be read in isolation but in the context of the relevant sections of the report as a whole.**

There is inevitably overlap between chapters as each was intended to be self-contained. The first four chapters describe what happened to Mr Isaacs.

As organ retention after Coroners' post mortems proved to be much more extensive than envisaged when I was asked to undertake this work, I have concentrated on the retention of brains for research. The Chief Medical Officer's survey had shown that brains comprised almost half of all retained organs. In the time available I have not investigated the scope of other organ retention.

The joint programme

Much of the report addresses the research programme jointly arranged and undertaken by staff of the Departments of Psychiatry and Physiology of Manchester University. For ease of reference, and to distinguish this programme from other contemporary research in Manchester, this is referred to as the **"joint programme"**.

Main findings

These will be found in the chapter on "Conclusions" but there are many subsidiary findings in the summaries at the end of each chapter. These, while of lesser significance, deserve attention in their own right.

Documents referred to in the report

The correspondence and other relevant documents are included in separate volumes of annexes and appendices. The short documents are listed as annexes, while larger documents, including relevant statutes, are separately listed as appendices.

Acknowledgements

Responsibility for the content of the report, its conclusions and recommendations are entirely mine. In its preparation I wish to acknowledge the support and assistance I have had throughout the Investigation from Mr Jim Connelly, whose experience of investigative undertakings has been indispensable. I also wish to express my thanks to Miss Lesley Knight, Mrs Judith Peachey and Miss Patricia Browne, whose help with the preparation of the report has been invaluable. Many of the events I needed to investigate took place between 10 and 20 years ago and entailed the recovery of archived documents and papers.

I wish to record my particular thanks to Mrs Diane Turnbull, Clinical Governance Manager, Mental Health Services of Manchester; Mr Stanley Wilson, Pathology Services Manager at North Manchester General Hospital; and Mr Colin Carr, Pathology Manager at Addenbrooke's Hospital, for their assistance in retrieval of documents and arranging for me to see others who could provide relevant information.

Jeremy Metters

Dr Jeremy S Metters CB
HM Inspector of Anatomy

MAIN CONCLUSIONS

Introduction

This chapter highlights the main conclusions from my investigation, which should not be read isolation but in the context of relevant sections of the report as a whole.

At the end of each chapter is a summary of my findings on individual subjects. Some of these findings are more important than others. To bring all the points together would obscure the most significant conclusions. This chapter is, therefore, restricted to those findings that I consider are the most important. That is not to say that the other findings in the individual chapter summaries do not deserve attention in their own right.

Changing public attitudes

The events that I have investigated took place mainly between 1985 and 1995. Public and professional attitudes to post mortems and to the retention of organs and tissues were then very different to the present time. In 1985 the public was largely unaware of what happened during a post mortem and of the possibility of organ and tissue retention. Pathologists, morticians and others were aware of the details but rarely discussed these with relatives.

Those who knew about organ retention after Coroners' post mortems did not consider their actions were in any way unethical, let alone unlawful. Many consent forms for hospital post mortems did not make any reference to retention. There was a widespread belief that organ and tissue retention was in the "public interest" and that retention was lawful because the post mortem was carried out for the Coroner.

Over the last decade there has been a radical change in public knowledge and attitudes to these matters. The publication of the Redfern[1] and Kennedy[2] reports marked a turning point, but even before these reports attitudes were changing. People wanted to know more about what had previously happened "behind closed mortuary doors".

There is now a lot of information available for those who wish to know about post mortems, but there are still many who do not wish to be told in detail. Their right "not to know" should be respected.

Interface between Coroners' and hospital post mortems

My Terms of Reference were directed to organ retention from Coroners' post mortems and from community mortuaries. In reality, many Coroners make extensive use of NHS mortuaries. The events I have investigated in Manchester, Cambridge, Nottingham and elsewhere took place in NHS mortuaries. Organ retention after Coroners' post mortems cannot, therefore, be considered entirely in isolation from NHS mortuary procedures and practices.

Consent

The ethical imperative in medical practice and research

The guiding ethical principle of medical care and practice has been that a doctor must obtain the consent of his patient for any treatment or care and that consent must be freely obtained after the relevant information has been given to the patient.

The Nuremberg Code and subsequent codes governing the ethical practice of doctors set out the principle that patients must have autonomy to agree or refuse to take part in any medical research. Medical research, with a few well defined exceptions, must only take place with the patient's consent. These ethical principles have been further developed and refined in the last 50 years.

When the patient is unable to consent it has been common practice to seek the views of relatives, although in life the consent of relatives gives no legal authority. The relatives, however, are usually well placed to know whether the deceased had expressed any views on the use of organs for research.

The legal requirement

The consent of the relatives was given legal standing in the Human Tissue Act, 1961. Appendix 2
Section 1(1) of the Act makes clear that Parliament intended the wishes of the deceased to be taken into account when parts of his body were to be used for medical research. However, Section 1(2) makes it clear that the objections of relatives should be recognised and that tissues and organs should not be used for medical purposes when the relatives object.

To collect brains or other organs specifically for research without attempting to discover the views of the relatives is an abuse of the privilege, authorised by the Act, for the use of human organs and tissues with consent for medical purposes, including transplantation, research and teaching.

The requirement for consent from the relatives for research also applies when organs and tissues have been initially retained in Coroners' cases for diagnosis. The fact that a post mortem is carried out for the Coroner does not mean that the relatives' consent to carry out research can be assumed once the Coroner's need to retain organs has ended.

During the 1980s, a number of other research teams visited during the course of this Investigation were scrupulous in observing the legal requirements for consent by the relatives as required by the Human Tissue Act. In Manchester the Cerebral Function Unit (CFU), which is part of the Department of Neurology, had always obtained the consent of the relatives for any post mortem research on a deceased patient's brain.

Findings

Mr Isaacs' brain and the collection of brains in Manchester

The retention of Mr Isaacs' brain was part of a system set up in mortuaries in the Manchester area that during the twelve years from 1985 retained more than 225 brains from Coroners' post mortems for research without the knowledge of the relatives who had no opportunity to express their objections. Before the post mortem examination, Mrs Isaacs had emphasised the family's religious objections to a post mortem. She was unaware that organs were retained from post mortem examinations.

The research programme that received Mr Isaacs' brain was run jointly by the Department of Psychiatry and the Department of Physiology of Manchester University. Dr Bill Deakin led the research programme within the Department of Psychiatry and Dr Alan Cross and Dr Paul Slater within the Department of Physiology.

The referral of brains from the North Manchester Coroner's office began in November 1985 following telephone calls from the University received by Mrs Joyce Langan, the senior member of the Coroner's office staff.

Between 1985 and 1997, at least 311 brains were collected for this programme. Almost three-quarters of the brains were obtained from Coroners' cases. Of the 225 brains from Coroners' cases, 112 were identified through the North Manchester Coroner's Office. One hundred brains from Coroner's cases were collected for the programme by the mortician in the North Manchester General Hospital (NMGH) mortuary.

The relatives were not aware or asked for their consent when a brain was retained from a Coroner's case for research in the joint programme.

On an unrecorded date, probably in 1986, Dr Slater visited the offices of the Coroner for the North Manchester district in Rochdale. This impromptu visit occurred when Dr Slater was collecting a brain from Rochdale public mortuary. Mr Bryan North, the Coroner, was not in the office at the time and Dr Slater left him a letter. Mrs Langan's recollection is that, following this visit, Mr North reconfirmed that Dr Slater could be notified of cases, from among deaths reported, where the brain might be of interest to the joint programme.

Mr Isaacs' brain was identified through this system. Forty-five other brains were similarly collected from Prestwich mortuary. Sixty-six further brains were collected from Coroners' cases in mortuaries at Bury, Oldham and Rochdale.

The mortician at NMGH was led to collecting brains from Coroner's and hospital cases by a letter from Dr Deakin that stated the research had Ethics Committee approval. This letter had followed telephone calls from the joint programme to Mr Leatherbarrow.

The post mortem reports submitted to Mr Gorodkin, the Coroner for Central Manchester, and other Coroners did not, with one or two exceptions, mention the fact that brains had been retained for research. In particular, Mr Gorodkin and his staff had no means of knowing that brains were being collected from the NMGH mortuary.

There was confusion in some mortuaries as the separate research programme of the Cerebral Function Unit was also collecting brains, but these were collected with the knowledge and consent of the relatives.

The joint programme

This programme collected brains specifically for research. Diagnostic histology was only undertaken in 37 cases. Reports on the research were not made to the Coroners or to the doctors who had looked after hospital in-patient cases.

In seeking research funds for the programme, the consent of the relatives was emphasised in applications to funding bodies and in protocols to the local Ethics Committees (ECs).

Ethics Committees and research funding bodies were not told that most of the brains collected in the programme were from Coroners' cases.

Applications to ECs were made by Dr Deakin on behalf of the joint programme. Although the Ethics Committees had not been told about collection of brains from Coroners' cases, letters sent to general practitioners requesting medical details of their deceased patient stated that the studies *"had ethical approval"*. The GMC guidance, current at the time, was that information should only be released for research that had ethical approval.

The letters also misinformed general practitioners by referring to *"brain samples"* when, in most cases, the research team had the whole brain.

The collection of brains of long-stay patients in mental hospitals who had no relatives was, in one letter, encouraged in the following terms: *"Often chronic patients don't have next of kin, in which case there is no difficulty"*. This disregards the need for consent from those responsible for vulnerable patients who had no one else to speak for them.

In correspondence to consultants, the need for the use of local consent forms for hospital post mortems was included. However, these forms are not relevant to the majority of brains collected from Coroner's cases.

Professor Deakin states that he did not intend deliberately to mislead anyone.

Brain collections in other locations

Research on brains retained was widespread in the 1980s. Scrupulous care was taken by the CFU and by some research teams elsewhere to ensure that the consent of the relatives was obtained when brains were collected from hospital cases.

The distinction between hospital and Coroners' post mortems became blurred in many locations and with it the research use of brains from Coroners' cases was deemed to be acceptable. Brains from Coroners' cases were frequently obtained as "controls", as "normal" brains were difficult to obtain.

In most locations brains from Coroners' cases used in research had first been retained for diagnosis. Once the Coroner's purposes had been completed, these brains were used in research rather than being sent for disposal.

Of the locations visited in this investigation, the collection of brains from Coroners' cases specifically for research, without any requirement for diagnostic histology, took place only in Manchester and Cambridge.

Questionnaire to centres not visited

A questionnaire to centres that were not visited during the investigation showed that more than 21,000 brains collected between 1970 and 1999 were still held. The majority of these had been retained from Coroners' cases, and in a few locations the brains had been collected specifically for research.

All those involved in research on brains from Coroners' cases considered the research was "in the public good". It was not recognised that brain retention for research, without the knowledge of relatives, did not comply with the Human Tissue Act. Covert research on retained brains is offensive to many relatives, particularly those of faith groups, who ask why they had no opportunity to voice their objections.

Why was brain retention so common in Coroners' cases?

My enquiries at other locations and the responses to the questionnaire sent to centres that were not visited, show that retention of brains, and of other organs, from Coroners' cases had taken place on a very wide scale. Why?

After the Human Tissue Act in 1961, a circular about the implications of the Act was issued by the Ministry of Health. This was to encourage Corneal donation. A further circular was issued later to encourage collection of Pituitaries as part of the national collection programme. These circulars stated that, while the body was on hospital premises, the NHS authorities were *"in possession of the body"* and could therefore consent to removal of tissue during the post mortem.

The circulars helped to establish the belief that consent of the relatives to tissue removal was not required once they had consented to a hospital post mortem. Pathologists carried out all post mortem examinations in the same way and to the same standards.

It was widely assumed that the circulars to the NHS applied to Coroners' cases where the post mortem was carried out in an NHS mortuary.

Many pathologists, morticians and researchers assumed that the Coroner had the authority to retain any organ, irrespective of whether the examination of that organ had a bearing on the cause of death.

There was a widespread belief that consent was not needed from the relatives for further retention of brains after the Coroner no longer needed the brain for purposes of determining the cause of death.

The retention of the brain of Mr David Webb from a Coroner's post mortem for a research project on suicide illustrates what can happen when the distinction between hospital and Coroners' post mortems becomes blurred. In this case, as in the case of

Mr Isaacs, it was assumed that relatives had no objections to organ retention for research.

Objections to post mortems

There have always been objections to post mortems from some faith groups, in particular those of the Hindu, Jewish and Moslem faiths. Similar objections are held by some Christian groups and by individuals.

There will always be some deaths where a post mortem is required for legal reasons. The Coroner must have the right to order a post mortem in such cases.

However, there are measures that can be taken to respond to those who object to post mortems. These include limiting the extent of the post mortem or adopting other methods of identifying the cause of death, such as Magnetic Resonance Imaging (MRI).

Distress to relatives from organ retention

While some relatives have no objections to post mortems or organ retention, the discovery by others that the brain of a close relative has been retained without the knowledge of the family has, on many occasions, been the cause of great distress. These relatives, had they been asked, would have objected. Some relatives who might have agreed to organ retention also feel deceived in that they were not asked

Many relatives believed they had buried or cremated their loved one's body complete. They feel an acute sense of being deceived and cheated. Their grievance is even more intense when a Coroner's post mortem was carried out despite their objections.

For those whose religious beliefs require that all organs should be returned to the body, the added discovery that the brain, or other retained organ, has been subsequently disposed of without their knowledge adds to their distress and sense of betrayal.

Even for relatives who are not, in principle, opposed to organ retention, the uncertainty of "not knowing" whether organs had been retained has caused prolonged anxiety and anger because, in many places, no disposal records were kept.

Benefits to society of post mortem research

There is no doubt of the advances in medical knowledge and, more importantly, the benefits and improvements that have resulted in the care of patients from discoveries made by research on retained organs. Research in this country has been at the forefront of international achievement in neuropsychiatric research. The importance of research on retained organs cannot be underestimated and steps must be taken to encourage organ donation for research, but this must always be with the safeguard of informed consent by the relatives in every case.

Responsibility and audit in Coroners' post mortems

There is at present no system of quality assurance or audit of Coroners' post mortems.

In some locations there was confusion about who is responsible for an NHS mortuary and the staff involved when irregularities occur during a Coroner's post mortem.

Public confidence

Many pathologists have indicated that, to avoid distress to the relatives, they had not mentioned organ retention in post mortem reports. The pathologists' motives were well intentioned but are no longer acceptable or compatible with the culture of openness which must now prevail.

Although the pathologists' intentions were to avoid distress, the covert retention of organs from Coroners' post mortems for research and teaching has seriously undermined public confidence and jeopardised benefits from research for the future.

For the future

It is essential that steps are taken to re-establish public confidence that research will only be undertaken with consent.

The present references in the Human Tissue Act to *"lack of objection"* have not prevented unauthorised retention of organs and tissues. In future, consent by the relatives must be the rule, not the exception.

For public confidence to be restored, complete openness is required from all involved in post mortem procedures.

Nevertheless, there will be some relatives who do not wish to be informed of the details. For those, unwelcome information must not be forced upon them.

References

1. The Royal Liverpool Children's Inquiry Report, 2001.
2. The Bristol Royal Infirmary Inquiry Report, 2000.

UNANSWERED QUESTIONS ABOUT THE JOINT PROGRAMME

At the end of my investigation of the joint programme in Manchester, a number of questions remain for which I consider no satisfactory explanation has been provided. These questions should not be read in isolation but in the context of relevant sections of the report as a whole. These are:

1. From the start of the joint research programme the brains of Coroners' cases were collected. Why were the Coroners not explicitly asked for their agreement to retention of brains for the research programme?

2. Why were brains collected before January 1986? This was the first date that any ethical approval was given. Any brain collection prior to that date for research purposes should have had ethical approval.

3. Why were Ethics Committees not explicitly informed about the joint research programme's plans to use the brains from Coroners' cases? Why, in particular in July 1986 when the submission was made to the South/North Manchester Ethics Committees, did the protocol not refer to the obtaining of brains from Coroners' cases? In July 1986 the joint team knew (or should have known) that 20 out of the 24 brains collected were Coroners' cases.

4. Why was the intention to collect brains from Coroners' cases not explicit in the applications to research funding bodies? There were no references to Coroners' cases in the 1988 application to the North West Regional Health Authority (NWRHA) when the team knew (or shown have known) that 52 out of the 61 brains collected by the programme before that date had been obtained from Coroners' cases?

   Similarly, in the subsequent applications to the NWRHA and the first to the Medical Research Council (MRC), why was there no reference to Coroners' cases when an even higher proportion of the brains already collected were obtained from Coroners' post mortems?

   The question of obtaining consent for "control" brains was obscured in the protocols submitted to Ethics Committees in 1986 and subsequently.

5. The main sources of brains for the joint programme were Coroners' cases. Professor Deakin, in correspondence to me dated 10 January 2003, has emphasised that at the time of the applications to the ECs, he believed that *"the sources of the brains were legal and ethical"*.

   If this was his belief at the time, why was the use of Coroners' cases as the main source of brains not made clear in the applications? The same applies to the three research applications to the NWRHA and to the first two applications to the MRC.

6. Why had the team encouraged morticians to provide brains of index and "control" cases without the knowledge or consideration of any objections from the relatives, by referring to Ethical Committee approval? The Ethics

Committees had only partial knowledge about brain retention procedures when they were asked for their approval.

7. Why in the 1980s when the team wrote to general practitioners did the letter about cases obtained from Coroner's post mortems:

   (a) refer to *"brain tissues"*, when what had been collected was the whole brain and
   (b) state that *"these studies have ethical approval"* when the Ethics Committees had not been given all the relevant information?

8. When the Salford and North Manchester Ethics Committees considered the applications from the joint team in January and July 1986 respectively, why were the Committees not told that brains from Coroners' cases were to be collected?

   The General Medical Council's guidance at the time was that:

   "information may be disclosed if necessary for the purpose of a medical research project which has been approved by a recognised ethical committee".

   Were the research team aware that the letters sent to the general practitioners led them to provide information for a research project where details had not been disclosed to the relevant Ethics Committees?

9. Why were no progress reports submitted to Ethics Committees?

10. In 1991, the guidelines to LRECs specified that research on *"the recently dead in NHS premises"* should be referred for LREC approval. Why was no action taken to inform the LRECs that Coroners' cases in NHS hospitals were included in the research programme?

11. Why were in patients in mental hospitals who had no relatives described as *"often chronic inpatients don't have next of kin in which case there is no difficulty"* when the NHS guidance circular required consent from the Hospital Secretary/Chief Executive, who should have made his own investigations before agreeing to the post mortem?

12. Why are there no consent forms in the hospital patients' notes that are still available?

13. Why do none of the documents about the programme state that two-thirds of the brains were obtained from Coroners' cases?

14. Why was the letter from Dr Deakin to Mr Leatherbarrow drafted in terms that could be regarded as providing inducements?

15. In 1994, Mr Leatherbarrow received payments from the University for more than 40 brains obtained from the North Manchester General Hospital mortuary

for the joint programme. Why, in that year, are only three brains from this mortuary recorded in the brain books?

16. Why did the joint programme become so reliant on Coroners' cases, although the applications to funding bodies had emphasised the requirements for consent?

17. Why were the Coroners of the Central Manchester and Cheshire districts not asked about retention of brains?

RECOMMENDATIONS

Introduction

This chapter sets out the action and recommendations that in my view should follow from my findings. It is important to remember that this investigation followed the chance discovery by Mrs Elaine Isaacs in April 2000 that the brain of her late husband had been retained for research in February 1987.

Had Mrs Isaacs not come across the letter sent to Mr Isaacs' general practitioner by the joint research team, she would never have known that her husband's brain had been retained, and the widespread retention of brains, and other organs, from Coroners' post mortems might have remained undisclosed.

Most of the brains from Coroners' cases in the 1980s and 1990s were initially held for entirely proper diagnostic investigation into the cause of death. A very much smaller number were retained specifically for research or teaching. The feature that unifies both these categories is that very few relatives were aware of the practice and I found no evidence that any were asked for their consent for later research or teaching use. In this way the requirements of the Human Tissue Act were consistently disregarded.

I have not investigated the extent to which relatives who signed consent forms for hospital post mortems were aware of the possibility of organ retention and that research or teaching use might follow. Among the limited number of consent forms that I have examined, few specifically mention organ retention. It appears the assumption was made that a signed post mortem consent form also indicated agreement to organ and tissue retention. It will never be known how many relatives were aware that organs might be retained from hospital post mortems without their knowledge.

Parallel investigations and policy reviews

Two major Government initiatives and the Shipman Public Inquiry have been in progress since my investigation began. These each have areas of common interest with the events I describe in this report:

> The Retained Organs Commission (ROC) was established as a Special Health Authority by the Secretary of State for Health in April 2001 in the aftermath of the Redfern Report. The ROC's Terms of Reference are at Annex 6. Annex 6
>
> The Home Office Fundamental Review of Death Certification and Coroner Services in England, Wales and Northern Ireland was announced on 23 March 2001. The Terms of Reference for the Review are at Annex 7. Annex 7
>
> The Shipman Public Inquiry, chaired by Dame Janet Smith, was announced on 31 January 2001. The Terms of Reference are at Annex 8. Annex 8

The recommendations set out below follow from the Terms of Reference I was given and the findings made during this investigation. I have endeavoured to take account of the consultation papers and interim reports of these important bodies and my recommendations are not intended to anticipate or detract from the recommendations of their work.

In particular, the first report of the Shipman Inquiry has illustrated the vital importance of evidence that can be obtained from retained organs, tissues and other post mortem specimens.

The objectives of these recommendations

My recommendations have four objectives:

1. **The primary and overriding objective must be the introduction of legal, administrative, ethical and other requirements designed to ensure that organs and tissues retained from Coroners' post mortems will not be retained for or used in research or teaching without the knowledge and consent of the relatives.**

2. The second objective is to restore public confidence in post mortem procedures and practices to enable organs and tissues to be used in research that cannot be undertaken during life, to improve treatment and care for the benefit of future generations **but only with the full and proper consent of relatives.**

3. Third, to ensure that the objections of those who do not agree to post mortem examinations or organ retention are recognised and, in respect of Coroners' post mortems, to facilitate religious observances to the extent that these are compatible with the Coroner's investigations.

4. To clarify those features of the current Rules and procedures that have created uncertainty.

The recommendations below are intended to restore public confidence that organs and tissues will not be used in research or for teaching without the knowledge and consent of relatives. To achieve these objectives a series of changes are needed to administrative and other procedures in professional and employment practices and to the law.

I. To prevent unauthorised organ and tissue retention

Review of relevant law relating to unauthorised removal of organs and tissues

The unauthorised removal and retention of organs and tissues from Coroners' post mortems for research, without the knowledge or agreement of the relatives, is the central issue of my investigation. The Human Tissue Act refers simply to "lack of objection" rather than "consent" **but retention of organs and tissues for research without the knowledge and consent of the relatives must never be permitted to recur.**

The most certain way to ensure there is no recurrence of unlawful organ and tissue retention is through a change to strengthen the law. The Department of Health has recently issued a consultation document on possible changes to the Human Tissue Act and the Anatomy Act.

The Shipman Inquiry has issued a discussion paper "Developing a new system for death certification".

The Home Office Fundamental Review of Coroners Services has conducted a separate consultation which outlines alternative arrangements for certifying death and for possible changes in Coroners' services.

The Retained Organs Commission is considering many issues that bear on the retention of organs and tissues.

From their interim reports and consultation documents, these inquiries and reviews are likely to recommend changes in the law that will affect post mortem procedures and practice.

Human Tissue Act

In my view there are serious weaknesses in the Human Tissue Act. Unlike the Anatomy Act, there are no record-keeping requirements in the Human Tissue Act and no penalties for those who disregard its provisions.

The lack of penalties is a serious weakness. In my opinion, when the opportunity arises to amend or replace the Human Tissue Act, the following changes are needed:

Recommendation 1a

- the retention of organs and tissues from post mortems, without legally defined and valid consent, should be made an offence;

1b

- there should be appropriate penalties for unauthorised retention in the legislation;

1c

- the term "lack of objection" should be replaced by "with consent of".

Until the law can be changed, there are other steps that will deter anyone who might be tempted to retain organs and tissues without proper consent. Therefore, unauthorised organ and tissue retention should become:

Recommendation 2

- a disciplinary offence within the Terms and Conditions of Service for (i) local authority staff working in public mortuaries and (ii) NHS staff working in hospital mortuaries;

Recommendation 3

- the General Medical Council should specify in professional guidance to medical practitioners that unauthorised organ and tissue retention will be subject to professional discipline.

Retention of "material" under Coroners Rules 9 and 12

These sections of the Coroners Rules have caused confusion to Coroners, pathologists and researchers.

Recommendation 4

- To resolve this confusion, the Rules need to be revised or clear guidance provided to clarify the legality of organ and tissue retention in the following circumstances:

  (a) when criminal legal action will or is likely to follow completion of the Coroner's action;
  (b) when civil legal action may follow after the Coroner's action has ended;
  (c) in the absence of instructions from the Coroner, for how long the pathologist may hold the retained material before it is disposed of in accordance with the instructions of relatives.

II. To ensure that consent for retention is properly obtained

Consent forms and retention of organs and tissues

The relatives' consent is not required for a Coroner's post mortem. However, the possibility of organ or, more probably, tissue retention should be explained and the reasons for this. This already happens in many districts.

The relatives should be asked for their wishes regarding disposal of any retained tissues; one option might be to delay the cremation or funeral until the retained tissues can be returned to the body. This should always be explained.

Recommendation 5

- The relatives should be routinely asked for their wishes for disposal of any organs or tissues retained from a Coroner's post mortem and systems put in place to ensure that these wishes are carried out.

Recommendation 6

- Organ and tissue retention forms, similar to those already in use in many districts, should be introduced everywhere.

Recommendation 7

- All post mortem reports should include full and accurate details of all organs, tissues and other tissue samples retained.

Recommendation 8

- Relatives, unless they decline, should be informed about what samples have been retained.

Recommendation 9

- Relatives should be given the opportunity to indicate whether eventual disposal of retained tissues should be (a) a delayed cremation or funeral to allow the tissues to be returned to the body; (b) returned to them after disposal of the body; (c) undertaken by the hospital; (d) donated for medical research.

<u>In respect of hospital post mortems</u>:

Recommendation 10

- Post mortem consent forms should have separate sections seeking (a) consent to the examination and (b) additional consent for organ and tissue retention. Relatives must know that they can refuse consent to the examination and they can separately consent to the post mortem but not to retention, if that is their wish.

Recommendation 11

- Relatives must never be pressured to agree to a hospital post mortem under the threat that if they do not agree the death will be reported to the Coroner.

III. <u>To ensure relatives are fully and properly informed when decisions are taken</u>

<u>Information and support for relatives following deaths reported to Coroners</u>

The sudden death of a relative is among the most stressful of life's experiences and the closer the relative the greater the distress. The same usually holds true for the relatives of those whose deaths are reported to the Coroner for other reasons.

Many who are suddenly bereaved are "in shock" in the days that immediately follow. More ready access is needed to the advice, support and counselling that is available for the relatives of those who die in NHS hospitals. In the community, similar help is provided by many voluntary organisations and faith groups, but many relatives do not know to whom to turn.

Recommendation 12

- Information about "what will happen next" during the Coroner's investigations should always be explained fully and with sympathy. The relatives should be told of their rights.

Recommendation 13

- When there is likely to be a Coroner's post mortem, the reasons for the examination should be explained unless the relatives do not wish to be given details.

Recommendation 14

- When for the Coroner's purposes a formal statement is needed, there should be no pressure on a relative for its urgent completion or duress over the contents. While "in shock", erroneous information may too easily be included.

Recommendation 15

- As many relatives do not, at first, take in details of what is explained to them a written summary should be provided.

Recommendation 16

- Support from NHS and voluntary sector bereavement services should be made more accessible to relatives of those whose deaths are reported to Coroners, particularly after sudden death. The range and availability of such local services should be more widely advertised.

Research and teaching use of retained organs and tissues

When the relatives are asked for consent to organ or tissue retention for diagnosis it must not, as in the past, be assumed that consent extends to research or teaching. In a hospital post mortem, when the relatives consent to diagnostic organ or tissue retention, separate consent is needed for research or teaching use. The same principle applies to consented research on organs and tissues from Coroners' post mortems.

The nature of the research should be explained. If organs or tissues are retained for research that has not yet been planned, this must be explained. Blanket consent for any research is not enough. In particular, if genetic or other research which may affect other members of the family is planned, the relatives should be asked specifically about this.

If there will be tissues for disposal at the end of the research, the relatives should be informed and asked about their instructions for disposal.

Recommendation 17

- Consent forms for research or teaching use should be specific to the purpose and investigation for which the organs or tissues have been retained.

Recommendation 18

- Genetic or other research that could affect other family members must be carefully explained before consent is requested.

IV. Role of NHS Trusts in organ and tissue retention

There are particular problems about consent where a person dies in the NHS without known relatives or next of kin. Guidance circulars place on NHS authorities "in possession of the body" the authority to consent to a post mortem and to organ and tissue retention after the death of a patient without known relatives.

It is not axiomatic that all those who die in NHS hospitals and have no next of kin would agree to their organs being retained for research. This is particularly relevant to patients who have been long-stay residents in hospital care.

Recommendation 19

- An independent authority should be given the responsibility for deciding whether a hospital post mortem and/or organ retention for research should follow the death in hospital of a person who has no known relatives or next of kin.

Coroners' post mortems in NHS mortuaries

There is confusion in some locations over who is responsible for the inappropriate actions of NHS mortuary staff when a post mortem is carried out in an NHS mortuary.

Recommendation 20

- The confusion over who is responsible for the conduct of NHS staff during Coroners' post mortems in NHS mortuaries should be resolved urgently.

V. Ethical approval and supervision of research on retained organs and tissues

Ethics Committees, organisations that fund research, Universities and other bodies that host research should all have procedures in place to ensure that all the projects they facilitate have received appropriate ethical approval.

Ethics Committees

There must now be no lingering doubts about the importance of Ethics Committee approval for research on retained organs and tissues. All such research, including the use of archived material, should be considered by a properly constituted Ethics Committee.

Ethics Committees should ensure that changes to research protocols are notified to them and that progress reports on research reach them by the due date.

Recommendation 21

- Ethics Committees should give particular attention to the consent forms that are proposed for any research using retained organs and tissues.

Research funding organisations

Research funding organisations have rightly requested information about the ethical approval of research applications submitted to them for funding. However, the ethics approval quoted in support of some research applications investigated had been given for a different project.

Recommendation 22

- Organisations that provide funds for research on retained organs and tissues should include in their procedures steps to check that the ethical approval quoted relates directly to the research that is under consideration.

Recommendation 23

- In complex areas of research on retained organs and tissues, research funding organisations should consider establishing their own Ethics Review Committees.

Universities and organisations that host post mortem research

Universities and other institutions that host research on retained organs and tissues on their premises should be aware of the special sensitivities of this research.

Recommendation 24

- Universities and other institutions should establish their own Ethics Committees which must be notified of all external grant support and Ethics Committee approvals obtained by their staff.

VI. Staff training

There are limited training opportunities for staff in Coroners' offices and also for mortuary staff. Many staff learn their duties through in-service experience without prior structured training. Coroners' Officers, staff of Coroners' offices and public mortuaries meet bereaved people at a time of great stress.

Recommendation 25

- Staff in Coroners' offices, Coroners' Officers, morticians and other staff involved in Coroners' post mortems should be given training better to assist and help the relatives and to explain the reasons for a Coroner's post mortem.

Recommendation 26

- Guidelines should be developed on all aspects of public mortuary practice and for NHS mortuaries where Coroners' post mortems are carried out.

Recommendation 27

- Systems for the audit and quality assurance of Coroners' post mortems are required, and similarly for the procedures and practices in public mortuaries.

VII. Recognition of the views of those who oppose post mortem examinations and organ retention

While the majority of the community may not hold firm views on post mortems and organ retention, there are some who regard these procedures as abhorrent and incompatible with their sincerely held beliefs. When a death is reported to a Coroner it is important that the sincerely held beliefs of the deceased or his relatives are rapidly identified. To acknowledge and, where possible, respect those who hold these beliefs:

Recommendation 28

- enquiries should be routinely made about the religion of the deceased, which should be stated in the papers that accompany each body to the mortuary and/or included in the information obtained by the Coroner's Officer;

Recommendation 29

- in the interval between death and burial or cremation, religious ceremonies and rituals that do not interfere with the Coroner's investigation should be permitted;

Recommendation 30

- a post mortem should not be carried out routinely where the cause of death can be established without one. Also, a limited post mortem procedure will be more acceptable than a full procedure to some faith communities;

Recommendation 31

- alternative methods for establishing the cause of death, such as Magnetic Resonance Imaging, require further evaluation to see if these will provide an alternative to post mortem examinations in a proportion of sudden deaths;

Recommendation 32

- use of toxicology may identify the cause of death in some cases and avoid the need for a post mortem examination;

Recommendation 33

- as the retention of organs and tissues poses major religious difficulties for some faith communities, these procedures should be avoided if possible.

Return of retained organs to faith communities

There are collections of retained organs which are known to include those of persons of the Jewish or Muslim faith. In some locations there are simple ways of identifying persons from these faith communities, either from the Mortuary Registers or by other means.

Recommendation 34

- In locations where retained organs and tissues from those of the Jewish or Muslim faiths are known to exist and can be identified, these organs should be returned to the religious authorities for burial, even when their return has not been requested by the relatives of the deceased.

SECTION 1

What happened after Mr Isaacs' death

CHAPTER 1

The death of Cyril Mark Isaacs

Introduction

This chapter describes the circumstances of Mr Isaacs' death and events that followed in the interval before his burial the following day.

Sources of information

- Mrs Isaacs' statement for the Chief Medical Officer's Summit; Annex 1
- witness statements at the inquest into Mr Isaacs' death; Annexes 9-13
- records provided by Greater Manchester police;
- recollections of Mrs Isaacs, Dr Rosenberg, Dr Farrand and Mr Walkden.

Background

Although the starting point of this investigation is the death of Mr Isaacs on 26 February 1987, aged 54, it is important to include in the record some relevant details of his mental health shortly before his death. This is to provide the context for concerns expressed later by his family. It is also important to emphasise Mr Isaacs' and his family's religious beliefs. The disregard of Mr Isaacs' mental health problems before his death, and of his religious beliefs, became the cause of great distress to Mrs Isaacs and her son, Austin.

Mr Isaacs' health

In the five months before his untimely death, Mr Isaacs had experienced depressive mental illness and had been under medical care from a number of both private and NHS doctors. He had taken three overdoses, two of these in the same weekend within one month of his death. Mr Isaacs had also received in-patient psychiatric care as a voluntary patient. He had been prescribed medication at the time of his death and was due to see his general practitioner, Dr Rosenberg, on 27 February. Annex 1

Mr Isaacs' religious beliefs

Mr Isaacs and his family are Orthodox Jews and follow the observation of Jewish Law.

The afternoon of Thursday 26 February 1987

In the early afternoon of 26 February Mrs Isaacs made an emergency call to the police, as she had been frightened after her husband had grabbed her wrists. The police had had to trace the telephone call after Mr Isaacs pulled the telephone plug from its socket whilst Mrs Isaacs was starting to speak. Calm was restored by the time the police arrived. Mrs Isaacs shortly after telephoned a friend, Mrs Eunice Foster, who came to see both Mr and Mrs Isaacs. Not long after Mrs Foster had left, Mr Isaacs for the second time that day grabbed his wife's wrists. Mrs Isaacs decided she would stay that night at Mrs Foster's house as she lived nearby.

Later that afternoon Mrs Isaacs needed to return home to collect some overnight clothes. As she was concerned about going home on her own, she asked the late Mr Clive Lingard, a relative, to accompany her to the house.

On arrival Mrs Isaacs noticed that the downstairs rooms were in darkness but there was a light on upstairs. After entering the house Mrs Isaacs asked Mr Lingard to go upstairs and switch the light off. Mr Lingard proceeded up the staircase as requested, but immediately turned round and guided Mrs Isaacs into the kitchen saying at the same time there had been a terrible accident, or words to that effect. Mr Lingard immediately telephoned for the police and while awaiting their arrival prevented Mrs Isaacs from going to the staircase.

Two police officers attended in response to Mr Lingard's 999 call at 7.00pm, arriving at the house within minutes. WPC Sharon Rigby, one of the officers, later wrote the report of the visit and provided a statement for the Coroner. This statement formed part of the evidence considered at the inquest. Although every effort was made to identify the second police officer in attendance, this has not been possible. The documents that still exist do not mention the name or number of the second officer.

Soon after the arrival of the police Mrs Isaacs was told that her husband was dead. His body, which had been found suspended through the hatch into the loft, was taken down. At 7.50pm Dr Abendstern, the duty police surgeon, confirmed that life was extinct. Annex 9

A fuller account of events as recalled by Mrs Isaacs is at Annex 1. Annex 1

First mention of a post mortem

While awaiting the arrival of the police surgeon, Mrs Isaacs was required to remain in the kitchen in the company of WPC Rigby. When Mrs Isaacs tried to leave the kitchen she was restrained from so doing. During this time, the probability of a post mortem to determine the cause of death was first mentioned.

Mrs Isaacs replied that Jewish Law forbade post mortems and, as the cause of death was obvious, no post mortem was needed to find out why Mr Isaacs had died.

When Mrs Isaacs was informed that Mr Isaacs' body would be removed to the mortuary she pointed out that in accordance with Jewish Law his body should remain in the house so that prayers could be said. A person of the Jewish faith should also be present to sit with Mr Isaacs' body during the night prior to burial, which must take place the following day.

Mrs Isaacs also asked the police if they would be contacting the hospitals where her husband had been a patient. The police asked her for details of Mr Isaacs' general practitioner. Mrs Isaacs advised that Dr Bethel Rosenberg was the family general practitioner. Mrs Isaacs believed that Dr Rosenberg would be able to confirm to the police and the Coroner that no post mortem was necessary because of Mr Isaacs' mental illness prior to and at the time of his death and in view of Mr Isaacs' religious beliefs.

Monday 2 March 1987 was mentioned by the police as the likely date of the post mortem. Mrs Isaacs stressed to the police that her husband had to be buried as soon as possible the following day, Friday 27 February, in order to meet the requirements of Jewish Law.

Mrs Isaacs spoke to Dr Rosenberg on the telephone. He was unable to attend and recommended that Mrs Isaacs should have an injection so that she would sleep. Dr Rosenberg would have arranged for this but Mrs Isaacs did not wish to receive sedation.

While the police records of what was said to Mrs Isaacs no longer exist, in the interval before Mr Isaacs' body was removed from the house, Mrs Isaacs was asked a number of questions by the police and a statement was obtained from her.

It was Mrs Isaacs' wish that their son, Austin, should arrive home before his father's body was removed. While the police were continuing their immediate investigations, arrangements were made through a relative for Austin to return home from University in London. However, he was not able to arrive until the early hours of the following morning due to distance and time factors. Austin was distressed when he arrived home and angry that his father's body had been taken from the house without the permission of the family.

Removal of Mr Isaacs' body to Prestwich mortuary

Once the police had fully documented the scene of Mr Isaacs' death, his body was removed to the mortuary at Prestwich Hospital which at that time served both as a hospital and public mortuary. The firm of local undertakers on duty for the police were called to convey the body to the mortuary. The time of arrival was logged in the mortuary at 20.45(1). Mrs Isaacs was unaware that undertakers had been called to transfer Mr Isaacs' body as she had assumed an ambulance would be called for this purpose.

As Mr Isaacs' death was "unnatural", the police reported his death to the office of the Coroner for North Manchester Police District.

Mrs Isaacs was later to complain that on the day of Mr Isaacs' death, her rights and those of her husband had been violated in the following ways:

- the police had unnecessarily restrained her in the kitchen while they investigated her husband's death upstairs;

- there was no justification for the removal of Mr Isaacs' body from the house until her son had returned home;

- removal of Mr Isaacs' body to Prestwich mortuary prevented the observance of the requirements of Jewish Law;

- she was required to sign a statement, the contents of which did not reflect the words she had used when speaking to the police. This statement was taken at a time when Mrs Isaacs was greatly distressed and she believes she signed under duress, as it contained information that was not factually correct;

- in respect of the foregoing point, Mrs Isaacs is clear that she did not see her husband's body before it was removed from the family home and therefore she could not have identified him as she had been prevented from going upstairs by the police before the removal of Mr Isaacs' body;

- no one told her that the Coroners Rules enabled her to have an independent representative at the post mortem.

These are not matters that come within the scope of my investigation, but Chapter 45 is relevant to the observance of religious rituals when these do not interfere with the investigation undertaken for the Coroner.

Friday 27 February 1987

Early in the morning the police contacted Mrs Isaacs to say that the post mortem would take place on Monday 2 March but that she should attend the Coroner's Court in Rochdale that morning for the opening of the inquest into the death of her husband.

Mrs Isaacs again pointed to the requirement in Jewish Law that the burial should take place that day. The fact that Mr Isaacs was Jewish must then have been recognised by a member of the Coroner's staff as arrangements were made for the post mortem to be brought forward, and the examination took place at 11.00am[1].

The Chazan from the Whitefield and Hebrew Synagogues, of which the Isaacs family were members, came round in the early morning to see Mrs Isaacs and her son, Austin. The Chazan also spoke to the Coroner's office to arrange a time for the burial. This call was made from Mrs Isaacs' home as she was leaving to go to the Coroner's Court.

Post mortem examinations undertaken for the Coroner at Prestwich mortuary were normally scheduled for 3.00pm. However, the rescheduling of the post mortem followed an established procedure when the deceased was Jewish, through which the Coroner's office in Rochdale would try to arrange for the post mortem to be brought forward to enable the burial to take place the same day, as required by Jewish Law.

Meanwhile, the synagogue at which Mr Isaacs worshipped, and the Burial Board to which he subscribed, had set in train the arrangements for his burial according to Orthodox Jewish Rites. As 27 February was a winter Friday, it would be particularly important that the burial was concluded before the start of the Sabbath.

Later in the morning Dr Rosenberg called at the family home.

The Coroner's office instructed Dr R J Farrand to carry out the post mortem. Dr Farrand was the pathologist who in 1987 carried out most of the Coroner's post mortems at Prestwich mortuary. Mr Isaacs' body was identified to Dr Farrand by WPC Rigby, who had been in attendance the previous evening. Mr Denis Walkden, the mortician at Prestwich Hospital, is the only other person known to have been present at the post mortem.

None of those who were present at the post mortem can now recall the examination of Mr Isaacs and the removal of his brain, see Chapter 2. The time of removal of Mr Isaacs' brain is, however, clearly recorded as 11.15am in the brain books held in Manchester University. It is clear that the brain was not returned to Mr Isaacs' body.

Goldfines, the Jewish undertakers in Manchester, were waiting at Prestwich mortuary to receive Mr Isaacs' body before the post mortem examination was completed. On completion, the body was released by the Coroner into the care of Goldfines so that the proper rituals of the Jewish faith could be undertaken before burial.

In accordance with practice in 1987, a telephone call would have been made from the mortuary to the Coroner's office to inform the Coroner that the cause of death had been established, before the body was released. No record exists of the time of this call.

Mr Isaacs' funeral took place in accordance with Jewish rites at 3.30pm.

When Mr Isaacs was buried his family were totally unaware that his brain had been inappropriately retained without their knowledge or agreement. Had the family been asked, consent would have been refused for retention of his brain for any purpose, in accordance with Mr Isaacs' religious beliefs and Jewish Law. In fact, as subsequent chapters describe, the brain had been retained solely for research at Manchester University, see Chapter 3. The legal position, including the Human Tissue Act, are described in Chapter 5.

Summary

Mr Isaacs was found dead by the late Mr C Lingard shortly before 7.00pm on 26 February 1987.

On hearing that a post mortem was likely, Mrs Isaacs pointed out that this conflicted with her husband's religious beliefs as an Orthodox Jew.

The post mortem examination ordered by the Coroner was brought forward in recognition of Mr Isaacs' Jewish belief to 11.00am on 27 February.

Mr Isaacs was buried before sunset that day in accordance with Jewish rites.

Mr Isaacs' family were unaware that his brain had been inappropriately retained for research at Manchester University.

References

1 Entry in the Prestwich Mortuary Register of Outside Deaths.

CHAPTER 2

Investigation of Mr Isaacs' death, the inquest and its aftermath

Introduction

This chapter describes the arrangements in the North Manchester Coroner's office in 1987, the staff involved and the procedures in place for investigation of sudden deaths in the community. Later paragraphs set out what happened in preparation for and at the inquest into Mr Isaacs' death.

Sources of information

The recollections of the Coroner, the Coroner's Officers and staff of the Coroner's office.

The Coroner and his office in 1987

Her Majesty's Coroner for the North Manchester jurisdiction was Mr Bryan North, who had been appointed in 1978. Mr North had previously served as Deputy Coroner for Lancashire from 1965 until the local government reorganisation of 1974 when he was appointed Coroner for Oldham.

Mr North's jurisdiction covered the boroughs of Oldham and Rochdale in addition to Bury, which included Prestwich and Whitefield districts. By agreement between the three boroughs, Rochdale Council took the lead in providing financial and administrative support for the Coroner as the Coroner's office is located in Rochdale. Mr North's office staff were employed by Rochdale Council. In 1987, in order of seniority, Mr North's office staff were Mrs Joyce Langan, Mrs Shirley Connolly and Mrs Gillian Williamson.

Coroner's Officers

In each of the three boroughs a police officer served as Coroner's Officer. PC Joe Cassells was Coroner's Officer for Bury, where he was responsible for investigation of deceased persons whose bodies were taken to the mortuaries in Bury and Prestwich. PC David Rigg and PC David Harrison were, respectively, Coroner's Officers for the Rochdale and Oldham boroughs.

The Coroner's Officers would generally, but not invariably, attend the start of a post mortem examination ordered by the Coroner, in order to identify the deceased to the pathologist. Thereafter the practice of the Coroner's Officers varied. In Rochdale, PC Rigg would almost always attend for the whole of the post mortem procedure. PC Cassells attended the vast majority of post mortems at Fairfield Hospital and usually, but not always, remained until the end of the examination.

After post mortems at Fairfield, PC Cassells would generally telephone or visit the family of the deceased to inform them of the cause of death and of arrangements for obtaining the death certificate.

PC Cassells attended only a few of the post mortems at Prestwich mortuary as the arrangements for examinations there were different. Dr Farrand would telephone the Coroner's office to inform the Coroner of the cause of death and the Coroner's office staff would communicate with the relatives.

In all mortuaries where the Coroner's Officers had not been involved in removal of the body to the mortuary, the police officer who had attended the scene of death would attend to identify the body to the pathologist. In the case of Mr Isaacs, identification of the body to Dr Farrand was WPC Rigby's responsibility.

Investigation of sudden deaths in the community

1. Deaths with no suspicious circumstances

When a sudden death was reported to the Coroner and there were no suspicious circumstances, an urgent responsibility of the Coroner's Officer or office staff was to contact the deceased's general practitioner or other recent medical attendant to ask if he was in a position to issue a death certificate. Where pre-existing disease was known to the doctor and a death certificate could be issued, there would then be no need for the Coroner to order a post-mortem examination.

2. Deaths in suspicious circumstances

In all deaths in suspicious circumstances, investigations are undertaken by the police who report their findings to the Coroner. A post mortem will invariably follow. In such cases the Coroner, after discussion with the police, will decide on the pathologist to carry out the post mortem examination.

Release of body

Where there are no suspicious circumstances, the body of the deceased can be released to the relatives once the Coroner is satisfied about the cause of death. The pathologist will normally convey his findings by telephone to the Coroner's office, to allow early release of the body. The written report will follow in time for the inquest.

Collection of evidence

It is the duty of the Coroner's Officers to interview witnesses, obtain statements from them for the Coroner and bring together other evidence that the Coroner might wish to consider before or during the inquest.

In preparation for the inquest into the death of Mr Isaacs, statements were obtained from:

- WPC Sharon Rigby; Annex 9
- Mrs Isaacs, his widow; Annex 10
- the late Mr Clive Lingard, who had found Mr Isaacs' body; Annex 11
- Dr Rosenberg, Mr Isaacs' general practitioner. Annex 12

No other statements were obtained for the inquest but Dr Farrand's written report on his findings at the post mortem was available to the Coroner. The report did not record that Mr Isaacs' brain had been retained at the end of the post mortem examination. Annex 13

The resumed inquest

On 16 March the Coroner, Mr North, reopened the inquest, which had been adjourned after evidence of identification had been heard on 27 February. Mr North, sitting without a jury, considered the written documents listed above. The record of the inquisition does not refer to other exhibits or documents entered as exhibits. Although in some cases of sudden death police photographs were taken of the scene, there is no record of any photographs being among the exhibits submitted to the Coroner. Annex 14

The resumed inquest was attended by Mrs Isaacs. She was represented by a solicitor and a barrister who asked a number of questions on her behalf. Mr Lingard and WPC Rigby attended the inquest to give oral evidence, but Dr Rosenberg and Dr Farrand did not. Dr Rosenberg's statement and Dr Farrand's report were part of the evidence considered by the Coroner.

After considering the written and oral evidence as presented to him, the Coroner summed up and recorded a verdict of *"Suicide"*. The inquisition records the cause of death as *"Hanging"* and that *"Cyril Mark Isaacs died of the aforesaid at his home. He was found hanging from the loft by an electric flex"*.

Immediate aftermath to the inquest

Mrs Isaacs and the family were devastated by the verdict. The stigma of suicide has profound implications to those of the Jewish faith and was to become an intolerable burden to the family.

Until the inquest, Mrs Isaacs was unaware of the contents of the statements submitted in evidence to the Coroner. In particular she was dismayed that, apart from her own statement, the Coroner had been told very little about the severity of Mr Isaacs' depression and other mental health problems. Mrs Isaacs had expected her husband's mental health, about which he had consulted a number of doctors in the last weeks of his life, would be fully described in Dr Rosenberg's witness statement. Annex 12

Mrs Isaacs believed that, if the Coroner had been fully informed of the extent of the Mr Isaacs' severe mental health problems and the medical care he had received prior to his death, the verdict would have been different.

The return of the kettle flex

Some days after the inquest the police called to return "property" to Mrs Isaacs. This property included medicines and the kettle flex which Mr Isaacs had used to cause his death. Mrs Isaacs has a receipt for the return of the medication dated 16 March 1987. This receipt does not refer to the kettle flex.

The police records of the case do not refer to this incident, but police practice at the time was only to return property involved in an unnatural death when this was requested. Mrs Isaacs and the family had certainly not asked for the flex to be returned. Mr Isaacs' clothes and personal effects had already been returned within days of his death.

The police property book in which the flex might have been recorded was destroyed several years ago in keeping with standard time limits on such documents. The definitive explanation for the return of the flex cannot be given. However, the police have told me that it is possible that a person representing Mrs Isaacs at the inquest was asked about the return of Mr Isaacs' property, as it was not the practice to approach the relatives direct. Without realising that the "property" in question was the means of Mr Isaacs' death, the reply given could have indicated that all property should be returned. Whatever was the explanation, the return of the flex was to cause unnecessary and avoidable distress to Mrs Isaacs.

Contact with official agencies

In the interval between Mr Isaacs' death and the inquest, the police were in contact with Mr Isaacs' family but no other official agency was involved.

Correspondence with the Coroner 1987-1991

On 23 March 1987 Mrs Isaacs wrote the first of many letters(1) to the Coroner requesting that he reconsider matters that had not been presented to him during the inquest. In his reply the Coroner emphasised that his verdict had been based on the evidence presented at the time of the inquisition.

Mrs Isaacs' correspondence with the Coroner continued until 1991. In her letters to the Coroner and to other authorities to whom she wrote challenging the verdict, Mrs Isaacs drew attention to aspects of Mr Isaacs' mental health that had not been included in the evidence presented at the inquest.

Discovery that Mr Isaacs' brain had been retained

On 5 April 2000, Mrs Isaacs was reviewing papers relating to the medical care of her husband, among which were some papers which Mrs Isaacs had not previously seen. The papers included an undated letter sent from the Department of Psychiatry at Manchester University to Dr Rosenberg, Mr Isaacs' general practitioner. The letter, reproduced at Annex 15, informed Dr Rosenberg that the University had collected samples of Mr Isaacs' brain and asked a number of questions about Mr Isaacs' mental health and medication prior to his death.

Annex 15

Mrs Isaacs and her family were greatly shocked by this discovery. It was an affront to Mr Isaacs' religious beliefs and those of his family. Mrs Isaacs immediately began to investigate why and how her husband's brain had been retained. This investigation is the direct result of the questions that Mrs Isaacs has asked.

Relevance of the evidence presented at the inquest to this investigation

While Mrs Isaacs' concerns about the inquest verdict, and other legal and financial aspects of the inquest on her husband, are specifically excluded from consideration in this investigation, the availability and presentation of relevant evidence at inquests is directly relevant to the fourth of my Terms of Reference. This is further considered in Chapter 43.

Matters in Chapter 2 that are developed in other chapters

Can more be done when a sudden death occurs in the community to ensure that the relatives are kept informed of what is to happen and why? In particular, when the relatives are firmly opposed to a post mortem for religious or other reason, what steps can be taken to explain to them why one is necessary and to respond to their concerns? Chapter 45.

Is it possible to modify the necessary investigative procedures of sudden death without prejudice to their effectiveness, in order better to accommodate the religious beliefs of the deceased and his/her relatives? Chapter 43.

Where there are no suspicious circumstances in a case of sudden death in the community, steps should be taken to find out if the deceased's general practitioner, or other recent medical attendant, is in a position to certify the cause of death before a Coroner's autopsy is ordered, Chapter 43.

Can more be done to ensure that all relevant medical factors are presented in evidence to the Coroner? Chapter 43.

The importance of recording the retention of any organs and/or tissues in the pathology report sent to the Coroner, Chapter 35.

The letter to Dr Rosenberg asking for information about Mr Isaacs' mental health, Chapters 6, 18 and 20.

Summary

The inquest into Mr Isaacs' death took place on 16 March 1987.

Mr Isaacs' previous mental health difficulties received little attention in the statement provided by Dr Rosenberg.

A verdict of hanging was recorded.

Mrs Isaacs in correspondence to the Coroner drew attention to Mr Isaacs' mental health problems. This correspondence continued for four years.

Mrs Isaacs' distress was added to when the police returned the kettle flex to her. This was the flex from which Mr Isaacs had been suspended. The reasons for returning the flex have not been explained. The practice of the police returning objects of this kind should, in my view, be reconsidered.

The police were the only official agency in contact with Mr Isaacs' family during a time of great distress.

References

1 Correspondence between Mrs Isaacs and the Coroner.

CHAPTER 3

Investigation of the post mortem examination of Mr Isaacs at Prestwich mortuary

Introduction

This chapter describes what took place during the post mortem examination of Mr Isaacs' body and the procedures in place at Prestwich hospital and mortuary in 1987.

Sources of information

This chapter is based on the Prestwich Mortuary Registers, other documents available from Prestwich Hospital and the recollections of those involved in the post mortem in 1987.

Background

Prestwich Mortuary

In 1987 Prestwich mortuary served as a community mortuary for the North Manchester districts of Prestwich and Whitefield. The bodies of those who died unexpectedly in the community or in accidents, and other deaths reported to the Coroner from these districts, were taken to Prestwich mortuary for post mortem examination.

The mortuary also served Prestwich hospital both for the conduct of hospital post mortems and to provide for the recently dead when there was no post mortem. As a hospital mortuary, Prestwich would occasionally receive the bodies of patients who had died in local nursing or residential homes when a limited hospital post mortem was requested or needed.

In August 1989 post mortem examinations at Prestwich mortuary ceased. Thereafter all post mortems on Coroners' cases and deaths in Prestwich hospital were carried out in the mortuary at Fairfield Hospital, Bury, which had served as the other community mortuary for the northern part of the Borough before 1989.

Prestwich Hospital

In the 1970s, Prestwich Hospital was a large, predominantly long-stay mental hospital. While one ward was allocated to the care of acute medical admissions, the patients in the other wards were there for mental illness or mental handicap. Many were institutionalised, having been in hospital for decades.

In the early 1980s and into the 1990s, the gradual transfer of long-stay patients to community care led to a progressive reduction in the number of inpatients in Prestwich Hospital which is now a shadow of its former size.

In the 1980s and earlier decades, a proportion of the long-stay patients had lost touch with their families. When long-stay patients with no known next of kin died, one of the administrative staff of the hospital appointed by the Hospital Secretary, later the Chief Executive, undertook the responsibilities that would normally fall to the relatives, including giving consent for a hospital post mortem if one was requested.

Procedures at Prestwich mortuary at the time of Mr Isaacs' death in February 1987

To reflect its dual function, two separate registers were maintained for the bodies of persons taken to Prestwich mortuary - the Register of Outside (Police) Deaths and the Register of Hospital Deaths.

The Register of Outside Deaths records the particulars of each body received at Prestwich mortuary, including the name, address and age of the deceased, the time the body was received and the person removing the body to the mortuary. This in most cases was a police officer. The second page of the register records the name and signature of the undertaker removing the body, the date and time of removal and the place of burial or cremation.

In cases where a post mortem was carried out, the register records whether this was a Coroner's or hospital post mortem.

The Mortuary Register of Hospital Deaths is no longer available. It is believed to have been destroyed, along with other records, when a record store was flooded. However, a register of all patients admitted to Prestwich Hospital survives. This document records details of all discharges and deaths from Prestwich Hospital between January 1982 and December 1989. From the in-patients register it is possible to identify the patients in Prestwich Hospital whose deaths were reported to the Coroner. The register does not, however, record why the death was reported.

The register entry for the body of Mr Isaacs

The transfer of Mr Isaacs' body to Prestwich mortuary is recorded in the Outside Deaths Register. The body was received at the mortuary at 8.45pm on 26 February 1987[(1)]. As Mr Walkden, the mortician, was not on duty when Mr Isaacs' body was taken to the mortuary, one of the hospital porters would have unlocked the mortuary door and filled in the first page of the register.

The date of Mr Isaacs' death, his age and address are correctly shown. His body was received from WPC Rigby. The second page records that a Coroner's post mortem was carried out. Mr Isaacs' body was removed by Goldfines (the Jewish undertakers) on 27 February 1987 for burial at Agecroft Cemetery. The removal entry is signed "*B Goldfines*" and initialled by the mortician, Mr Walkden, but the time is not recorded[(1)].

Other relevant documents

In addition to the Mortuary Register, the police "751 report"[(2)] and Dr Farrand's report to the Coroner on the findings of the post mortem examination provide contemporaneous information about the post mortem. Annex 13

Persons at the post mortem examination of Mr Isaacs

The post mortem examination took place at 11.00am on 27 February. Dr Farrand and Mr Walkden were present throughout and WPC Rigby was present at the start of the examination. If others were present, their names are not recorded in any surviving documents.

Dr R J Farrand

Dr Farrand holds an NHS appointment as Consultant Pathologist (Microbiology) at Bolton General Hospital. In addition to his NHS duties, Dr Farrand had regularly undertaken Coroners' post mortem examinations at Prestwich Mortuary since 1975. In that year Dr Farrand was asked to carry out post mortems by Mr Leonard Gorodkin, who was then Coroner for North Manchester. Dr Farrand continued to undertake post mortems at Prestwich when Mr North was appointed Coroner in 1978. He still acts as pathologist for Mr Barrie Williams who was appointed Coroner for the district in 1995.

Mr Dennis Walkden

Mr Dennis Walkden was the mortician at Prestwich from 1973 until 1988 when he transferred to Fairfield Hospital, Bury. He still works as the senior mortician at Fairfield Hospital. Apart from a short period in the 1970s, Mr Walkden was the only mortician at Prestwich Hospital. Mr Walkden and Dr Farrand had worked together since 1975.

WPC Sharon Rigby (now Mrs Dunn)

Having supervised the removal of Mr Isaacs' body to the mortuary, it was WPC Rigby's duty to identify the body to Dr Farrand. Dr Farrand's report to the Coroner, dated 27 February 1987, records that she did so. Annex 13

Recollections of those present

No one present at the post mortem now has any recollection of this particular post mortem examination. This is not surprising as both Dr Farrand and Mr Walkden have attended numerous similar examinations in the 15 years since February 1987. At the time there was nothing unusual about the examination of Mr Isaacs' body.

Retention of Mr Isaacs' brain

While both Dr Farrand and Mr Walkden acknowledge that Mr Isaacs' brain could not have been returned to his body at the end of the examination, neither specifically recalls this.

In fact, the records show that Mr Isaacs' brain was removed at 11.15am. It is clear from the entries in the Manchester University brain book that the brain was retained for the purpose of research. There is no suggestion in the post mortem report that retention was needed for any purpose related to determining the cause of death, or that Dr Farrand needed histological examination of the brain in order to notify the Coroner of the cause of Mr Isaacs' death. In these circumstances, to satisfy the requirements of the Human Tissue Act, consent for retention should have been obtained from Mrs Isaacs prior to the post mortem. Consent would have been refused.

The retention of Mr Isaacs' brain was, however, not unusual at Prestwich mortuary. Many brains had already been retained in similar circumstances following instructions received from the Coroner's office, as described in Chapter 10.

WPC Rigby has no recollection of the examination, although she does distantly remember what happened when she attended Mr Isaacs' house on 26 February 1987.

Dr Farrand's report to the Coroner

This report states the cause of death as "*Hanging*" and that the brain appeared "*normal*". The report, however, does not mention the retention of Mr Isaacs' brain. Annex 13

Was Mr Isaacs' brain the only organ retained?

In view of the family's concerns that other organs might have been retained, Dr Farrand and Mr Walkden were both asked about any other practice of organ or tissue retention. Neither has any recollection of other organs being retained for research, Chapter 4.

Other brain retentions at Prestwich mortuary

Chapters 10, 12 and 21 describe the retention of brains for the joint programme in the Departments of Physiology and Psychiatry at Manchester University.

Chapter 26 sets out the arrangement through which a small number of brains were retained and transferred to the brain bank at Addenbrooke's Hospital, Cambridge, before the joint programme began at Manchester University in 1985.

Chapter 8 outlines the separate system for retaining brains for research in the Cerebral Function Unit of the Department of Neurology at Manchester University.

Organs retained for diagnostic reasons

In principle, there could have been situations when retention of a whole organ was needed for further tests to establish the cause of death. The brain was the organ most often retained for diagnosis, but in Mr Isaacs' case his brain was not retained for this reason.

Retention of lungs

The retention of lungs was the only other example of systematic organ retention at Prestwich mortuary that either Dr Farrand or Mr Walkden could remember. This occurred when a Coroner's post mortem was ordered because the cause of death was related, or possibly related, to an industrial lung disease. In these post mortems the lungs were retained and forwarded by courier to a designated centre for specialist examination. This system was not limited to Prestwich mortuary and was reported to me by pathologists, morticians and Coroners' Officers in many places.

Other organ retention for research

When asked about other organ retention practices, Dr Farrand, Mr Walkden and PC Joe Cassalls, the Coroner's Officer, all replied that in the 1980s there were no other research teams, apart from the Cerebral Function Unit, Chapter 8, who obtained organs for research from Coroner's post mortems at Prestwich mortuary.

Tissue blocks

While retention of whole organs to determine the cause of death was rare, tissue blocks were retained more frequently for histology. In view of his findings as reported to the Coroner, Dr Farrand considers he would have had no reason to retain any tissue blocks after the post mortem on Mr Isaacs.

What followed the post mortem?

After the post mortem, Mr Isaacs' brain would have been placed in the mortuary fridge to await collection by a member of staff of the Department of Physiology of the University. Mr Walkden completed a form for the University, including Mr Isaacs' name, age, date and time of death, and the time the brain was removed (11.15am). Annex 16

Other information recorded on the form are the cause of death (Hanging) and the names of Mr Isaacs' general practitioner (Dr Rosenberg) and the pathologist (Dr Farrand). Dr Rosenberg's address, written in different handwriting, appears to have been added later. Mr Walkden confirmed that most of the handwriting on this form is his own. He completed a similar form for each brain that was collected for the joint programme.

Later on 27 February, Mr Isaacs' brain was collected by an unidentified member of the University.

Summary

The surviving documents provide contemporary details of the post mortem examination of the body of Mr Isaacs on 27 February 1987. These do not mention retention of his brain, except for the note completed by Mr Walkden which shows that **Mr Isaacs' brain was undoubtedly retained for use at the University.**

At Prestwich mortuary in the 1980s some brains were retained from Coroner's cases for diagnostic reasons. Apart from these, brains were retained for three different research activities – two at Manchester University and, until 1985, for the Cambridge brain bank, Chapter 26.

The retention of lungs for confirmation of industrial disease was the only other systematic example of diagnostic organ retention from Prestwich mortuary.

References

1 Entry in Prestwich Mortuary Register of Outside Deaths.
2 "751 police report".

CHAPTER 4

Were other organs of Mr Isaacs retained for use at Manchester University?

Background

This chapter describes the investigations undertaken to see if any of Mr Isaacs' other organs had been retained for research at Manchester University.

Sources of information

The chapter is based on contemporaneous records of a number of departments of Manchester University and the recollections of staff involved.

Background

The undated letter to Dr Rosenberg discovered by Mrs Isaacs on 5 April 2000 was signed by M Simpson on behalf of Dr J F W Deakin, Senior Lecturer in Psychiatry at the University of Manchester. The letter, inter alia, states *"We collect post-mortem brain samples and these are analysed in the department of physiology in the Medical School"*. Annex 15

Mrs Isaacs' first enquiries at Manchester University

Though greatly distressed and angered by this discovery, Mrs Isaacs began her own enquiries soon after she found the letter. She approached several individuals and agencies. She telephoned Dr Farrand who, in a message on Mrs Isaacs' answering machine, confirmed that her husband's brain had been retained. She then approached Manchester University where she initially contacted Professor Deakin. Several meetings and telephone conversations with him then followed.

(At the time of the start of the joint research programme Dr Deakin had been Senior Lecturer in Psychiatry based at the University Hospital of South Manchester. He was appointed Professor in the Department of Psychiatry in 1990.)

Professor Deakin confirmed Mrs Isaacs' and Dr Isaacs' worst fears, that Mr Isaacs' brain had been destroyed. Professor Deakin remembers he apologised to Mrs Isaacs that her husband's brain, without her knowledge or consent, had been obtained for use in research by the University.

Subsequently, in a letter to Mrs Isaacs dated 28 July 2000, Professor Deakin emphasised his regrets:

"I do fully understand and sympathise with the additional distress this discovery has caused you. I very much regret that current standards and safeguards about post-mortem tissue that would have prevented this occurrence today, were not in place 13 years ago. At that time there was little awareness that a relative might have strong views or legitimate rights concerning the removal of tissue and this was overshadowed by a strong desire to assist research. While not in any way condoning these attitudes,

it is worth reflecting that this UK research led directly to understanding the causes of Alzheimer's disease and to entirely new treatments for this incurable condition". Annex 17

My enquiries have subsequently confirmed that no research had been undertaken on Mr Isaacs' brain, which had probably been disposed of in 1993[1]. The date of disposal was not recorded.

The realisation that her husband's brain had been destroyed added to the family's distress. In accordance with Jewish Law, if Mr Isaacs' brain or any other organ or part of an organ had been retained after the post mortem and was still in existence, then all the retained organs or parts should be buried with or near to Mr Isaacs' body in a Jewish burial ground.

Dr Austin Isaacs' letter to Sir Martin Harris

On 29 January 2001 Mrs Isaacs' son, Dr Austin Isaacs, wrote to Sir Martin Harris, Vice Chancellor of the University, demanding a full explanation of why his father's brain had been taken and of what had subsequently happened. Annex 18 Sir Martin replied on 7 February *"I was very sorry to read your letter dated 29th January 2001. I can understand how distressing this situation must be for you and your family*". Annex 19

Sir Martin ordered *"a full investigation into these events"*. He added *"We all agree that this matter must be reviewed as a matter of urgency so that I can respond to you in detail as quickly as possible"*. Further correspondence between Mrs Isaacs and Sir Martin Harris followed.

On 14 March 2001 Sir Martin wrote to Mrs Isaacs summarising the results of his further enquiries and replying to specific questions Mrs Isaacs had raised. Annex 20 Sir Martin's reply to Mrs Isaacs indicates the scope of the investigations undertaken.

On 28 March 2001 Sir Martin in a further letter to Mrs Isaacs again confirmed *"I have indicated to you that the University will co-operate fully with any official investigation that may be undertaken into this matter"*. Annex 21

Scope of my investigation at Manchester University

In October 2001, after I had received the Terms of Reference for this investigation, I wrote to Sir Martin Harris to take up the assurances given in his letter of 28 March to Mrs Isaacs. A meeting with Sir Martin Harris and Professor David Gordon, the Dean of the Faculty of Medicine, Dentistry, Nursing and Pharmacy, was held on 12 November 2001. At this meeting the scope of and the results from the internal investigation about which Sir Martin had written to Mrs Isaacs on 14 March were not mentioned. However, I was assured that full co-operation would be given by all staff of the University.

The search at Manchester University for other organs retained from Mr Isaacs

The Terms of Reference for this investigation refer to the retention of *"organs"* and not only to the retention of Mr Isaacs' brain. This wider scope had been decided as Mr Isaacs' family was concerned that other organs may have been retained and sent for research at Manchester University.

To explore whether any other organs had been sent to the University, I asked Sir Martin Harris and Professor Gordon for access to the records of any University department that might have used, or had access to, human organs and tissues for research and/or teaching programmes. This was immediately agreed.

Inventory of organs and tissues held by Manchester University

Following the meeting with Sir Martin Harris, Professor Gordon made arrangements for me to see Professor Anthony Freemont first. Professor Freemont had, since March 2001, been responsible for checking the completeness of the lists of organs and tissues held by the University. This inventory was required by the Retained Organs Commission, for a separate purpose.

Meeting with Professor Freemont on 28 November 2001

At this first meeting with Professor Freemont, he identified the University departments that held retained organs and tissues. These included the Medical School Departments of Anatomy, Neurology (including the Cerebral Function Unit), Pathology, Physiology including Psychiatry, and a number of specialist surgical departments.

The first inventory of retained organs and tissues had been carried out in May 2000 to respond to the Chief Medical Officer's Census. As there had been misunderstandings in some parts of the University about the coverage of the Census, the University had repeated the Census in September 2000. Since Professor Freemont had been given responsibility to ensure the completeness of the inventory, he had revisited the returns from a number of departments.

To ensure the validity of the returns made, Professor Freemont had worked closely with Mr Tony Armstrong, who had the same responsibility for identification of retained organs held by the Central Manchester NHS Trust, and with Mr Peter Sullivan, Chief Technician in the University Pathology Department.

Coverage of the inventory

The inventory had identified over 5000 organs and tissues held at four locations. These were:

i. the University Medical School in Oxford Road ;
ii. the Central Manchester Hospital site (including the Children's Hospital);
iii. the Salford (Hope) Hospital site;
iv. the South Manchester Hospital (Wythenshawe/Withington) sites.

A full list of specimens is held at each site, with a copy held centrally. Among these specimens were 473 brains in brain collections that had been reported to the Chief Medical Officer's Census.

Almost all the retained organs and tissues, including post mortem and surgical specimens held by the University, would have first entered via the Pathology

Department. A minority of tissue specimens would have been sent as tertiary referrals to specialists in Manchester because of their particular expertise in the diagnosis of rare conditions.

The exceptions to the route of entry via pathology were those organs and tissues that were obtained directly from researchers who had set up direct links with surgical departments or mortuaries outside central Manchester.

Search for any mention of Mr Isaacs' organs in the records of the University

Mr Peter Sullivan, the Chief Pathology Technician in the Medical School, is responsible for the records of all specimens (surgical and post mortem) that are received in the University Pathology Department. The records include specimens received for neuropathology which are allocated numbers in the Neuro Special Pathology (NSP) series.

While most of the University pathology records are kept in the Medical School by Mr Sullivan, some records, including the Mortuary Registers, are held at Manchester Royal Infirmary.

At a meeting with Mr Peter Sullivan on 19 December 2001, the inventories and pathology records of organs ever held by the other University departments were scrutinised. These lists were searched for any mention of Mr Cyril Isaacs in the years 1987-1995. No such reference was found.

At a meeting at Manchester Royal Infirmary on 11 January 2002, Dr Benbow, Honorary Consultant Pathologist at Manchester Royal Infirmary, provided access to the relevant records of the Infirmary. During a careful search no record of Mr Isaacs was found anywhere in these papers.

Other checks

To see if other research at Manchester University had made use of organs other than brains that were obtained from community mortuaries, an attempt was made to identify relevant studies from the research literature. In 1987 the number of publications by members of the University was very large. At that time the University did not hold a list of all research undertaken by staff in clinical, pathology or other departments that used human organs or tissues in research. This approach was not pursued once the staff of Prestwich mortuary had been interviewed.

Four collections of brains and parts of brains

At the meeting with Professor Freemont and Mr Sullivan on 28 November, the records indicated the existence of four separate collections of brains in different departments of the University, located in:

> The Department of Physiology - jointly held with the Department of Psychiatry (the joint programme). **It was this collection to which Mr Isaacs' brain had been transferred, Chapters** 9-18.

The Cerebral Function Unit of the Department of Neurology – this research unit and brain collection is now located at Hope Hospital, Salford, having transferred there from the Medical School in 2001, Chapter 8.

The Neuro Special Pathology (NSP) collection held at Manchester Royal Infirmary - a diagnostic collection where the specimens were all referred for specialist neuropathological diagnosis to Dr Helen Reid or her predecessors in post, Chapter 8.

The Department of Anatomy where all the brains held there had been collected for use in the teaching of medical students. See below and Chapter 36.

What happened to Mr Isaacs' brain?

The "brain books" maintained for the joint research programme of the Departments of Physiology and Psychiatry show that the brain of Mr Isaacs was obtained from Prestwich mortuary on 27 February 1987, Chapter 12.

What happened after Mr Isaacs' brain reached the University?

After Mr Isaacs' brain reached the Department of Physiology it would have been prepared for research use within one to two hours of arrival in accordance with a standard protocol. The hand writing in the brain book indicates that preparation was carried out by Michael Simpson. In 1987 Mr Simpson was one of the Research Fellows working in the Department of Physiology.

The prepared pieces of brain were then carefully labelled and placed in one of the storage freezers in the department. The objective was to place the prepared brain in the freezer as rapidly as possible.

Could Mr Isaacs' brain have been transferred within Manchester University?

The Cerebral Function Unit did not collect brains of cases that were not already patients known to the unit. The unit would have had no interest in receiving Mr Isaacs' brain and their records do not include any mention of anyone named "Isaacs".

I have scrutinised the records of the Neuro Special Pathology Collection held in the University Pathology Department and at Manchester Royal Infirmary. There are no references in these records to Mr Isaacs' brain in 1987 or in subsequent years.

The records of brains obtained by the Anatomy Department no longer exist. The department never obtained brains from Prestwich mortuary, and a consent form had been routinely used. Annex 22

The researchers and clinicians in these teams have all been interviewed and have each assured me that on no occasion did they receive any brain, or parts of brains, prepared for research use in the Department of Physiology.

I am satisfied from these enquiries that Mr Isaacs' brain was not transferred to the Cerebral Function Unit, the Neuro Special Pathology Section or the Department of Anatomy.

Obtaining Mr Isaacs' medical history

When Mr Isaacs' brain was received, the department knew nothing about him except for his age and cause of death. To find out more of Mr Isaacs' medical history and mental health problems, if any, the undated letter (found by Mrs Isaacs in April 2000) was sent to Dr Rosenberg, who did not reply to this letter. Dr Rosenberg has no recollection of receiving any further communication from the Department of Psychiatry at Manchester University. Annex 15

It would have been usual practice for a medically qualified member of the research team to follow up unanswered letters with a telephone call to the general practitioner. This almost certainly happened, as the brain book includes a hand-written note dated 4 March 1988 to the effect:

"Took several overdoses several brief contacts with psychiatrists* after o.d. on medical wards. No formal psychiatric* history."*

NB: The words marked * are symbolised and the signature is not legible.

This note[2] indicates that some additional information about Mr Isaacs' mental health had been obtained by an unidentified member of the research team and is the last entry about Mr Isaacs' brain in the brain book.

What happened later?

Was Mr Isaacs' brain transferred within Manchester University?

As mentioned above, there is no evidence or reason to believe that Mr Isaacs' brain was transferred to other parts of Manchester University.

Was Mr Isaacs' brain transferred to a research team in another institution?

In the brain books there are a small number of references to brains that were of no relevance to the joint research team being sent or offered to researchers elsewhere.

In phase three of the investigation, contact was made with all the researchers named in the brain books. With their help their records were searched for any reference to Mr Isaacs after 1987. Each of these research teams was also asked if they had ever received any brain specimens from Manchester. These enquiries have not discovered any mention of Mr Isaacs or reference to a sample from his brain.

While it is impossible to prove that Mr Isaacs' brain was not transferred from Manchester, in the light of what I have been told I believe this did not happen.

Was Mr Isaacs' brain disposed of by Manchester University?

Three different members of the Manchester research team have stated that from time to time the contents of the research freezers were reviewed. Space in these was limited and brain specimens that were unsuitable for research were disposed of by incineration following these reviews.

Mrs Isaacs had herself been told by Professor Deakin in 2001, based on information provided by other members of the joint programme team, that her husband's brain had probably been disposed of after a review of the freezer contents in 1993.

In the knowledge that the research team had failed to obtain any definite information about Mr Isaacs' health prior to his death, I put the same question to three members of the research team. Each replied that it was most likely that Mr Isaacs' brain samples had been removed and disposed of after one of these periodic reviews. Professor Deakin referred to 1993 as the probable date. Michael Simpson commented that he was surprised that the date of disposal had not been entered in the brain book.

Summary

Mr Isaacs' brain was obtained from Prestwich mortuary on 27 February 1987 for use in research. It was then taken to the Department of Physiology in the University, prepared for research use and held in a research freezer for an unrecorded period of time.

Attempts were made to find out details of Mr Isaacs' mental health from his general practitioner, Dr Rosenberg. These were not successful.

What eventually happened to Mr Isaacs' brain cannot be firmly established. I am nonetheless satisfied from my discussions with members of other departments, and examination of their records, that no part of Mr Isaacs' brain was referred to the Cerebral Function Unit, the Neuro Special Pathology collection or to the Department of Anatomy.

From my enquiries in other locations, I consider it is most unlikely that parts of Mr Isaacs' brain were transferred to research teams at other Universities or Institutes.

While it cannot be proven, the most likely outcome was the disposal of Mr Isaacs' brain by incineration some time in the early 1990s.

There is not one reference to Mr Isaacs' other organs or tissues in the Inventory of Retained Organs or in the records shown to me of other departments of the University from 1987 onwards. This serves to support the conclusion I reached after investigating the procedures at Prestwich mortuary and from speaking to the staff who worked there in 1987.

I am satisfied that, with the exception of his brain, none of Mr Isaacs' other organs or tissues was sent to Manchester University.

References

1 Recollections of Professor Deakin and Dr Michael Simpson.
2 Entry in the brain books of the joint programme.

SECTION 2

Research on brains retained at post mortem

CHAPTER 5

The legal framework: guidance to the NHS on organ retention and the collection of pituitary glands, and Home Office advice to Coroners

Background

This chapter describes the statutes, circulars and other official guidance that were relevant to organ and tissue retention in the late 1980s.

In the late 1980s the legislation that bore directly on the retention of body parts from post mortem examinations were the Human Tissue Act, 1961, and the Coroners Rules, 1984. (The Corneal Tissue Act (1986) deals only with the removal of eyes.) Appendix 2

The Human Tissue Act, 1961

This Act applies to all bodies and made provision for the removal of body parts for medical purposes.

Before this Act, only the Anatomy Act of 1832 and the Corneal Grafting Act of 1952 had specifically regulated the use of bodies or body parts for medical purposes, research and teaching.

The Human Tissue Act gives authority to *"the person lawfully in possession of the body"* to consent to the use of a body or parts of the body for therapeutic purposes or for medical education or research. The reference in the Act to *"any part of a body"* clearly implies that the part in question will be separated from the body and retained.

Importantly, this consent was subject to the requirement that the deceased in life had expressed "no objection" and that the surviving relatives did not object.

The authority to give consent did not extend to bodies that might be subject to the jurisdiction of the Coroner. In these cases Section 1(5) requires the prior consent of the Coroner.

The key point of Section 1 of the Human Tissue Act is that the person in possession of a body must first make reasonable enquiries to make sure there are no objections. This cannot be assumed.

Section 1 is relevant to this report as it refers to bodies lying in hospitals or other institutions. While a body is in a hospital *"the person having the control and management"* has the authority to consent to removal of body parts *"if, having made such reasonable enquiry as may be practicable, he has no reason to believe –*

(a) that the deceased had expressed an objection to his body being so dealt with after his death, and had not withdrawn it; or

(b) that the surviving spouse or any surviving relative of the deceased objects to the body being so dealt with."

The Human Tissue Act repealed the Corneal Grafting Act (1952). This Act had permitted the removal of the eyes of deceased persons subject to very similar authority and consent requirements. The Corneal Grafting Act required that there was "no objection" from the deceased or surviving relatives.

The Coroners Rules (1984)

The Rules are a Statutory Instrument, deriving their authority from Sections 26 and 27 of the Coroners (Amendment) Act 1926.

Rules 7, 9, 10 and 12 are relevant to the issues described in this report. Rule 7 sets out who should be notified that a post mortem is to take place, Rules 9 and 12 relate to the preservation of material (body parts), and Rule 10 to the post mortem report to the Coroner.

Rule 7 "*Coroner to notify persons of post mortem to be made*"

7(1) requires the Coroner to notify a number of persons of the time and place of a post mortem that he has ordered, *"..unless it is impracticable to notify any such persons or bodies or to do so would cause the examination to be unduly delayed".*

7(2) lists the persons to be notified and includes, *"any relative of the deceased who has notified the coroner of his desire to attend, or be represented, at the post- mortem examination"* and *"the deceased's regular medical attendant*".

Rule 9 "*Preservation of material"*

9 *"A person making a post-mortem examination shall make provisions, so far as possible, for the preservation of material which in his opinion bears upon the cause of death for such period as the coroner thinks fit".*

Rule 10 "*Report on post-mortem*"

10(1) *"The person making a post-mortem examination shall report to the coroner in the form set out in Schedule 2 or in a form to the like effect".*

10(2) *"Unless authorised by the coroner, the person making a post-mortem examination shall not supply a copy of his report to any person other than the coroner".*

Rule12 *"Preservation of material"*

12 *"A person making a special examination shall make provision, so far as possible, for the preservation of the material submitted to him for examination for such period as the coroner thinks fit".*

Guidance to the NHS

HM(61)98 Human Tissue Act, 1961

This Ministry of Health memorandum was distributed to the NHS in England and Wales on 21 September 1961. Its purpose was to describe *"the effect of the Human Tissue Act, 1961, on the law relating to the use of parts of bodies for therapeutic purposes, medical education or research, and to post-mortem examinations..."*

Paragraphs 5, 8 and 10 are relevant to this report. The memorandum is at Appendix 3. Appendix 3

Paragraph 5 draws attention to the authority vested in the person in control of the body while it is in a hospital or other institution to give consent to removal of tissue so long as the body is in the hospital: *"Where the deceased person has not requested that his body or a part or parts of it be used, the Act empowers the person lawfully in possession of the body to authorise the removal of any parts, for use for the purposes specified in the Act".*

Paragraph 8 emphasises the need for the relatives to be consulted about the use of body parts by the person lawfully in possession of the body: *"The nearest relative available should be asked if he objects or has reason to believe that any other relative would object."*

Paragraph 10 requires the consent of relatives to a post mortem: *"Even if the deceased has expressed a wish that there should be a post-mortem examination on his body, the examination may not be authorised if there are objections from relatives... The coroner's consent must be obtained if there is reason to believe that he may require an inquest or post-mortem examination".*

One purpose of this memorandum was to reassure NHS hospitals that it remained lawful under the Human Tissue Act to remove eyes for corneal transplantation despite the repeal of the Corneal Grafting Act provided there were no objections expressed by the relatives. Appendix II of the Memorandum addresses the Enucleation Storage and Transport of Eyes.

HSC(IS)156 Guidance circular to NHS Authorities: Human Tissue Act, 1961

This circular was issued in June 1975 to clarify the uncertainty that had arisen over the interpretation in HM(61)98 over who is *"the person lawfully in possession of the body"*. The circular reinforces the advice in HM(61)98. Paragraphs 6, 11, 12 are relevant. Appendix 4

Paragraph 6 states: *"If a person dies in hospital, the person lawfully in possession of the body, at least until the executors or relatives ask for the body to be handed to them, is the Area Health Authority or the Board of Governors responsible for the hospital".*

Paragraph 11 reinforces the need for the person in possession of the body to ensure the relatives do not object to removal of tissue: *"A person lawfully in possession of the body of a patient who has not requested that his body or parts of it be used may only authorise removal of parts if, having made such reasonable enquiry as may be practicable, he has no reason to believe that the donor would have objected or that the surviving spouse or any surviving relative objects to the body or the specified part being so dealt with. Specific consent is not necessary, merely a lack of objection".*

Paragraph 12 emphasises that the retention of parts of the body removed with the authority of the person in possession at the time the removal took place continues to be lawful after the body is returned to the relatives:

"In cases where the Health Authority is the person lawfully in possession of the body, and an authorisation under Section 1 (of the Human Tissue Act) *has been given, the relatives or executors may subsequently ask that the body be handed over to them; but this action does not revoke the authorisation which continues to be legally effective".*

The circular includes paragraphs on kidney transplantation, corneal grafting and human materials used in treatment, diagnosis or monitoring of therapy.

<u>HC(77)28 Removal of human tissue at post mortem examination – Human Tissue Act 1961</u>

This circular was issued in August 1977. The first paragraph sets out its purpose to facilitate *"the removal of human organs and tissue, eg pituitary glands, during post mortem examination for subsequent use for the treatment of other patients and for medical education and research".* The same paragraph comments *"It would be tragic if insufficient pituitary glands became available, since it is at present impossible to synthesise human growth hormones".* Appendix 5

Paragraph 3 repeats the advice previously given in HSC(IS)156 with regard to the *"person lawfully in possession of the body".* Health Authorities were asked to designate officers to undertake their responsibilities in this respect. The same paragraph states: *"Specific consent is not required by the Act".*

<u>Collection of pituitary glands</u>

To set the context of HC(77)28, a short account of the pituitary collection programme is included at the end of this chapter.

<u>DA(82)9 The national pituitary collection and treatment with human growth hormone</u>

This circular letter, dated 11 May 1982, to District Administrators drew attention to a shortage of the number of pituitary glands becoming available for the growth hormone treatment programme. In substance, the letter repeated the advice in HSC(IS)156, that Health Authorities should designate officers for ensuring that the necessary enquiries were made for authorising the removal of organs or tissue. Appendix 6

Other circulars on related matters

HN(83)3/HN(FP)(83)4 Introduction of brain death check list

This circular was issued with a revised code of practice on the removal of cadaveric organs for transplantation, and the introduction of a check list for diagnosis of brain death. The circular did not alter the advice on tissue removal that was not related to transplantation.

Home Office newsletter to Coroners 1989

The Home Office newsletter to Coroners included the following paragraph: *"Post mortem examinations: We still receive representations from MPs and members of the public about the fact of post mortem examinations or their extent. Invariably our reply is that the post mortem examinations are required only to establish the precise cause of death, that they are not requested or granted gratuitously and are limited in extent to that necessary for the purpose. You will wish to remind your pathologist that Ministers are concerned that tissue and organs should not be taken for teaching or research purposes from Coroners post mortem examination cases"*[(1)].

The pituitary collection programme

This programme was started in the 1950s as a research project supported by the Medical Research Council. The initial objective was to discover if the height of children who were very short for their age could be increased by treatment with growth hormone. Growth hormone is a complex of molecules produced naturally in the pituitary gland which is attached to the underside of the brain, deep inside the skull.

The research project was successful and this prompted an increased demand for growth hormone so that the treatment could be provided for more short-of-stature children. Until synthetic growth hormone was successfully manufactured, the only source of the hormone was by extraction from the pituitaries obtained at post mortem.

As only minute amounts of growth hormone could be extracted from each pituitary gland, very large numbers of glands were required. Between the start of the programme and its discontinuation in 1985, small glass jars containing acetone were to be found in mortuaries across the country. The pituitary glands were collected in these jars until a sufficient number had accumulated. The full jars were then sent centrally for extraction and purification of growth hormone.

It was the intention of HC(77)28 to increase the number of pituitaries collected. In practice, the glands were usually removed by the morticians at the end of post mortem examination. To encourage the collection of pituitaries, a small payment was made for each gland by the Medical Research Council.

This was initially one shilling and six pence for each gland but had increased to twenty new pence by 1980.

The Medical Research Council continued the growth hormone research programme, with the backing of the Department of Health and Social Security (DHSS), until 1980 when the DHSS took over responsibility for its management. A letter dated 25 April 1980 was sent to all NHS hospitals in England to explain the transfer arrangements and encourage the continued collection of pituitary glands. Annex 23

With the transfer of responsibility from the MRC to the DHSS the payment per gland to NHS morticians was discontinued. Instead, the work involved in retaining pituitaries was consolidated into a new Whitley salary scale. This payment change did not apply to morticians working in Local Authority mortuaries who continued for a period to receive payment for each gland.

The pituitary collection programme continued until 1985 when treatment with growth hormone obtained from pituitaries ceased following the discovery that Creutzefelt Jacob Disease (CJD) had been unwittingly transmitted to some of the children who had been treated with growth hormone.

Fortunately, a synthetic form of growth hormone became available within a few months of this discovery.

Summary

In the late 1980s the Human Tissue Act and Coroners Rules were the relevant legislation. Guidance circulars from the Ministry of Health and DHSS provided further advice.

The National Pituitary Collection Programme encouraged the collection of pituitary glands at post mortem.

References

1. Home Office newsletter to Coroners, August 1989.

CHAPTER 6

Ethics Committees and access to health records for post mortem research

Introduction

This chapter describes the guidance on Ethics Committees and on access to medical records for research purposes.

Background

The establishment of Ethics Committees within the NHS began following recommendations within the Report of the Medical Research Council for 1962/63. This was presented to Parliament in July 1964. The Report of the Royal College of Physicians of London followed in July 1967. The first Ethics Committees were set up to give guidance to staff in hospitals only.

Appendix 7
Appendix 8

In these early documents the emphasis was on the rights of patients freely to accept or refuse procedures that were of no direct benefit to their care. From these beginnings the responsibilities of Ethics Committees have evolved progressively, but it was not until 1991 that Ethics Committees were specifically made responsible for considering research on the dead.

Ministry of Health, DHSS and Department of Health Circulars on Ethics Committees

HM(68)33: "Supervision of the Ethics of Clinical Investigations"

This first circular about Ethics Committees, issued on 13 May 1968 to Regional Hospital Boards, Hospital Management Committees and Boards of Governors by the then Ministry of Health, referred to the earlier reports of the Medical Research Council and the Royal College of Physicians of London.

Appendix 9

HSC(IS)153: "Supervision of the Ethics of Clinical Research Investigations and Fetal Research"

This was issued in June 1975 and cancelled HM(68)33. HSC(IS)153 emphasised that *"all proposed clinical investigations should be referred to an ethical committee"* and included specific references to fetal research, research on minors and on mentally handicapped adults. There was no mention of research on the dead.

Appendix 10

Following HSC(IS)153, all researchers who planned to investigate patients during life and to correlate in-life findings with later results obtained from post mortem examinations should have submitted their research protocols for ethical review.

HSC(91)15: "Local Research Ethics Committees"

On 19 August 1991 the Department of Health issued HSG(91)5 to cover distribution of the guidance booklet, also entitled "Local Research Ethics Committee" but colloquially referred to as "the Red Book". This guidance set out the role and responsibilities of Local Ethics Committees. Appendix 11 Appendix 12

HSC(91)15 cancelled HSC(IS)153 and for the first time brought research on the dead into the list of research that should be referred to Local Research Ethics Committees (LRECs). The Red Book on page 5 states "An *LREC must be consulted about any research proposal involving the recently dead, in NHS premises."* Annex 24

The Red Book also drew particular attention to the need for LRECs to be consulted on research on children and those with mental illness. On page 17, the Code of Practice prepared by the Royal College of Psychiatrists was commended to LRECs as a source of advice when research on mentally ill patients is being considered. Annex 24

From 1991 onwards, LRECs considering research proposals on patients with Alzheimer's disease, schizophrenia and other neuro-psychiatric diseases had the benefit of this Code to assist their evaluation of the research protocol.

The Red Book also contained sections on access to health records, which are discussed in the next section.

Medical records: obtaining health and lifestyle data about the deceased

HSC(IS)153 does not mention access to records. In the 1980s the position of a researcher who wished to obtain information from records of the dead was not clear cut. There was uncertainty about what, if any, ethical clearance a researcher required when he had had no contact with or consent from the deceased during life, but wished to obtain information about the deceased's previous health or life style in order to correlate post mortem findings with health and life events.

For many studies, researchers planned to retrieve health and personal information from the records of dead patients, from the recollections of general practitioners, other doctors or from relatives of the deceased. This access posed questions about who should give consent for the researcher to see the records.

As a result, before 1991 practice varied. Some Ethics Committees expected researchers to submit protocols that involved retrieval of clinical data on dead persons who had not given their consent to collection of their personal or health information. Other Ethics Committees were less concerned about the retrieval of data about deceased persons.

A further complexity occurred when the dead person's health or lifestyle data was to be accessed by a researcher to check whether the deceased was suitable as a research "control".

General Medical Council guidance on "Professional Conduct and Discipline: Fitness to Practise"

The following excerpts provided by the General Medical Council from guidance issued to registered medical practitioners between 1980 and 2000. Appendix 13

August 1980

A section of this guidance, headed *"Professional Confidence"*, states: *"The following guidance has been given on the principles which should govern the confidentiality of information relating to patients:*

i. It is a doctor's duty (except as below) strictly to observe the rule of professional secrecy by refraining from disclosing voluntarily to any third party information which he has learned directly or indirectly in his professional relationship with the patient. The death of the patient does not absolve the doctor from the obligation to maintain secrecy.

ii. There are some exceptions to this principle ... (e) information may be disclosed for the purposes of a medical research project. In such a case the project should have been approved by a recognised Ethical Committee appointed for such a purpose".

August 1983

The same heading of the updated guidance states: *"The death of the patient does not absolve the doctor from the obligation to maintain secrecy".*

The exception in relation to disclosure for medical research states:

"h. Information may also be disclosed if necessary for the purpose of a medical research project which has been approved by a recognised ethical committee".

August 1985

The introductory section and section h, as above, has not changed, but there is a new section in relation to disclosure after the death of the patient:

"6. The extent to which disclosure of medical information after the death of a patient is regarded as improper will depend on a number of factors, for example:

(i) the nature of the information disclosed;
(ii) the extent to which such information has already appeared in published material;
(iii) the circumstances of the disclosure, including the period which has elapsed since the patient's death.

The Council feels unable to specify an interval of years to apply in all such cases, and a doctor who discloses such information without the consent of the patient or a surviving close relative of the patient may be required to justify his action".

There was further revision of the guidance in 1992 which did not affect the principles of disclosure after the death of an adult patient, set out in the 1985 guidance.

2000

The GMC's advice *"Confidentiality: Protecting and Providing Information"* contains a new section on medical research, but the prohibition on disclosure after the death of a patient remains similar to the 1985 guidance.

Access to Health Records Act (1990)

This Act provided the right of access by an individual, or in some circumstances his representatives, to his own health record and to correct any inaccurate information in that record. Section 3 lists those who may apply for access to a health record, but the list does not refer to any right of access by researchers to health records of living or dead people. Appendix 14

In addition, the Red Book on page 5 states *"an LREC must be consulted about any research proposal involving access to the records of past or present NHS patients"*. This clarified for the first time the need for researchers to obtain Ethical Committee approval for access to the health records of dead NHS patients. Paragraphs 3.12 and 3.13 in the 1991 book impose a duty on LRECs to consider research that involves access to records where "individual consent" is impossible, as will clearly be the case where the data subject is dead. Annex 24

Coroners Rules (1984)

Records

For Coroners' cases, access to the post mortem report is regulated by Rule 10 which requires the Coroner's agreement to any disclosure of the report. However, the Coroner has discretion to disclose other documents.

Rule 56: "*Retention and delivery of documents*": *"...Provided that the coroner may deliver any such document to any person who in the opinion of the coroner is a proper person to have possession of it."*

Rule 57: "*Inspection of, or supply of copies of, documents etc"* is similarly worded to rule 56 and allows access to documents at the discretion of the Coroner.

Data Protection Act

In 1998 the legal position of data access was clarified in the Data Protection Act (1998), and by the appointment of the Data Protection Commissioner (now Information Commissioner).

NHS confidentiality: Code of Practice

Discussions are currently proceeding on the scope and content of a Code of Practice on confidentiality for the NHS.

Involvement of Ethics Committees in research on the dead in Manchester University

As Chapter 8 records, all research studies on patients undertaken by the Cerebral Function Unit were submitted for and received approval from Ethics Committees.

Chapters 12, 13, 14 and 15 discuss the protocols submitted to Ethics Committees by the joint research team from the Departments of Psychiatry and Physiology.

Ethics Committee involvement at other locations is discussed in the chapter on each location.

Summary

Ethics Committees were first established in the 1960s since when their role has evolved.

Until 1991 Ethics Committees were not required to consider research on the dead. From 1980 the General Medical Council gave guidance on the confidentiality of medical records, including records of dead patients.

CHAPTER 7

The retention of brains after post mortem and the origins of brain research and brain banks

Introduction

This chapter describes the purposes of brain retention, the different categories of brain collections and the origins of the arrangements by which brains were transferred from Prestwich mortuary to the Cambridge brain bank.

Sources of information

The information was provided from a number of neuropathology centres and from documents in the Cambridge brain bank.

The Chief Medical Officer's Census

The Report of the Census of Retained Organs, published by the Chief Medical Officer in January 2001, showed that brains accounted for 44% of all retained organs for the years 1970-1999. The Census included returns from all NHS Trusts in England. The definition of a retained organ used for the Census was that the organ had been retained after diagnostic examination had been completed.

Appendix 15

Why is it necessary to examine the brain in the first place?

For many years it was routine practice for the brain to be removed and a naked eye examination made in almost all post mortem examinations, Chapters 40 and 42.

Prior to 1985, removing the brain during post mortem enabled access to the pituitary gland in the years that these were being collected as part of a national programme for therapeutic purposes, Chapter 5.

At the end of the post mortem it was usual for the brain to be returned to the body with the other organs that had been removed during the examination.

Why is it necessary to retain the brain at the end of the post mortem?

During a post mortem it is not always possible to identify the cause of death from the naked eye appearance of the internal organs. In such cases it is important to take tissue samples to study the microscopic structure to detect disease processes that cannot be seen with the naked eye.

When this is necessary small pieces of tissue, usually referred to as "blocks", are taken as part of a post mortem examination. The rest of the organ is then returned to the body. The tissue blocks are stabilised in a process called "fixation" after which very thin slices of tissue are cut and placed on glass slides for study under the microscope. This process is referred to as "histological examination". As brain tissue is very soft, fixation is essential before microscopic examination can begin.

It takes between four and six weeks for the brain to be properly fixed. This delay means that it is not possible to return the brain to the body at the end of the post mortem. If the brain is to be returned to the body, the funeral or cremation will necessarily be delayed. The delay will be longer if the blocks and slides are also to be returned to the body.

What happens to the brain after the diagnostic examination is finished?

Once the histological examination is complete and the pathologist is satisfied that no further diagnostic review will be needed, the brain is usually set aside. Disposal by incineration as clinical waste takes place when a sufficient number of brains have accumulated. (The method of disposal of retained organs, including brains, is an important subject that the Retained Organs Commission has under consideration.)[1]

Brain accumulations, brain collections and brain banks

The returns submitted by NHS Trusts in 2000 for the Chief Medical Officer's Census and the discussions during the course of this investigation show that brain collections, including parts of brains, fall into three general categories, depending on their origins and purpose. The categories are:

Brain accumulations

Some hospital pathology departments hold large numbers of brains that were retained for diagnostic reasons and histological examination. There was, however, no plan for further use of these brains for research or teaching.

The number of brains in this category has increased as no instructions have been given or received about disposal. Collections of this type may include brains from Coroners' cases. The overall result has been that the number held has increased over time. These brains awaiting a decision on disposal can be regarded as accumulations.

A decision is needed about the disposal of identified brains about which NHS Trusts have received no enquiries from relatives. This is a matter that is also under consideration by the Retained Organs Commission.

Brain collections

The brains in this category are held in diagnostic pathology departments. The collections have similarities to accumulations in that the brains were retained initially for diagnosis. However, after the diagnostic process has been completed the brains have been intentionally retained for:

i diagnostic review at a later date;
ii research, either as an index or control case;
iii teaching use.

Brain banks or archives

Some brain banks are linked to clinical pathology departments while others are located in University departments and research centres; the brains have been intentionally obtained for research or teaching use.

Brains taken to banks may have come either directly from mortuaries or from diagnostic pathology departments after the diagnostic process has ended. A histology report will usually have been made before a brain is referred to the bank from a diagnostic department (or a decision may have been made that no diagnostic examination is necessary).

Where brains are referred direct to a brain bank, some routinely carry out histology and send a report to the doctor responsible for the medical care of the deceased. Others banks do not undertake histology or send any report to the deceased's doctor.

Some brain banks are highly specialised and these are of national importance. For example, when the first cases of variant CJD were reported in 1996, brain banks and archives were checked to see if there had ever been a case with similar findings. If brain banks and archives had not existed, it would have been impossible to know if variant CJD was a new condition or the re-appearance of one that had been seen before(2).

The origin of brain collections

In England, the deliberate retention of brains for research after diagnostic investigations began at Runwell Hospital, Chapter 33. As brains accumulated, the potential of brain collections in the investigation of specific neuropsychiatric conditions was recognised. Brain banking, as it is now known, had begun.

Between the 1950s and 1980s, many brain banks for research had been set up in other countries. By 1987, when Mr Isaacs' brain was retained, brain collections for research and teaching were active in several universities and centres of neuropsychiatric research in this country.

The Corsellis (or Runwell Hospital) collection

The first large collection of brains in England was started in 1950 by Dr Corsellis, who was then Consultant to the Pathology Department of Runwell Hospital. This collection is now held at the West London Mental Health NHS Trust. The Corsellis collection is discussed in Chapter 33, and a further description is at Appendix 16. Appendix 16

From diagnostic collection to research archive

The Runwell or Corsellis collection started as an accumulation of brains retained after diagnosis, but over the next four decades became an invaluable research archive.

Two features must be emphasised:

i. the collection started 11 years before the Human Tissue Act (1961) when the procedures for collecting brains were entirely consistent with medical and legal requirements of that time;
ii. discoveries of major clinical importance have been made possible through research based on the number and diversity of the Corsellis collection.

The significance and importance of the Corsellis and other brain collections is referred to in Chapter 46.

Other brain collections and banks

Other collections followed the pattern pioneered by Professor Corsellis. Some were condition specific. Others collected brains of patients with many different neuropsychiatric diseases and "control" brains from those who had died without any such disorders. Some banks acted as repositories from which research teams could request brain samples of the conditions they were investigating.

Chapters 26, 28, 30 and 32 report on the collections visited during this investigation.

Collections for teaching

Most retained brains were held for research use, but a smaller number were retained for undergraduate and postgraduate teaching, Chapter 36. This is an important objective of some collections.

The Cambridge brain bank

Between 1972 and 1985, brains were regularly referred from mortuaries in the Manchester area, including the Prestwich mortuary, to the Cambridge brain bank. Chapter 26 describes my investigations at Cambridge.

Huntington's disease brains sent to the MRC Neurochemical Pharmacology Unit

In the 1970s, the Medical Research Council provided support for the Neurochemical Pharmacology Unit (NCPU) which, as its name implies, was established to undertake research into the chemistry of the brain. The Head of the Unit was then Dr, now Professor, Leslie Iverson.

Dr E D Bird

Dr Ted Bird, a medically qualified American citizen, was a member of the scientific staff of the unit. In the early 1970s, Dr Bird became interested in neurochemical factors in Huntington's disease. When this research was first mooted, there were doubts about the feasibility of finding enough willing patients and relatives for a meaningful investigation.

Dr Bird was undeterred. He explained his research to relatives, psychiatrists and pathologists and began to collect the brains of patients who died from this progressive and incurable condition. His research attracted the enthusiastic support of many relatives. Some became very active in identifying patients with early symptoms of

Huntington's disease. As a result, Dr Bird received referrals from many parts of the country[3].

Referrals of brains from Prestwich mortuary to Cambridge

Dr Rockley, a Consultant Psychiatrist at Prestwich Hospital, on hearing of Dr Bird's research, wrote to him on 26 October 1972: Annex 25

"We are, of course, agreeable to co-operating in your proposed research, and I suggest that you write to our Consultant Pathologist – Dr. R. Pell-Ilderton – at Crumpsall Hospital".

In 1972 the pathology services at Prestwich Hospital were provided from Crumpsall (North Manchester General Hospital).

While there is no record of a letter of reply from Dr Bird to Dr Pell-Inderton, further communication must have followed as in April 1973 Dr de Kretser, one of Dr Pell-Ilderton's colleagues, sent Dr Bird the brain of a patient who had died from Huntington's Disease. Dr Bird later wrote requesting the patient's case notes which were sent on 9 July 1973[4].

This referral was the first of at least 28 brain referrals from Prestwich and other mortuaries in North Manchester to Dr Bird and other researchers at the Cambridge brain bank. The records at the Cambridge brain bank show that most of these referrals were made by Dr Farrand after he started working at Prestwich mortuary in 1975. He continued to refer to Cambridge the brains of patients who had died with a diagnosis of Huntington's disease and, at a later date, schizophrenia.

The last referral from Prestwich mortuary to the Cambridge brain bank took place on 11 November 1985[5]. This death had been referred to the Coroner, and the telephone number of the Coroner's office in Rochdale and the name "Joyce Langan" are found in the records at Cambridge. This brain was referred by the pathologist and there is no evidence that the Coroner's office staff were involved in the referral.

Publication on Huntington's disease

In 1974 Dr Bird and Dr Iverson published the first results of their research on Huntington's chorea[3]. The methods section of this report records:

"Several consultant psychiatrists and pathologists throughout the United Kingdom provided invaluable assistance by seeking permission for post-mortem examinations of the brains of patients with Huntington's chorea and in the initial handling of the brain material.

Controls consisted of coroners' cases and hospital cases of various ages, on which necropsies had been performed in the University Pathology Department at Addenbrooke's Hospital, Cambridge. Cause of death was widely variable..."

This article resulted in more brains being referred for study in the Neurochemical Pharmacology Unit at Cambridge.

Later, the Cambridge brain bank diversified its programme and by 1979 was requesting referrals not only of the brains of patients who had died from Huntington's disease but from cases of Parkinson's disease, schizophrenia, dyskinesias and related disorders[5].

Summary

The brain is the organ most frequently retained at post mortem.

Most brains are retained only for diagnosis.

The brain has to be "fixed" before it can be examined under the microscope.

The fixation process takes 4-6 weeks.

After the diagnostic process is complete most brains are disposed of as clinical waste.

Brains for research use are obtained either after the diagnostic process is finished or specifically retained for research.

Brains can be retained for teaching.

The first brain collection for research in England was started in 1950 by Professor Corsellis in the Pathology Department of Runwell Hospital, a long-stay mental hospital.

Other brain banks were later set up and brain banks or archives evolved to become an important research resource.

The brain bank at Cambridge began as an investigation into Huntington's disease initiated by Dr E D Bird.

The referral of a brain taken from a patient who had died from Huntington's disease started the link between Prestwich mortuary and the Cambridge brain bank.

Where brain accumulations are now held, a decision on their disposal will be needed after the Retained Organs Commission has given advice on disposal arrangements for both identifiable and unidentified organs.

References

1. Terms of Reference for the Retained Organs Commission.
2. Requests by the Department of Health to the Department of Neuropathology at Queen's Medical Centre, Nottingham. Personal communication from Professor J Lowe.
3. Huntington's Chorea: Post-mortem Measurement of Glutamic Acid Decarboxylase, Choline Acetyltransferase and Dopamine in Basal Ganglia: Brain 1974; Vol 97, part iii: pp 457-472.
4. Case records held by the Cambridge brain bank.
5. Data from the Cambridge brain bank files.

CHAPTER 8

The Cerebral Function Unit and the Neuro Special Pathology Collection at Manchester University

Introduction

This chapter describes the Cerebral Function Unit (CFU) and the brains collected for the unit's research programme and the Neuro Special Pathology (NSP) collection. These collections are mentioned in Chapters 3 and 4.

Both collections were reviewed to exclude the possibility, however remote, that Mr Isaacs' brain might have been transferred to one or other collection. These collections have different procedures from the joint programme of the Departments of Psychiatry and Physiology.

Sources of information

This chapter is based on contemporaneous registers, other documents and the recollections of staff involved at the time.

The Cerebral Function Unit

The history of the Cerebral Function Unit

In 1982 the CFU was set up within the Department of Neurology. The unit was planned by Dr, now Professor, David Neary as a regional tertiary referral resource for investigation of patients with progressive neurological degenerative conditions such as Alzheimer's disease.

The unit was located at Manchester Royal Infirmary until transferred in 2001 to Hope Hospital, Salford. Professor Neary and Professor David Mann, the neuropathologist of the unit, are now based at Hope Hospital, as are the unit's laboratories and brain collection.

Reasons for exploring the procedures of the Cerebral Function Unit

There were a number of reasons for including the CFU in my investigation:

i. to ensure that the brain of Mr Isaacs had not been transferred to the Unit. I am satisfied this did not happen, Chapters 3 and 4;

ii. between 1985 and 1994, the CFU was collecting brains from the same mortuaries as the joint programme;

iii. nineteen brains recorded in the brain books are listed as being obtained from Professor Mann. However, only fifteen of these are among the brains regarded as part of the joint programme[1];

iv. a number of research protocols submitted to funding bodies or to Ethics Committees by members of the joint programme had included references to brains being collected and shared between the two programmes[2&3];

v. morticians from four local mortuaries had referred to the checks that were made before any brain was obtained for the CFU research programme.

Meetings with Professor Mann and Professor Neary

To clarify the procedures of the unit and its research programme, meetings were held with Professor David Mann on 19 December 2001 and 11 January 2002 and with Professor Neary on 20 March 2002. These discussions confirmed the recollections of morticians at four hospitals, data in the Prestwich Mortuary Register and extant patients' records that the CFU only collected brains from patients with dementing conditions who were already known to the unit.

The procedures of the Cerebral Function Unit

All patients in the unit's care are seen and assessed in life. Multidisciplinary care programmes are tailored to the needs of each patient. The patient's relatives are kept fully informed of the unit's purpose and of the progress of the patient's condition. When a patient is considered to be nearing the end of life, the relatives are asked if they are willing to consent to post mortem study of the patient's brain.

The relatives are given time to reflect on this request. If they agree, a written consent form for post mortem study of the brain is signed and placed with the patient's notes. Written consent forms have been in use since the CFU research programme started. If the relatives do not agree, the unit's clinical care of the patient is unaffected.

When a patient dies, arrangements are made for the brain to be removed soon after death. It was frequently the patient's relatives who informed Professor Mann of a patient's death.

After the body reaches the mortuary, the consent form is checked before the brain is removed. This procedure was independently reported by morticians at four hospitals. In many cases the extent of the post mortem is limited to removal of the brain. Professor Mann always collects the brain from the mortuary himself.

The removal of the brain in the early years of the programme took place as soon as possible after death. This sometimes required the mortician and Professor Mann to attend the mortuary in the middle of the night.

Professor Mann also undertook neuropathological investigations with other research workers on the brains of patients with Down's syndrome and Huntington's disease. This work was not related to the CFU research programme.

Each brain was examined by Professor Mann and the results of the examination are correlated with in-life clinical findings. Letters are then sent to the relatives explaining the results of the brain examination.

Other information and features of the CFU programme

The research undertaken in the unit has all been approved by Local Research Ethics Committees.

The only brains obtained from Coroner's cases were those of patients already known to the CFU whose deaths had been reported to the Coroner for unrelated reasons.

Copies of the earlier CFU consent form were found in patients' records at Prestwich Hospital. A copy of the current form is at Annex 26. Annex 26

Copies of standard letters similar to those sent to relatives of patients enrolled in programme were provided. Annex 27

Co-operation with the joint programme of the Departments of Psychiatry and Physiology

There was very limited co-operation between the CFU programme and the joint programme. Professor Neary, on behalf of the members of the CFU, states that:

"None of the members of the CFU, including myself, had any knowledge of the contents of the research protocols submitted to funding bodies and Ethics Committees by the Psychiatry Group (i.e. the joint programme). *We had taken no part in engendering protocols and had no knowledge of research aims or methodology. We were certainly not aware of any intention for brains to be 'shared' with us".* See also Chapter 9.

Although the programmes were different, parts of 19 brains collected by Professor Mann were provided for the joint programme. The first sample was provided in January 1986 and the last in June 1995. Sixteen of these brain samples were from cases with Alzheimer's disease, two with Down's syndrome and one Huntington's disease. Four of the samples were not subsequently used by the joint programme. Histology had been undertaken by Dr Mann in all these cases.

No brains or parts of brains were transferred in the reverse direction from the joint programme to the CFU.

Several mortuaries were involved in providing brains to the CFU and the joint programme. This confused staff in at least two mortuaries, Chapters 13 and 15. In all mortuaries the morticians were aware that the CFU had no interest in collecting brains from Coroner's cases or cases of sudden death who had not previously been assessed within the CFU's programme.

Summary

All CFU patients were seen and assessed in life.

Brains obtained by the CFU were all retained with the knowledge and consent of the relatives.

The CFU did not receive any brains from cases of sudden death reported to Coroners, unless the deceased had been assessed in life within the CFU programme.

The research programme of the CFU and the post mortem retention of the brains of patients investigated in the unit received Ethics Committee approval.

There was very limited overlap between the CFU and the joint programme but in at least two mortuaries there was some confusion about the differences between the two.

I am satisfied that the CFU's procedures for obtaining consent from the relatives were robust and designed to comply fully with the requirements of the Human Tissue Act. Consent was obtained in all cases where the brain was removed. If the relatives changed their minds, the brain was not removed. In addition, the research undertaken by the Unit had obtained ethical approval after disclosure of all relevant matters.

The Neuro Special Pathology Collection

Introduction

The Neuro Special Pathology (NSP) collection was identified during the meeting with Professor Freemont on 28 November 2001 as one of the collections that Manchester University had reported to the Chief Medical Officer's Census. Brains held in the collection were included in the lists prepared by the University to enable the return of organs and tissues by the Central Manchester Hospitals NHS Trust to relatives who requested this.

Reasons for including the NSP collection

The reason for investigating the records of the NSP was to see if these contained any reference to Mr Isaacs' brain.

I am satisfied from these checks that Mr Isaacs' brain was not referred to the NSP collection, Chapter 4.

Meetings held

To clarify the purposes and procedures of the NSP and to scrutinise the NSP records, meetings were held with Dr Helen Reid on 19 December 2001 and later that day with Mr Peter Sullivan who holds the records of all specimens sent to the University Pathology Department, including the NSP. A separate meeting was held with Dr Emyr Benbow at Manchester Royal Infirmary on 11 January 2002.

Purpose of the NSP

The origin and purpose of the NSP collection is very different to both the CFU and the joint programme. The NSP is a diagnostic accumulation of brains. No research has been undertaken on brains in the collection.

Dr Helen Reid

Dr Reid is the only medically qualified Consultant Neuropathologist in Manchester. Her nearest colleagues in the same specialty are in Liverpool and Preston. Dr Reid provides a diagnostic clinical service for surgical and post mortem specimens from a very wide geographical area well beyond the boundaries of the City of Manchester.

All specimens are allocated an NSP number. Most are surgical but some whole brains are referred among which are a number from Coroners' cases. For the latter, Dr Reid ensures her report on the neuropathological findings is available to the Coroner in time for the inquest.

When whole brains have been referred, each brain is stored until Dr Reid is satisfied no further diagnostic examination is required.

Location of the NSP

The NSP collection was held in the Department of Pathology in the Medical School until the Department of Clinical Neuropathology moved to Hope Hospital, Salford, in 2001. At that time the NSP collection was transferred to the Pathology Department of the Central Manchester Hospitals NHS Trust.

Summary

Mr Isaacs' brain was not referred to the NSP.

Brains are only referred to the Neuro Special Pathology collection for diagnosis.

The collection includes a number of brains from Coroners' cases.

No research is carried out but diagnostic review may sometimes be required.

There is no overlap and there were no transfers between the NSP collection and the joint programme.

References

1. Entries in the brain books of the joint programme.
2. Protocol dated 17 July 1986 submitted to the North Manchester Ethics Committee.
3. Application for research funds dated 2 May 1985 to the North West Regional Health Authority.

SECTION 3

The research programme of the Departments of Physiology and Psychiatry of Manchester University (the "Joint Programme")

CHAPTER 9

Origin of the joint programme, funding application to the North West Regional Health Authority and progress 1985 -1988

Introduction

This chapter describes the origins and objectives of the joint programme, the leadership of the programme, the initial research application and the sourcing of brains in the first three years.

It was to this research programme that the brain of Mr Isaacs was taken on 27 February 1987 after the Coroner's post mortem examination at Prestwich mortuary.

Prior to the start of the joint programme, Dr Slater had begun research into Alzheimer's disease for which brain samples had been obtained from a number of sources. Some of these samples appear to have been listed in the first of the brain books. See below.

The joint research programme, organised by the Departments of Psychiatry and Physiology, started in 1985.

Leaders of the joint research team

The research programme was jointly led by Dr J F W Deakin, Senior Lecturer, later Professor, in the Department of Psychiatry, Dr Paul Slater, Reader in Physiology, and initially also by Dr Alan Cross, Lecturer in Neurochemistry in the Department of Physiology.

Dr J F W Deakin

Dr Deakin was appointed Senior Lecturer in the Academic Department of Psychiatry of Manchester University in the autumn of 1983.

Before moving to Manchester Dr Deakin had, from 1978, held a Joint Clinical-Scientific Member of Staff appointment at the Clinical Research Centre (CRC). The Centre was a major MRC research institute attached to Northwick Park Hospital. Dr Deakin had held an Honorary Senior Registrar appointment at the hospital while his research was almost entirely laboratory-based.

For his clinical responsibilities in Manchester, Dr Deakin worked at the University Hospital of South Manchester.

Dr Paul Slater

Dr Slater was appointed Reader in Physiology at Manchester University in 1983.

Dr Alan Cross

Dr Cross was appointed Lecturer in Neurochemistry in the Department of Physiology at Manchester University in 1984. Before taking up this appointment, Dr Cross had also worked at the CRC as a post-doctoral scientist from 1979 until 1984. Dr Cross left the team early in the joint programme and before the first progress report.

Origins of the joint research programme

In 1985 there were a number of research programmes in this country and abroad that collected brains. Before moving to Manchester both Dr Deakin and Dr Cross had been involved in brain research at the CRC. The CRC programme, which had included the collection of brains, was led by Dr Tim Crow, Head of the Mental Illness Division, and Dr Eve Johnstone.

After Dr Deakin and Dr Cross moved to Manchester, they had a shared research interest in neurochemical research on the brain with Dr Slater. From that shared interest the joint brain research programme was planned and developed.

Objectives

The main focus of the joint research programme was the investigation of neurochemistry in different parts of the brains of patients who had exhibited in life well defined psychiatric or neuro degenerative conditions. In 1985 brain neurochemistry had not been investigated in many psychiatric disorders.

Alzheimer's disease and schizophrenia were the conditions identified in the first applications to the North West Regional Health Authority (NWRHA) and the Medical Research Council.

There were a number of large hospitals, for patients with neuropsychiatric disorders and mental handicap conditions, in and near Manchester in 1985. Many were long-stay patients with Alzheimer's disease, schizophrenia and other mental conditions.

The joint research programme was planned to study these patients in life and link in-life findings to post mortem neurochemistry of the brain.

Methodology

Brains were to be collected to provide a bank of specimens for the joint programme. The method of brain collection was expected to adopt procedures similar to those of the brain research programme at the CRC, with which Dr Deakin and Dr Cross were familiar.

One CRC programme, for example, had collected the brains of patients with schizophrenia who died in Shenley, a long-stay mental hospital. Similar clinical and post mortem arrangements were already in use in Manchester by the Cerebral Function Unit as described in Chapter 8.

The collection method in Manchester was therefore planned to follow methods used in contemporary research elsewhere in this country.

The CRC research programme is discussed in Chapters 31 and 32 but two features should be noted:

1) the consent of the relatives for brain retention had been obtained routinely in the CRC schizophrenia study of patients at Shenley Hospital. The only exceptions had been for deceased patients with no known relatives. In accordance with HM(61)98 the Hospital Secretary was approached for his consent;

2) the brains of persons who had died of unrelated diseases were not collected by the CRC research team. Instead "controls" were obtained from the Corsellis collection, Chapters 31-33.

No histological report

A significant difference between the joint research programme and the methodology of the Cerebral Function Unit was that no histological examinations were undertaken. Dr Slater has indicated that some samples were sent by Dr Cross to the Pathology Department, adding *"with the dearth of neuropathologists the delays in getting answers just took far too long and we were forced to abandon attempts"*. Both Dr Slater and Professor Deakin emphasised that histology in schizophrenia would not be informative. Professor Deakin states that *"histology could not have been the primary reason for retention of the whole brain in any post-mortem brain programme researching schizophrenia in the UK"*. However, some other contemporaneous programmes undertook histology as a matter of routine.

Another significant difference between the methodology of the Cerebral Function Unit and the joint programme was that no reports were sent to the doctor who looked after the deceased before death. Dr Slater states that *"the fact is that we never intended to do this and had never been asked by anyone to do so"*.

Dr Slater recollects, however, that on more than one occasion messages were received from the relatives via the Coroner's office to ask if anything unusual had been discovered during examination, as there had been doubts about old diagnosis or possible exposure to occupational diseases. The circumstances of these enquiries are not mentioned in the brain books.

Research proposals

The first of three research applications submitted to the Locally Organised Clinical Research Scheme of the North West Regional Health Authority in May 1985 describes the initial proposals of the joint programme. Appendix 17

This application, entitled *"An Investigation of Amino Acid Neurotransmitters in the Temporal Lobe of Brain in Alzheimer's Disease and Schizophrenia"* was submitted by Dr Deakin, Dr Cross and Dr Slater. A grant for three years, to start in October 1985, was requested.

A preambular paragraph states *"At present there is no funding for collaborative projects between Psychiatry and Physiology"*.

Features of the application that are common to later applications to the NWRHA

Normal and diseased brains would be studied:

"It is proposed to apply these techniques to study amino acid neurotransmission in the human temporal lobe of post-mortem brains of those without brain disease and those with Alzheimer's disease and schizophrenia".

Brains would be obtained from a number of hospitals in or near Manchester:

"... studies of normal brain will be an essential part of the investigation. Brains from subjects with no history of neuropsychiatric disorders will be obtained from Manchester Royal Infirmary (MRI). We have secured a formal arrangement with the Department of Pathology which allows us access to brains removed at post-mortem examination and within a few hours of death. We have, in storage, brains from patients with pathologically-confirmed Alzheimer-type dementia that are obtained via the Pathology Department. These will be supplemented for this project by brains from subjects with Alzheimer's disease from the Pre-Senile Dementia Unit at Prestwich Hospital. Arrangements have been made with Dr D Neary (MRI), the administrator of the Unit and Dr I Stout, the Consultant in charge for the supply of brains whenever pre-mortem consent has been obtained. A similar arrangement exists with Dr S D Soni, Consultant Psychiatrist at Prestwich Hospital, for brains from subjects with clinically-confirmed schizophrenia ... Post-mort em brains may also be obtained from Withington Hospital."

This extract is taken verbatim from the application submitted to NWRHA. However, it is contested by Professor Neary and Dr Stout.

Professor Neary states in a letter to me dated 3 January 2003 *"that the CFU and the schizophrenia groups were and are seen in practice to be independent is attested by the decision of clinicians such as Dr Ian Stout, who has supported my work in dementia for over 20 years, not to take part in the schizophrenia project.*

I do not consider myself as having taken part in a collaboration and I remain uninformed about the workings of the schizophrenia group. The latter has, I understand, sought some pathological assistance from David Mann, which was minimal and non-reciprocal".

Dr Stout in a letter dated 10 January 2003 states *"At no time that I can remember was I ever approached to participate in a formal research study"*.

On the matter of consent by the relatives, Dr Stout emphasises *"the only such examinations that I was aware of were on those patients whose families had already provided me with written consent that they would be investigated thereafter by Professor Neary and Professor Mann and colleagues, but* *<u>no other</u>"*.

Dr Stout adds *"I have absolutely no idea whatsoever as to what was meant by the statement 'arrangements have been made with Dr D Neary (MRI), the administrator of the Unit, and Dr I Stout' "*.

Dr Stout does not recall any subsequent request in the late 1980s from the joint research team to provide clinical material or extract information from case notes.

For further details of the CFU programme, see Chapter 8.

<u>The brain collection and investigations would be in the neurochemical laboratories in the Department of Physiology</u>

The brains would be held in the neurochemical laboratories of the Department of Physiology in the Medical School.

<u>Clinicians would be contacted and case records would be accessed</u>

"The post-doctoral worker will be expected to liase with the clinicians and mortuary staff who are providing the clinical material for the project, and to extract the information relevant to the diagnoses from the case notes".

In practice, for patients who died in hospital the case notes were later obtained by the research team. When brains were obtained from cases of sudden death reported to the Coroner, the deceased's general practitioner would usually be identified through the information available to the pathologist at the time of the post mortem. The mortician would include the name of the GP in the form that accompanied the brain to Manchester University. Annex 16

Where the general practitioner was not known at the time of the post mortem, the research team would write to the relevant Family Practitioner Committee in order to identify the general practitioner who would then receive a copy of the letter requesting details of the deceased's mental health and medication. Annex 15

<u>Two relevant matters were not included in the first application</u>

<u>Ethics Committee Referral</u>

Ethics Committee referral was not mentioned in the first application to the NWRHA but was included in a later application to the authority for an extension of the original grant. Ethics Committee applications are described in Chapters 12-15.

<u>Coroners' Cases</u>

The inclusion of brains obtained from post mortems ordered by the Coroner is not mentioned in this or subsequent applications to the NWRHA. The retention of brains from Coroners' cases from the North Manchester coronial district is described in Chapter 10.

Award of the NWRHA grant

The research application was approved after scientific referees had been consulted and the project began in October 1985.

Progress October 1985 - February 1988

Brains collected

The first brain collected for the joint programme and coded in the brain book as 85/01[1], was obtained from Prestwich mortuary on 1 November 1985. The number of brains obtained in the first three years of the programme by mortuary were:

Brains received	Prestwich mortuary	NMGH mortuary	Other mortuaries	Total
1985	5	0	0	5
1986	29	6	6	41
1987	9	2	1	12

The last brain collected in the first phase of the programme was obtained from Prestwich mortuary on 18 May 1987. There was then an interval of over nine months as no further brains were collected from any mortuary until 29 February 1988. When collection resumed, the brains were obtained mainly from other mortuaries and only nine more from Prestwich.

The available documents provide no explanation for this suspension of brain collection from 18 May 1987 until 29 February 1988. Members of the team were asked but could not remember why brain collection was interrupted. However, Professor Deakin has suggested the interval *"corresponds to the period between the end of a Research Clinician's (Dr C Royston) six-month Wellcome Registrar appointment (February 1987) and their 3 year appointment as a Wellcome Trust Training Fellow in 1988 (Oct 88)".*

However, these time intervals do not correspond or explain why brain collection resumed in February 1988, but almost entirely from NMGH.

Storage of brains

The brains collected were stored in temperature-controlled freezers in the neuro chemical laboratory of the Physiology Department. The freezers were attached to an emergency power supply to prevent damage to the brain specimens in the event of a power cut. Dr Slater had responsibility for the laboratory arrangements in the Department of Physiology. Dr Slater states that for this reason his name was included in all applications made by the joint programme.

Appendix 1

Status of brains collected

In the first three years of the programme the status of the brains obtained for the research programme is set out in the following table.

Brains received	Coroners' Cases	Hospital Cases	Total
1985	5	0	5
1986	34	7	41
1987	10	2	12

This illustrates the heavy predominance of Coroners' cases in the first three years of the programme, which continued in the following eight years. The inclusion of Coroners' cases was not mentioned in the applications to the NWRHA and the MRC in 1988 and 1989. However, the involvement of the *"Rochdale Coroner"* was referred to in the 1989 application to the Mental Health Foundation.

Research reports and subsequent applications to the NWRHA

June 1987

A progress report on the research grant awarded following the application made in May 1985, was submitted to the NWRHA by Dr Deakin and Dr Slater. This included a request for additional funds to take account of new developments and stated *"We have made considerable progress towards the aims set out in the original application". "Recently, we have secured a large number of samples from the Cambridge Brain Bank and work on schizophrenia will therefore be expanded".* Appendix 18

February 1988

A further progress report stated *"We have obtained brain samples from control subjects and from subjects with clinically diagnosed schizophrenia from the Cambridge Brain Bank laboratory"*. The report recorded *"very exciting findings and we have been fortunate in securing from the Clinical Research Centre, Northwick Park Hospital, brain samples from a particularly well-defined group of schizophrenic subjects"*. It is not clear in this report whether the control samples were obtained from the Cambridge brain bank or collected locally. Appendix 19

The award of a Wellcome Trust Fellowship was also reported.

March 1988

A second grant application was submitted to the NWRHA. Appendix 20

Plans to expand the programme

Between November 1985 and March 1988, the promising results reported in the two progress reports to the NWRHA encouraged the team to expand the work. This expansion required:

i. additional research funding, Chapter 11;
ii. an increase in the number of brains obtained for the programme. Action taken to increase the number of brains collected is described in Chapters 14 and 15.

Summary

The joint research team began working on the programme in 1985. The team leaders were Dr Deakin in the Department of Psychiatry, Dr Cross and Dr Slater in the Department of Physiology.

The system for brain collection was planned to adopt the procedures that had been in place at the Clinical Research Centre, Northwick Park, where Dr Deakin and Dr Cross had previously worked.

The programme would involve the collection of brains of patients with Alzheimer's disease and schizophrenia who died in mental hospitals in the Manchester area.

Pre-mortem consent from relatives was planned.

Brains from "normal" persons without any evidence of mental or neurological disease were to be collected as "controls".

Where the deceased's general practitioner was not identified at the time of post mortem, the Family Practitioner Committee would be asked for this information.

Initial funding was obtained from the NWRHA. A brain bank was established in the Department of Physiology.

Good scientific progress followed. Novel and *"very exciting findings"* encouraged the team to develop their work and apply for further NWRHA grants.

Some brain specimens were obtained from the Cambridge and Northwick Park brain banks.

Referral to Ethics Committees was not mentioned in the 1985 application or the 1987 and 1988 reports to the NWRHA.

The collection of brains from Coroners' cases was not mentioned in any of the applications or reports to the NWRHA between 1985 and 1988.

The collection of brains from Coroners' cases, set out in Chapter 10, was a major feature of the programme and, in view of the large proportion of brains collected from Coroners' cases, should have been mentioned in the reports to the NWRHA.

Reference

1 Entry in the brain books.

CHAPTER 10

Brain collection at Prestwich mortuary 1985-1989 and arrangements with the Coroner's office

Introduction

This chapter describes the arrangements that were in place between 1985 and 1989 to collect brains from Prestwich mortuary in which the Coroner's office had a central role.

Sources of information

The chapter is based on the recollections of staff in the Coroner's office, Prestwich mortuary and Manchester University.

Collection systems that influenced the procedures adopted for the joint programme

Dr Deakin and Dr Cross had both worked at the Clinical Research Centre (CRC). The CRC's procedures for collection of brains are outlined in Chapter 9 and are also described more fully in Chapters 31 and 32. The Corsellis collection, Chapter 33, had provided control brains for the CRC programme.

The Cerebral Function Unit in the Department of Neurology had collected brains from hospitals in the Manchester area for its research programme since 1982.

The brain collection system for the joint programme described in the first application to NWRHA

The brain collection methodology has been described in Chapter 9 and is also set out in Appendix 17. Three points should be noted: Appendix 17

- consent of the relatives would be obtained, and this was emphasised;
- control brains would be collected but consent for these was not mentioned;
- collection of brains of Coroners' cases was not referred to.

The collection system as it evolved at Prestwich mortuary

Between November 1985 and May 1987 the brains of only three cases were obtained from hospital or "brain only" post mortems at Prestwich mortuary. The other 40 brains all came from Coroner's cases. Eight of these were deaths of patients in Prestwich Hospital reported to the Coroner. The remaining 32, including Mr Isaacs', were deaths in the community.

Involvement of the Coroner's office

The links that were in place before 1985, through which brains had been transferred from Prestwich and other mortuaries in North Manchester to the brain bank at Cambridge, are described in Chapter 7.

The link between the Coroner's office in Rochdale and the identification of suitable cases for the joint programme is illustrated by one of the first entries in the brain books, dated 30 January 1986. This entry includes the telephone number of the Coroner's office in Rochdale, and Mrs Langan's name. The relevant death had been referred to the North Manchester Coroner [(2)].

Earlier entries in the same brain book show that between 1 November 1985 and the end of January 1986, five brains of patients with a diagnosis of schizophrenia or other psychiatric diseases had been obtained from Prestwich mortuary.

1986

During 1986 the brains of 26 patients from Prestwich mortuary were obtained by the joint programme from post mortems ordered by the Coroner. Six of these were on inpatients. Three brains were obtained from hospital post mortems with which the Coroner's office had no involvement.

How the system at Prestwich mortuary worked

Early in the investigation it became clear that the Coroner's office in Rochdale was centrally involved in identifying suitable brains for the joint programme in its early years. The arrangements were described during separate meetings with Mrs Langan, three other staff members of the Coroner's office, Mr Walkden, Dr Farrand, and by Dr Slater and Dr Simpson who was a member of the Department of Physiology from 1985.

When the death of a patient with Alzheimer's disease, schizophrenia or other psychiatric disorder was notified to the Coroner for the North Manchester Police District, Mrs Langan, the senior member of the office staff, would herself telephone the Department of Physiology at Manchester University, or ask another staff member to do so. The message conveyed was that a brain that might be suitable for the research programme would become available later in the day.

The Rochdale Coroner's office held for this purpose two telephone numbers. The first number was Dr Slater's extension; if unanswered, the call would be transferred to the neurochemical laboratory in the Department of Physiology. Dr Deakin's extension number was held as a reserve. However, the Coroner's office staff report, and Dr Deakin has confirmed, that he was rarely telephoned.

Once a call had been received in the Department of Physiology, Dr Slater or one of his staff would telephone Prestwich mortuary to ask Mr Walkden, the mortician, when the brain would be ready for collection.

Mr Walkden would notify the pathologist that the brain was to be retained for the joint programme. Most of the Coroner's post mortems at Prestwich were undertaken by Dr Farrand. Once the brain had been removed, Mr Walkden would place it on ice in the mortuary refrigerator where it would remain until collected.

Mr Walkden would also complete a short note giving basic details of the deceased, including name, age, date, the time of death, the time the brain was removed and the cause of death. The name and address of the general practitioner of the deceased would be included if this was known.

At Prestwich mortuary these particulars were always written on a piece of thin, pale yellow paper of A5 size. Copies of these notes are still held in the brain books and are characteristic of brain referrals from Prestwich mortuary. Annex 16

Dr Slater, sometimes accompanied by another member of staff, would visit Prestwich mortuary to collect the brain. If Dr Slater was unavailable, another member of staff or the University courier would be sent. Whoever went to the mortuary would take a cold box designed to transport the brain safely.

On some occasions the Coroner's office would inform the mortician, Mr Walkden, before letting the Department of Physiology know there was a brain to be collected, but this was more unusual.

All the staff involved in the Coroner's office, and Dr Farrand, Mr Walkden, Dr Slater and Dr Simpson all described these arrangements in similar terms. I have no doubts about the reliability of their descriptions.

Investigation of the origins of the arrangement with the Coroner's office

I have been unable to discover when and how the first contact was made between the joint research team and the North Manchester district Coroner's office in Rochdale as there is no agreement between the recollections of those directly involved at the time.

Both Mrs Langan and Dr Slater confirm there were a number of telephone calls between them and a visit by Dr Slater to the Coroner's office in Rochdale, but their detailed recollections differ.

What is certain is that in the autumn of 1985 there must have been some contact between the University and Mrs Langan. Mrs Langan recollects telephone calls received from Dr Slater before any brains were identified. The first two brains, regarded as part of the joint programme, were both from Coroner's cases and were collected on 1 November 1985 from Prestwich mortuary. Three other brains were collected during 1985 from Prestwich mortuary, all from Coroner's cases. All five were from deaths outside hospital.

Mrs Langan's recollection

Mrs Langan is clear that Dr Slater initiated the first telephone calls to the Coroner's office and that these were made before any cases were identified to the joint programme. Mrs Langan's recollection is that Dr Slater's visit to the Coroner's office in Rochdale was not as early as 1985 and could have been much later. What is clear is that Mr North was not in the office at the time of Dr Slater's visit and a letter was left for him, which Mrs Langan had typed for Dr Slater. The letter was then placed on Mr North's desk.
Mrs Langan is also clear that the letter was a request to the Coroner to agree that brains from suitable cases, whose deaths had been referred to the Coroner, could be made available for the joint research programme.

Mrs Langan states that in keeping with the procedures at the time, she and other members of the Coroner's office staff would have taken no action without the agreement of the Coroner. Mrs Langan assures me that no cases were identified to the joint programme following the telephone calls she had received from Dr Slater until Mr North had indicated his agreement to Dr Slater's telephoned requests.

Dr Slater's recollection

Dr Slater agrees that he made telephone calls to the Coroner's office and that he had probably made the first call on behalf of the joint programme. He is unsure of the date. Dr Slater is convinced that the identification of suitable cases to the joint programme began as a result of the telephone calls and before his visit to the Coroner's office in Rochdale.

Dr Slater's recollection is that his visit to the Coroner's office was certainly not in 1985 but later, perhaps as late as 1988. The visit was, he recalls, "*on the spur of the moment*" when he was in Rochdale to collect a brain from the public mortuary. The brain in question had been identified through the arrangements with the Coroner's office. Dr Slater also believes this was not the first brain that he had collected from Rochdale public mortuary.

As there were only three brains collected from Rochdale public mortuary in the first five years of the joint programme, Dr Slater's recollection would pinpoint his visit to the Coroner's office on 30 January 1986, 16 October 1986 or 19 October 1988.

Dr Slater recollects that, during his visit, he left a letter and confirms that this was typed for him by Mrs Langan. Although he never received a reply, the referral of suitable cases continued.

Other recollections

The Coroner, Mr North, states that he was unaware of the arrangement and has no knowledge of Dr Slater's phone calls or of Dr Slater's visit to the Coroner's office in Rochdale.

Apart from Mrs Langan, the other members of Mr North's office staff remember that Dr Slater had visited the office in Rochdale. They confirm that Mr North was not in the office at the time, but no one can remember the date of the visit. Their recollections tend to support those of Mrs Langan.

There are no documents or correspondence about the origin of the referral arrangements, or other information that helps to date Dr Slater's visit. The present staff of the Coroner's office have searched for any relevant papers but have found nothing.

Visit to Prestwich Hospital and mortuary

Dr Deakin, Dr Cross and Dr Slater visited Prestwich Hospital and mortuary in 1985. Dr Deakin suggests the date was either 19 or 22 April, although this date is unconfirmed. The visit was intended to meet the consultant psychiatrists at the hospital and explain the research programme to them. The team also visited the mortuary. They did not meet Dr Farrand, the pathologist who undertook most of the Coroner's post mortems at Prestwich in the late 1980s, but did see the mortician Mr Walkden. The visit is also remembered by others who travelled in Dr Deakin's Vauxhall car[3].

Collection of brains from "normal" individuals

While the collection system at Prestwich began with the intention of obtaining brains from patients who had died in Prestwich Hospital from neuropsychiatric conditions, the records of the programme and the entries in the brain book show that from February 1986, brains of "normal controls" were also being collected from Prestwich mortuary. In that year at least 18 brains, described as "controls", were obtained from Prestwich mortuary.

Professor Deakin's comments in 2001 on the origin of the system

In a letter dated 11 June 2001 to the General Medical Council, Professor Deakin set out his recollection of the start of the brain collection system[4]:

"Dr Slater initially set the system up for Alzheimer's disease but I began collaborating with him with schizophrenia sometime afterwards. The local mortuaries and coroner's offices would telephone Dr Slater's laboratory if possible cases of Alzheimer's disease or schizophrenia were undergoing post mortem and also if non-psychiatric control subjects were.

This system continued an earlier one in which brains from all over the country were supplied to The Medical Research Council Brain Bank at Addenbrooke's Hospital. My understanding is that in Coroners' cases of non-patient deaths in the community, consent was not routinely sought in the 1970s and early 80s. In contrast, where deaths occurred in hospitals, removal of tissue could not happen without written consent of the relatives. We continued existing practise (sic) *in the NW. As far as I could see, this did not differ from practises* (sic) *in the previous research institute where I trained or from practice in other hospitals at that time".*

Chapters 31 and 32 describe the brain collection arrangements at the CRC, where the collection of Coroner's cases was authorised under Coroners Rules 9 and 12, which are not mentioned anywhere in the documents of the joint programme.

Brains collected through Prestwich mortuary

November 1985 - May 1987

Five brains were collected in 1985, all from Coroner's cases.

The collection of brains from Prestwich mortuary was brisk throughout 1986 and continued until May 1987 when the whole collection programme for the joint programme came to a halt. No further brains were collected from any mortuary until 29 February 1988. When brain collection resumed, this was mainly from North Manchester General Hospital (NMGH), Chapter 13.

1988/89 until the closure of Prestwich mortuary

There were only five further brains collected from Coroner's cases in Prestwich mortuary when the programme restarted. The last brain was collected on 18 July 1989. Three of these five cases were inpatient deaths referred to the Coroner. The remaining two were categorised as "controls".

Prestwich mortuary closed for post mortems in August 1989 but continued for hospital use. Any post mortems required on patients who had died in Prestwich Hospital were carried out at Fairfield Hospital, Bury.

Mr Walkden, the mortician at Prestwich, transferred to Fairfield Hospital in 1988.

1986-1996 – Bury, Rochdale and Oldham mortuaries

Although brains for the programme obtained from these mortuaries were mainly taken in the later years of the programme, these mortuaries are discussed in this chapter as the office of the North Manchester Coroner was involved.

Discussions with Mr Walkden on the arrangements since his transfer to Fairfield Hospital, Bury, and with Mr Paul Owen, the mortician at Rochdale mortuary, indicate that between 1986 and 1996 the same arrangements that operated originally at Prestwich had continued until 1996. Six Coroner's cases were referred from Oldham mortuary, 34 from Rochdale and 27 from Bury.

A difference was that these Coroner's cases had almost all suffered from psychiatric illnesses. Only three "control" cases were referred from Rochdale mortuary in 1994. After 1989 no "controls" were referred from Bury or Oldham mortuaries.

The last brains from Coroner's cases were collected from Bury mortuary in July 1996, from Rochdale mortuary on 5 September 1996 and from Oldham mortuary on 5 November 1996.

I have considered the possibility that some of the deaths of patients with neuropsychiatric disease were referred to the Coroner in order that the brain could be obtained for the joint programme. However, I have found no evidence that any of the deaths were inappropriately referred to the North Manchester Coroner in any of the cases where the post mortem examination was undertaken at Bury, Oldham or Rochdale mortuaries.

Request for brains from patients with epilepsy

Another feature at Rochdale is the letter dated 1 June 1994 signed by Mrs Joyce Langan to Dr Menon, Consultant Pathologist in Rochdale, which indicates plans for widening the brain collection programme to include brains from those who had been treated for epilepsy. Mrs Langan is certain that she would have cleared this letter with Mr North *"to keep him in the picture"*. Annex 28

Chronology of brains collected from Prestwich Mortuary

May 1985	First application to the NWRHA by the joint programme for research funding
October 1985	NWRHA funding awarded
1 November 1985	First brain collected from Prestwich mortuary
15 January 1986	Salford EC approval of research protocol submitted by Dr Deakin and Dr Soni
17 July 1986	Date of signature of research protocol later submitted to North Manchester and other Ethics Committees
26 February 1987	Mr Isaacs' death
27 February 1987	Post mortem examination at Prestwich mortuary
16 March 1987	Inquest into Mr Isaacs' death
23 March 1987	Mrs Isaacs' first letter to Mr North
16 April 1987	Mrs Isaacs' further letter to Mr North
18 May 1987	Collection of brains for the joint programme halted from all mortuaries
29 February 1988	Brain collection for the joint programme restarts with collection of a brain from NMGH mortuary
14 April 1988	Restart of brain collection from Prestwich mortuary
18 July 1989	Collection of last brain from Prestwich mortuary
August 1989	The last post mortem at Prestwich mortuary
Date uncertain (probably 1989)	Closure of Prestwich mortuary

Summary

The plan for brain collection described in the original research application of the joint programme and in subsequent documents recorded that brains would be collected after consent had been obtained from the relatives.

The collection programme was planned to be similar to that in use in the Cerebral Function Unit and to the procedures of the Clinical Research Centre, Northwick Park Hospital.

Professor Deakin in his letter of 8 November 2001 to me states that the brain collection system was set up to follow the practice that had been in operation in other centres in the 1980s[(5)]. The collection of brains of Coroners' cases did not, however, follow the procedures under Coroners Rules 9 and 12 that had been in place at the Clinical Research Centre.

When the programme started, an arrangement with the Coroner's office in Rochdale identified the great majority of the brains that were obtained.

It was the Coroner's office in Rochdale that identified suitable cases from Prestwich mortuary for the joint programme and later continued to do so from Coroner's cases at mortuaries in Bury, Rochdale and Oldham.

References

1. Case papers at the Cambridge brain bank.
2. Entry in the first brain book of the joint programme.
3. Letter from Professor David Gordon dated 1 March 2002.
4. Letter from Professor Deakin to Ms Alexandra Nall at the General Medical Council dated 11 June 2001.
5. Letter from Professor Deakin to Dr Metters dated 8 November 2001.

CHAPTER 11

Development of the joint programme at Manchester University from 1988: applications for research funds and awards

Introduction

This chapter describes some of the research grant applications made by the joint team.

Due to the passage of time it has not been possible to trace several of the applications made by the team. Those that are available are described in detail since they provide contemporaneous information about features of the programme that are directly relevant to my investigation.

The chapter also describes the application submitted to the Mental Health Foundation in 1988 which, for the first time, includes a direct reference to the involvement of the North Manchester Coroner's office in identifying suitable brains for the joint programme.

A: Applications for research funds to the NWRHA

March 1988 Second application

The title of the application was "*Neuropeptide Synthesis in Alzheimer's Disease and Schizophrenia*".

This application, Appendix 20, for a two-year grant was submitted by Dr Slater and Dr Deakin. The application referred to progress previously reported in June 1987 and February 1988. Appendix 20

While the basic plan for collection of normal and diseased human brains was unchanged, there were some differences from the first application. A new dimension was the inclusion of comparative studies of animal brains.

The procedure for brain collection from Manchester Hospitals was described as: "*Control human brains from subjects with no history of neurological or psychiatric illness will be obtained from hospitals in the Manchester area, via long-standing arrangements. Brains from subjects with Alzheimer's disease and schizophrenia will also be obtained from the Greater Manchester area. Pre-mortem consent is obtained for the removal of brains at post mortem examination*".

Expenses for "*Travel costs, materials and fees for collecting human brains*" of £250 per year were requested.

The application did not mention Ethics Committee referral or the fact that by March 1988 the majority of the brains already collected had been retained from Coroners' cases.

The NWRHA were informed that some funding had been secured from the Wellcome Trust and the Science and Engineering Research Council (SERC).

July 1990 Progress report

This report on the first research project grant applied for in May 1985 on *"An investigation of amino acid neurotransmitters in the temporal lobe of brain in Alzheimer's disease and schizophrenia"* stated that the brains of cases of Down's syndrome had been investigated in addition to Alzheimer's disease, and that: Appendix 21

"One of the benefits of the NWRHA project grant was the opportunity it gave us to establish a successful local brain collection scheme which provides tissue for both our present and future investigations".

20 August 1990 Third application

This application requesting support for two years was submitted by Dr Claire Royston, Professor Deakin and Dr Slater. In 1988 Dr Royston had joined as a junior member of the team funded as a Wellcome Research Fellow. She also held an Honorary Senior Registrar appointment in Psychiatry. Appendix 22

The title of the project was *"Computerized image analysis of the anatomy of glutamate and GABA systems in schizophrenia*".

This proposal was to build on novel research results obtained from the work supported by the two previous NWRHA grants. The scientific plan had been developed and modified in the five years since the first application.

Brain collection and Ethics Committee involvement

The procedure for obtaining human brains is set out for the first time in the plan of investigation, and the involvement of Ethical Committees is also mentioned:

"A system for the collection of whole brains from schizophrenic and control subjects is established in collaboration with ethical committees and hospitals within the Greater Manchester region".

"For the control subjects an exhaustive review of all available hospital case notes together with the General Practitioners case notes were made confirming that control subjects had no history of psychiatric or neurological illness nor had received any psychotropic medication. Collection of brains will continue to provide future tissue resources".

Coroners' cases

There is, however, still no reference to Coroners' cases although by June 1990 75 per cent of the brains obtained from mortuaries in the Manchester area had been retained from Coroners' cases, Chapter 16.

B: Applications to the Medical Research Council

In 1988 and 1989 the Medical Research Council (MRC) received three project grant applications from Dr Slater who was the sole applicant. These were considered and funded through the Council's competitive project grant scheme.

The three project grants

All three projects involved investigation of the neurochemistry of the brain and were planned to compare the results obtained in diseased brains with those taken from neurologically normal people.

March 1988

The title of the first project was: *"Cortical and basal ganglia neurotransmitters in Huntington's disease"*. Appendix 23

The application states: *"The study will be made using sections of frozen brain from normal (control) and HD* (Huntington's disease) *subjects"*.

"We have control brains from subjects with no history of neurological disease which were obtained from hospitals in Greater Manchester through long-standing arrangements".

December 1988

The second project's title was: *"Amino acid neurotransmitters in Alzheimer's disease brains"*. Appendix 24

The application states: *"The study will be made using frozen brains from normal subjects, from cases of advanced AD* (Alzheimer's disease) *and from subjects with DS* (Down's syndrome) *of middle age with AD"*.

"Brains are obtained through the cooperation of relatives, clinicians, pathologists, coroners' officers and mortuary staff in the Greater Manchester area. We have set up a brain collection scheme with teaching and long-stay hospitals which involves obtaining pre-mortem consent from patients and relatives for brain removal at death".

May 1989

The third project's title was: *"Calcium channel antagonist binding sites in normal and schizophrenic human brains"*. Appendix 25

The plan stated: *"The study will be made using frozen brain from normal (control) and schizophrenic subjects"*.

"We have whole brains removed at post-mortem examination. Brains from subjects with schizophrenia and from neurologically normal subjects have been obtained during the past 18 months from hospitals in Greater Manchester through long-

standing arrangements. Either the coroner's office or the hospital alerted us that a postmortem was taking place (with the consent of a close relative) on a subject with a psychiatric history".

This application was the second to refer to the involvement of the Coroner's office in identifying cases. The first such reference is in the application submitted in 1988 to the Mental Health Foundation, see below. In the application to MRC it is unclear if the reference to the "*consent of a relative*" is also intended to apply to Coroner's cases.

1993

The MRC did not, at any stage, provide funds for the other general activities of the joint programme's brain bank, but in 1993 the MRC funded a small project grant of one year's duration in the Department of Psychiatry. The grant was awarded to J Graham, C J Taylor and Professor Deakin. No other details are available.

C: The Wellcome Trust

1988-1991 A Wellcome Training Fellowship awarded to Dr Claire Royston on: *"The anatomy and development of amino-acid containing neurones and their role in schizophrenia"*[(1)].

Dr Royston had joined the research team as a junior Wellcome Research Fellow and Honorary Senior Registrar in 1988 to work with Dr Deakin and Dr Slater.

1991 A two-year project award to Dr Deakin on: *"Amino-acid receptors and the pathogenesis of Schizophrenia".*

This project was later extended for a third year.

D: The Mental Health Foundation

1988 Two project grant applications were made to the Mental Health Foundation.

One application entitled *"Quantitative and anatomical studies of receptors for psychotomimetic drugs and of glutamate systems in schizophrenia"* was made by Dr Deakin and Dr Slater. This was for a 3 year project grant on which Dr Simpson, a junior member of the team, would be the chief investigator. The grant was requested to start in September 1988. Appendix 26

The summary of the project states: *"It is proposed to use immunocytochemical and autoradiographic methods to study glutamatergic systems in sections of schizophrenic and control brains in which neuroanatomy is preserved".*

The source of brains is described in the section of the application headed *"The Investigation. Control brains, from subjects with no history of psychiatric or neurological illness, will be obtained from hospitals in the Manchester area through long-standing arrangements. The GP is automatically contacted to exclude cases with dementia, a previous psychiatric history or other relevant condition such as epilepsy or neurological diseases. A number of brains are presently stored in our laboratory and more will be obtained as needed.*

Brains from subjects with clinically diagnosed schizophrenia are obtained at regular intervals. We have the collaboration of clinicians and mortuary staff at Prestwich Psychiatric Hospital, North Manchester, in obtaining consent and brain removal at post mortem examination. Similarly, via the Rochdale Coroner, we obtain brains from the Lancashire area. We already have sufficient brains for the project to start.

The brain bank laboratory (Addenbrooke's Hospital Cambridge) have recently supplied us with samples of schizophrenic (and normal) brain and this source will be used again during the project."

This application is significant as it is the first by the joint team to make any reference to the involvement of the Coroner in obtaining brains for the programme.

The application does not mention whether the work had been referred to an ethics committee. However, the section on *"Consumables"* includes a request for *"mortuary & travel expenses for brain collection"* of £250 per year.

1988-1991 A second three-year grant application entitled *"Neurochemical Studies of Schizophrenia"*(1) was awarded by the Mental Health Foundation to Dr Deakin, M Simpson and Dr Slater, but the protocol for this application is not available.

E: Other NWRHA grants

1993 Faculty of Medicine/Regional Health Authority equipment grant.

1994 North West Regional Health Authority grant to Dr Slater and Professor Deakin for a project on: *"Cerebellar structures & neurochemical markers in schizophrenia"*(1).

F: The Stanley Foundation

1990-1992 Award to Dr Royston for: *" A morphometric study of the frontal cortex in schizophrenia"*(1).

For the grants and awards listed at C, E and F, only the titles and details recorded above are now available.

Summary

The successful results of the first research grant awarded in 1985 by the North West Regional Health Authority led to the award of two further grants in 1988 and 1990.

Three grant applications to the MRC by Dr Slater were awarded through the Council's competitive projects grant system.

The third of the applications to the MRC was the first to include any reference to the collection of brains identified by the Coroner's office.

The Wellcome Trust made two awards in 1988 and 1991.

Two grants were awarded by the Mental Health Foundation. One of these is notable as the first reference to a Coroner in any application made by the joint team to a research funding body. No details are available of the second application to the Mental Health Foundation.

Grants were obtained from a number of other funding organisations.

The award of these grants at a time when competitive research grants were becoming increasingly difficult to obtain indicates that the scientific quality of the research was highly regarded by the team's peers.

With these grants the team were able to expand the scope of the programme between 1988 and 1994.

Further grants were obtained after the period of this investigation.

References

1. Details of the grants and awards in paragraphs C, E and F were listed in the applications submitted to the NWRHA in August 1990. Appendix 22

CHAPTER 12

Prestwich mortuary
Application to the Salford Ethics Committee, January 1986

Introduction

This chapter describes the research protocol submitted to Salford Ethics Committee (SEC) that was considered on 15 January 1986, and the chronology of the brains obtained from Prestwich mortuary.

Sources of information

The chapter is based on documents provided by Professor Deakin and the minutes and papers of the SEC.

Background

Following the 1974 NHS reorganisation, Prestwich Hospital became part of Salford Area Health Authority. The SEC had responsibility for consideration of research projects that affected patients in Prestwich Hospital. (The designation Salford Ethics Committee changed in 1991 to Salford Local Research Ethics Committee (LREC)). For consistency, the earlier name is used throughout the rest of this chapter.

In 1987 Circular HC(77)28 was the most recent advice to the NHS on the "*Removal of Human Tissue at Post Mortem Examination*", Chapter 6.

Discussions and correspondence preceding the application to Salford EC

Dr Som Soni, consultant psychiatrist at Prestwich Hospital, had carried out research and clinical reviews of long-stay patients in Prestwich Hospital. His findings offered a unique opportunity to relate clinical features to post mortem changes.

Discussions in the spring of 1985 with Dr Soni and other clinical colleagues at Prestwich Hospital had indicated that the joint team would, in principle, be able to obtain the brains of patients who died in Prestwich Hospital with neuropsychiatric diseases. These discussions had been on the understanding that consent would be obtained from the relatives. As Chapter 8 documented, the Cerebral Function Unit was already obtaining brains from Prestwich hospital on the same basis.

Dr Soni wrote to Dr Deakin on 31 July 1985 enclosing: "*copies of the literature on getting consents for post mortem studies. Perhaps you would like to go through this and decide on a protocol, which we can then get printed for our patients at Prestwich* Annex 29 *Hospital*".

Dr Deakin replied on 2 October 1985: "*I enclose a draft submission to the Prestwich* Annex 30 *Ethical Committee. Do you think there might be some mileage in meeting groups of relatives ward by ward to speed things up?*"

The version of the protocol submitted to the SEC is no longer available. Annex 31 is a copy of the draft enclosed with Dr Deakin's letter. (Two pages are unfortunately missing from this document). Annex 31

The title of the project was: *"Brain Research in Schizophrenia and Tardive Dyskinesia".*

This includes a section headed *"Request for Brain Tissue"*: *"The consent for postmortem will be obtained in advance from the patient (if possible) and his relatives. It is not an easy matter to make a request of this nature, but is vital if progress in understanding and treating schizophrenia is to be made. It is important that relatives of patients with schizophrenia are involved in this decision; we must safeguard any wishes that patients may have but may not be able to express. Where possible, the decision will be discussed with patients and their relatives. Such requests have been successfully made in areas of research on other illnesses such as multiple sclerosis and Parkinsonism. A standard form has been prepared based on the forms used by the Multiple Sclerosis Society of Great Britain and by the Parkinsonism Research Group (copies of form and related documents enclosed)".*

As this research focussed on hospital inpatients with a diagnosis of schizophrenia, the draft protocol did not mention control cases or refer to collection of brains from Coroners' post mortems.

The SEC meeting and minutes

The application was considered by the SEC on 15 January 1986, as project number 8608. The title of the proposal had not changed from the draft.

The relevant minute reads: *"Brain research in schizophrenia and tardive dyskinesia"* Annex 32

"Dr Deakin and Dr Soni attended the meeting. The protocol explained that a programme of research has been set up, at Manchester University, to investigate brains of schizophrenic patients with a view to elucidating the abnormalities of biochemistry relevant to the illness. Researchers at the university are now able to study the chemistry of brain cells in remarkable detail. Very careful records have been kept at Prestwich Hospital of all patients but especially those with schizophrenia, (done in connection with a separate study on tardive dyskinesia, in progress since 1981). The records include not only detailed treatment profiles but also a chronological change in the clinical picture. These records should enable them to determine which brain systems are involved in schizophrenia but correlating the postmortem findings with the antemortem clinical pictures. It may also delineate the reasons why some patients develop dyskinesia and not others. This study is a long term project which will involve continuing clinical documentation on long stay patients at present resident in Prestwich Hospital. This will involve not only assessment of clinical parameters of schizophrenia but also documentation of psychological and psychometric tests on the population. When any of these patients die from any cause, the brain will be retrieved at postmortem as soon after death as possible. This will then be subjected to the research procedures at Manchester University. The consent for postmortem will be obtained in advance from the patient (if possible) and his relatives. Informed written consent will be obtained on a special

form submitted with the protocol".

The SEC: *"had no ethical objection to the study".*

Features of the SEC's minute

The minute refers to patients with schizophrenia but there is no mention of Alzheimer's disease.

The retention of brains from "normal" controls and from cases of sudden death reported to the Coroner are not mentioned.

SEC minutes after January 1986

There are no further references in the minutes of SEC to research applications using brain tissue from Dr Deakin jointly with Dr Soni. The SEC did not receive any progress reports and no changes to the protocol were notified to the Committee(1). The SEC did not receive any proposals from Dr Slater. Dr Soni submitted applications to the Committee on other matters until the 1990s.

Chronology of brains obtained from Prestwich mortuary 1985-1989

The Cerebral Function Unit had been collecting brains, with the knowledge and consent of the relatives, from Prestwich mortuary before the joint programme started.

The first brain for the joint programme was obtained from Prestwich mortuary on 1 November 1985. This mortuary was the source of 43 of the 58 brains obtained before brain collection was suspended in May 1987.

When brain collection recommenced in February 1988, the main source of brains was the mortuary at North Manchester General Hospital, Chapter 13. Five brains were obtained from Coroner's cases at Prestwich mortuary between April 1988 and 18 July 1989 when the last brain was received. Three of these were from in-patients with neuropsychiatric diseases whose deaths had been reported to the Coroner, and the other two from sudden deaths in the community.

Post mortem examinations at Prestwich mortuary ended in August 1989. After that date, further brains were obtained from in-patients who died in Prestwich Hospital but the post mortems were carried out at Bury mortuary(2).

Analysis of all brains from Prestwich mortuary

Fifty-three brains were obtained through Prestwich mortuary between 1985 and 1989.

Thirty-four brains, including Mr Isaacs', were obtained from Coroner's autopsies into cases of sudden death in the community. (These deaths can be easily distinguished as they are listed in the Mortuary Register of "Police Outside Deaths"). Twenty-one are categorised in the brain books as "controls".

Eleven brains were obtained from post mortems on in-patients at Prestwich Hospital whose deaths were reported to the Coroner. Most of these patients had some pre-existing neuropsychiatric disease.

Seven brains were obtained from post mortems on hospital cases without any involvement of the Coroner. In five of these, the brain was initially retained for the Cerebral Function Unit. Parts of these five brains were later transferred to the joint programme by Professor Mann.

The last brain collected from Prestwich was obtained on 18 July 1989.

Brain collection in relation to Ethics Committee consideration

Five brains recorded as part of the joint programme were obtained prior to 15 January 1986 when the SEC considered the protocol submitted by Dr Deakin and Dr Soni. These five were all Coroner's cases, including one in-patient whose death had been reported to the Coroner. In addition, there were 15 other brains collected before January 1986 which are not included in the list of brains collected for the joint programme. These brains were obtained for research without reference to any Ethical Committee.

Dr Slater, in commenting on the collection of brains prior to consideration by the SEC, has stated:

"It is a fact that in making grant applications in the UK one can be in an impossible situation. No project would ever get funded if there is doubt about securing the material, brain samples in this case, or if no pilot study has been made. I have already said that brain 'collection' was entirely random. Thus no brain samples and no pilot study equals no funding and no research on serious diseases. This is even more true today".

Summary

A research protocol was submitted to the SEC and considered by the Committee on 15 January 1986.

The protocol referred to studies of the brains of patients with neuropsychiatric conditions.

The patient and/or the relatives were to be asked to give consent to brain retention.

The protocol did not refer to collection of "control" brains or brains from Coroner's cases.

Five brains were obtained before the SEC had considered the protocol and a further 15 brains were collected that were recorded in the brain books but not considered a part of the joint programme.

Although these brains were collected for research, no Ethical Committee had been consulted.

Thirty-four brains were from sudden deaths in the community of which 21 are categorised as controls.

Eleven of the brains from Coroner's cases were from in-patients with neuropsychiatric diseases.

Seven brains were obtained from hospital post mortems, of which five were initially collected for the CFU programme.

Prestwich mortuary provided 43 of the 58 brains obtained for the joint programme before collection was suspended in May 1987.

After brain collection resumed, nine more brains were collected before post mortems at the mortuary ended in August 1989.

References

1 SEC minutes 1986-1996.
2 Data provided by Mental Health Services of Salford NHS Trust.

CHAPTER 13

North Manchester General Hospital mortuary
Application to the North Manchester Ethics Committee

Introduction

This chapter describes discussions in 1986 that preceded and followed consideration of the research protocol submitted by Dr Deakin and Dr Slater to the North Manchester Ethics Committee (NMEC). The chapter also sets out the chronology of brain collection from the mortuary of North Manchester General Hospital (NMGH). Annex 33

Sources of information

This chapter is based on documents provided by Professor Deakin at a meeting on 21 February 2002. Other sources are the registers and other documents obtained from NMGH, and the recollections of the pathologists and the mortician at the hospital.

Correspondence preceding the application to the NMEC

Dr Malcolm Green, Consultant Psychiatrist at NMGH, wrote to Dr A Theodossiades, Chairman of the Division of Psychiatry, on 17 February 1986 enclosing papers provided by Dr Deakin. Dr Green wrote: *"He requires post mortem brain tissue and already has an agreement with Prestwich Hospital to obtain this.... Can we agenda this item for the Division of Psychiatry so that it may be forwarded to the Ethical Committee if Division agrees".* Annex 34

Dr W G Brown, Consultant Histopathologist, wrote to Dr Deakin on 20 February 1986 concerning the research programme: *"I have already agreed to help in a clinical pathological correlative study on patients dying with pre-senile dementia, planned between the psycho-geriatricians in our hospital and the department of Neuropathology of the University of Manchester....* Annex 35

I would be agreeable to co-operate with your studies of schizophrenia along the lines you are pursuing with the psychiatrists at this hospital".

The reference in Dr Brown's second paragraph is to the research programme of the Cerebral Function Unit (CFU).

Dr Green in a letter to Dr Deakin dated 1 April 1986 reported that the research application had the unanimous support of the Division of Psychiatry. Dr Green added: *"you would need to send a detailed submission to the North Manchester Ethical Committee".* Annex 36

Dr Marshall, Consultant Psychiatrist with special interest in the elderly, wrote to Dr Deakin on 18 April 1986 to point out the overlap with the existing arrangements with the CFU. Dr Marshall suggested that: *"the two departments can collaborate or come to some mutual arrangement".* Annex 37

Dr Deakin replied to Dr Marshall on 30 June: *"The mortuary technician in North Manchester is willing to ring us whenever a post-mortem is carried out on a patient from psychogeriatric or other department in psychiatry".* Annex 38

"Perhaps you could clarify with me whether you or your firm routinely ask the next of kin after a patient has died for permission to brain material at post-mortem. All that is necessary is for a standard post mortem consent form to be signed".

The protocol submitted to the NMEC

Dr Deakin wrote to Dr Weller, Chairman of the NMEC, on 27 June 1986 enclosing a research protocol. He assures me this protocol was similarly worded to that signed on 17 July 1986, although the latter document is written on the South Manchester Ethics Committee (SMEC) form. Annex 39

In discussion, Professor Deakin has emphasised that this was the only protocol he sent to any Ethics Committee, with the exception of the one submitted to the Salford Ethics Committee in 1985. (The title of the protocol considered by the Salford Ethics Committee is quite different to that quoted by other Ethics Committees, Chapter 14.)

Features of the 17 July 1986 protocol

The protocol signed by Dr Deakin on 17 July 1986 states *" After a patient has died the Psychiatrists who have been looking after the patient will seek permission from the nearest relative to remove the brain tissue at post-mortem. This is already in operation at Prestwich Hospital and has been approved by the ethical committee. A standard post-mortem consent form will be used".* Annex 33

The protocol also refers to the collection of brains *"of patients who have died from medical conditions who have not suffered from mental illness",* but does not mention how consent for these will be obtained. These patients would not have been under the care of a psychiatrist. There is no reference to collection of brains of Coroners' cases.

Although Dr Slater's name appears as an applicant, Dr Slater states that he was not involved in seeking approval by Ethics Committees and he correctly points out that he did not sign the protocol.

Consideration of the protocol by the NMEC

Dr Deakin's letter to Dr Weller dated 27 June 1986 indicates the protocol was then circulated to all members of the Ethical Committee. Annex 39

The Chairman later asked Dr Deakin to comment on two matters raised by Dr Joyce Leeson on behalf of the North Manchester Health Authority in a letter to Mr Brown, the District General Manager for NMGH. Annex 40

Dr Leeson had commented: *"This does not present any problems of ethics, if consent for post-mortem is obtained... Are the histopathologists happy to collect and store the specimens?... What arrangements will be made for collecting relevant information from the notes"... "the information must be treated as confidential".*

Dr Deakin, responding to Dr Leeson's questions, wrote on 26 August 1986 to Dr Weller: *"Information from the notes is being collected by myself and concerns age, diognosis* (sic) *and drug treatment. The information abstracted is coded... The coded information stays in my office and is completely confidential".* Annex 41

The NMEC approved the protocol on 4 September 1986 and on 11 September Dr Weller wrote to Dr Deakin to confirm this. Annex 42

Dr Deakin wrote to Dr Theodossiades on 30 September 1986 suggesting that he should attend a meeting of the Division of Psychiatry to explain the programme to the consultants of the Division. Annex 43

Letter requesting brain collection from the NMGH mortuary

On 17 October 1986 Dr Deakin wrote to the Chief Technician at the NMGH mortuary, Mr Peter Leatherbarrow. This letter had a significant impact and was to lead to over 130 brains being collected from the NMGH mortuary for the joint programme. The following features should be noted: Annex 44

"I enclose a copy of the ethical committee submission that was recently approved by the North Manchester committee".

"We are keen to obtain brains from patients dying on the psychiatric wards or who have a history of mental illness. We also need normal control brains".

"We collaborate with Dr David Mann so just continue sending him brains which are for his attention and let us know of the others".

"We can arrange payment of £10.00 per brain before tax which is deducted at source".

Dr Slater states that he had no involvement in sending this letter to Mr Leatherbarrow.

Mr Leatherbarrow's concerns about the letter

When Mr Leatherbarrow received this letter he was uncertain about his position. The collection of brains by Dr Mann for the CFU research programme had been in place since 1982. The brains for the CFU were all removed with the consent of the relatives. The planned collection of other brains went further than the CFU programme.

In view of his concerns, Mr Leatherbarrow first asked for a copy of the protocol that the NMEC had approved. He discussed this and the letter he had received from Dr Deakin with the consultant pathologists. Dr Brown had noted there was potential overlap with the CFU programme, as he had referred to this in his letter of 20 February to Dr Deakin. Annex 35

The NMEC had nevertheless authorised the protocol. Mr Leatherbarrow was reassured by his discussions with the consultant pathologists, as well as by the references in the protocol to consent and to the collection of brains of patients without mental illness.

Referral of brains from NMGH mortuary

When a suitable index or "control" case was identified, Mr Leatherbarrow, as requested in Dr Deakin's letter, would telephone Dr Slater's contact number in the Department of Physiology. In practice, he never referred a brain without first asking the pathologist responsible for the post mortem.

Mr Leatherbarrow has told me that, with the knowledge he has now, he considers he was misled about the joint programme. He believed at the time that the brains collected had been consented to in the same way as the brains obtained for the CFU, and that the Coroner was aware of the brain collection programme.

Mr Leatherbarrow has kept all the payslips from the University for brains retained, Chapter 24.

Differences between the NMGH and Prestwich mortuaries

There were two significant differences between the brain collection systems at these mortuaries.

First, unlike Prestwich mortuary, there was no involvement of the Coroner's office in identifying suitable cases at the NMGH mortuary. Indeed, the Coroner and his staff were unaware that brains were being retained.

Secondly, Prestwich mortuary received the bodies of cases of sudden death in the community referred by the police. The NMGH mortuary did not act as a public mortuary or receive bodies referred by the police. There were, however, some post mortems on sudden death in the community as the mortuary received bodies of patients who were certified dead on arrival in the ambulance or at the NMGH Accident and Emergency Department.

Chronology and analysis of brains from the NMGH mortuary 1986-1994

Following the NMEC approval, the first brain (from a Coroner's case) was referred from NMGH on 28 October 1986. Between that date and the suspension of brain collection in May 1987, six brains were referred to the programme from Coroner's cases. Four of these were categorised as "controls".

When brain collection recommenced on 29 February 1988, the NMGH mortuary was the primary source of brains for the programme and continued as such until 1991. Between the period 1992 and 1994 the number of brains referred diminished.

The total number of brains obtained from the NMGH mortuary was 132, of which 100 were from Coroner's cases.

All but one of the brains obtained from NMGH mortuary in 1988 were from Coroner's cases.

Thirty-two brains were obtained from hospital or "brain only" post mortem examinations. Twenty-eight of these were retained in 1989 and 1990.

The last brains obtained from NMGH were two Coroner's cases in May 1994.

When brain collection for the joint programme ceased, Mr Leatherbarrow recalls he was told that no further brains were to be collected as "*there were problems about the arrangements*" or words to that effect. Mr Leatherbarrow was not told the nature of the problems. He does not remember which member of the team spoke to him at that time.

Summary

The Division of Psychiatry at NMGH were keen to support the joint research programme.

The potential overlap with brains collected for research in the CFU was pointed out.

The need to collect information from medical records in a confidential manner was emphasised by the Health Authority.

The NMEC approved the protocol in September 1986.

Dr Deakin wrote to the mortician on 17 October 1986 asking for referral of brains from patients who had died with psychiatric conditions. Control brains were also requested.

A fee of £10 per brain was offered.

The arrangement for collection of brains was dependent on the identification of suitable index and "control" cases by the mortician.

The mortician routinely asked the pathologists before any brain was referred to the joint programme.

The collection of brains for two different research programmes caused confusion.

From February 1988 when the programme restarted, NMGH provided index and control brains from Coroner's cases.

One hundred and thirty-two brains were obtained, the largest number from any mortuary, and included 100 brains from Coroner's cases. The other 32 brains were either hospital or "brain only" examinations.

Collection of brains from NMGH mortuary ceased in May 1994 after unspecified "problems" were identified.

CHAPTER 14

Action to enlarge the programme and increase the collection of brains from other hospitals: approaches to consultants and Ethics Committees

Introduction

This chapter sets out:

- the action taken to inform clinicians working in hospitals near Manchester of the aims of the programme and to increase the referral of suitable brains;

- approaches to Ethics Committees at the same hospitals.

Sources of information

The chapter is based on copies of contemporaneous correspondence provided by Professor Deakin. Other letters and documents were obtained from LREC records.

Background

By 1988 the research team had made good progress and had reported exciting findings to the NWRHA. An application for further funds had been made to the NWRHA. To build on their earlier work and to investigate the role of glutamate on the neurotransmitter systems, the programme needed more brains to investigate.

Disseminating information to clinicians in nearby hospitals

Dr Deakin's successful discussions with consultant psychiatrists at Prestwich Hospital and North Manchester General Hospital in 1985/86 had shown that, when the programme based on research on hospital inpatients was explained, clinicians would generally support it.

To encourage doctors in other hospitals to refer suitable patients, the research team prepared separate papers, one for doctors, the other an explanation for relatives. The latter described in less technical terms the purpose of their investigations of the neurotransmitter systems of patients with Alzheimer's disease and schizophrenia.

Letter for doctors

The letter explains: *"The physiology department had developed a way of assessing the integrity of the cortical glutamatergic neurone"* and requests: *"It would be a great help to our research if you would ask the relatives of a patient who has died, for permission to carry out a post mortem examination"*.

A copy of the letter for clinicians dated 17 October 1988, prepared by Dr Deakin, is at Annex 45. Annex 45

Explanation for relatives

To accompany this letter was a single page explanation which the doctor could give to the relatives of the patient when raising the question of consent for brain retention. The note explains: *"At Manchester University a programme of research has been set up to investigate the brain chemistry in people who have died and who suffer from Alzheimer's disease in life. Some significant new results have already emerged."* Annex 46

A similar note was prepared for the relatives of patients with schizophrenia. Annex 47

Approaches to Ethics Committees and consultants at "new" hospitals

Between 1988 and 1991 Dr Deakin wrote to consultants at hospitals in Bolton, Macclesfield, Oldham, Rochdale, Stepping Hill, Warrington and Wigan. There may have been approaches to other hospitals but any correspondence is no longer available.

The initial letters to a "new" hospital were sent to a consultant psychiatrist or, occasionally, to a consultant pathologist. These letters would follow the draft referred to above and would enclose a copy of the notes prepared for relatives.

Other letters followed to chairmen of the ECs. These invariably mentioned approval of the research by Salford EC and the Ethics Committees of North and South Manchester.

Form of acknowledgement for brains collected

The joint team introduced, on an unrecorded date, a form to acknowledge the collection of brains for the programme. The form appears to have been intended for pathologists and possibly morticians who had already provided a brain. Annex 48

The hospitals and ECs contacted

Bolton

Very little information remains available about the approach to consultants at Bolton.

Dr Deakin received a letter dated 20 April 1990 from Dr Mahadevan, Consultant Psychiatrist at the John McKay Clinic, Royal Bolton Hospital. Dr Mahadevan wrote: *"The Psychiatrists in Bolton would be happy to co-operate with your research, provided of course that the proposal is approved by our District Ethics Committee".* Annex 49

No brains were obtained from hospitals in Bolton.

Macclesfield

Dr Deakin wrote on 17 October 1989 to Dr Williams in the Department of Pathology at Macclesfield General Hospital: *"My psychiatric colleagues at Parkside Hospital have agreed to request academic post-mortems on any of their schizophrenic patients who die in hospital. However, this cannot go ahead unless the department of pathology and the mortuary staff are in agreement".* Annex 50

On the same date Dr Deakin wrote to Dr Walter Brodie (sic), Consultant Psychiatrist at Parkside Hospital. He enclosed a copy of the leaflet for patients' relatives. Annex 51

Dr Braude replied on 23 October 1989: *"Do we need to get specific written consent from relatives and if so, could you supply us with the relevant forms?"* Dr Braude also advised Dr Deakin to write to Dr Wills, chairman of the local Ethical Committee, to obtain approval for the research project. Annex 52

Dr Deakin wrote to Dr Wills on 9 February 1990: "*This application has been approved by the South Manchester Health Authority, by Salford and by North Manchester*". Annex 53

On 13 February 1990 Dr Deakin wrote again to Dr Braude: *"Written consent should probably be obtained from the next of kin"*. Dr Deakin added: "*Often chronic inpatients don't have next of kin, in which case there is no difficulty"*. Annex 54

In a letter to me dated 10 January 2003 Professor Deakin states *"This is the sole reference to patients without next of kin in correspondence with hospitals in the NW. The next paragraph refers to obtaining the necessary consent forms for the post mortem from the Pathology Department"*.

What was not mentioned in Dr Deakin's correspondence to Dr Braude is that in cases of patients who die in hospitals but without known relatives, guidance in HC(77)28 applies throughout the NHS, see Chapter 5. This guidance requires consent by the *"person lawfully in possession of the body"*. It should not have been assumed that consent would be given in every case, particularly when the patient was suffering from mental illness at the time of his death.

The reply and decision of the Macclesfield Ethics Committee are not available.

In the brain books there is a single reference to "Parkside" as the source of one brain but it is not clear if the brain in question came from Parkside Hospital, Macclesfield. No other brains are recorded coming from Macclesfield.

Oldham

On 10 September 1990 Dr Deakin wrote to Dr Wallis, chairman of the Ethics Committee for Royal Oldham Hospital, enclosing a copy of the protocol that had been submitted to the South Manchester Ethics Committee in 1986 and requesting the Oldham Ethics Committee's approval of the joint research programme. Dr Deakin had previously written to the Division of Psychiatry at Royal Oldham Hospital. Annex 55

Dr Deakin was invited to attend a meeting of the Ethics Committee on 18 October, but was unable to do so. On 2 November Dr Wallis replied giving the EC's approval adding: "*It was the considered opinion of the members that a direct approach to the relative was preferable to a telephone call and that contact should be made either by you or a senior clinician*". Annex 56

Brains obtained from Oldham

Oldham is part of the district of the Coroner for North Manchester.

Between 1986 and 1996 six brains were obtained from Coroner's cases. These were all from patients with schizophrenia or other psychiatric disease. No brains were obtained from hospital post mortems[(1)].

Rochdale

On 10 September 1990 Professor Deakin wrote to Dr Purnell, chairman of the Rochdale Ethics Committee. The Committee had responsibility for Birch Hill Hospital, Rochdale. Dr Deakin enclosed the protocol dated 17 July 1986, adding that "*The research is approved by the South Manchester Health Authority Ethics Committee and in Salford and North Manchester*". Annex 57 Annex 33

On 7 November Dr Purnell asked Dr Bowker, Consultant Psychiatrist at Birchill, how many patients would be involved and whether these patients would normally be submitted to a post mortem examination. Annex 58

Dr Bowker replied on 17 December that the number of patients involved would be not more than half a dozen in a year: "*It would not be our usual practice for these patients to have post mortem examinations*". Annex 59

Dr Deakin was invited to the Ethics Committee meeting on 15 February but was unable to attend.

Dr Purnell wrote to Professor Deakin on 22 February 1991 indicating that the study had been approved. The title referred to "*Brain Research in Schizophrenia (Trial No. 120)*". Dr Purnell asked whether a full post mortem would be carried out and "*whether your department would be paying for the post mortem examination*". Annex 60

On 5 March Professor Deakin replied: "*A full postmortem is not always carried out, this is at the discretion of the pathologist. We pay a small fee to the mortuary technicians and any undertakers fees.*" Annex 61

Brains obtained from Rochdale

Rochdale, like Oldham, is part of the district of the Coroner for North Manchester. The retention of brains from Coroner's cases, on the instructions of the Coroner's office, was confirmed by PC Rigg, the Coroner's Officer for Rochdale, and Mr Owen, the mortician at Rochdale mortuary.

Thirty-four brains from Coroner's cases were obtained from Rochdale mortuary between 1986 and 1996. Three of these were categorised as "controls". Many of the other cases had psychiatric conditions. Only one brain was obtained from a hospital post mortem in Rochdale.

Stepping Hill Hospital

Dr Deakin wrote early in 1990 to Dr Bhattacharyya, Consultant Psychiatrist at Stepping Hill Hospital. On 25 April 1990 Dr Bhattacharyya replied: *"Our Divisional Meeting approved your request regarding brain research into schizophrenia. I have written to Dr Dymock".* Annex 62

Dr Dymock was the chairman of the Stepping Hill Hospital Ethics Committee.

No other correspondence is available and there is no record of the Ethics Committee reply.

Brains obtained from Stepping Hill Hospital

Five brains were obtained from Stepping Hill Hospital between 14 April 1990 and 12 March 1992. Four were from hospital post mortems and one was a Coroner's case[(1)].

Warrington

The correspondence and retention of brains from Warrington General Hospital is described in Chapter 15.

Wigan

On 28 March 1990 Dr Deakin wrote to Dr Thomas, Chairman of the Division of Psychiatry at Billinge Hospital near Wigan, to inform him of the neurochemical research in schizophrenia.

Dr Thomas replied on 23 May indicating that the consultants in the Department of Psychiatry would support the programme after ethical approval had been given by the Wigan Ethics Committee. Annex 63

Dr Deakin wrote to Dr McGucken on 10 September requesting Ethical Committee approval and enclosing the protocol dated 17 July 1986. Annex 64 Annex 33

On 29 October the secretary of the Committee replied that approval had been given, subject to: *"satisfactory arrangements being made with the responsible Consultant for either yourself or that Consultant to approach the relatives for permission to carry out a post mortem".* The Committee asked for progress reports and enclosed a proforma for that purpose. Annex 65

There is no record that any brains were obtained from Billinge Hospital.

Central Manchester Health Authority

Dr Slater and Dr D'Souza, consultant in the University Department of Child Health, submitted an application to the Ethical Committee in April 1991 for a study entitled: *"The Development of Amino Acid uptake sites and receptors in human brain"(reference number 37/91(I) (d)).*

The Central Manchester Clinical Research Ethical Committee approved this application on 22 July 1991. In doing so, the Committee: *"wished to be kept informed of progress during the course of your research activity"*. Annex 66

After this study was approved, Dr Slater and Dr D'Souza approached Dr Barson, Senior Lecturer in Pathology, about obtaining brain samples for this investigation.

Dr Barson replied on 18 December 1992: "*I write to confirm that I am willing to supply samples of human brain tissue to you for the purposes of your medical research funded by the Medical Research Council subject to the constraints laid upon me by the Human Tissues* (sic) *Act"*. Annex 67

Although research on brains of children was not part of the joint programme, Dr Barson's reply is relevant as it should have reminded Dr Slater of the constraints of the Human Tissue Act. The Ethics Committee had emphasised the importance of the Committee receiving progress reports on projects that had been approved.

Approach to pathologists in 1995

On 28 March 1995 Professor Deakin wrote by fax to Professor John McClure at the Manchester Royal Infirmary to ask for his comments on a draft letter that had been prepared for circulation to pathologists in the Manchester area.

The draft letter entitled *"Research Programme on Neurodevelopmental Abnormalities in Psychiatry"* includes:

"At present, we are collecting brains from patients who undergo a hospital post-mortem. We are, however, also discussing with Local Coroners whether we can have access to tissue from Coroner's cases. We anticipate the number of brains collected from each hospital to be small – perhaps as little as one or two a month, as we have set very stringent criteria for the quality of the brains".[2]

The wording of this paragraph is notable as it implies that discussions with Coroners were a new initiative. This overlooks the fact that at the time this draft letter was prepared more than two-thirds of the brains already collected had been obtained from Coroners' cases.

Professor McClure replied to Professor Deakin by fax on 4 April 1995.

"Thank you for your recent draft letter regarding the above. I am afraid the matter is now not very simple. Several years ago it was relatively easy to allow materials from post mortem examinations to be used in the manner in which you describe. Unfortunately the vast majority of our cases coming through the mortuary are cases which the local Coroner has asked for the post mortem examination. It is, therefore, necessary for you to obtain from the Coroner permission for the use of brain tissue which you outline. I know from previous experience that he will probably say 'yes' but you will also have to obtain permission from the immediate relatives of the deceased and it is your responsibility to do so. This may not be particularly easy in cases of sudden and unexpected death in the community. For the very small number of cases which are not reported to the Coroner and which are hospital cases, then the

consent form which the relatives sign will allow you to have the materials which you requested. I and my colleagues (I have discussed it with them) would have no objection whatsoever to letting you have tissues from these cases. Unfortunately for you these cases are likely to be very small in number and you will not be able to collect at the rate which you suggest. The bottom line is that you need now to discuss your proposals with Mr. Gorodkin, the Manchester Coroner".[3]

Professor McClure's response appears to have led Professor Deakin to request the meeting with Mr Gorodkin which took place on 26 June 1995, see Chapter 22.

It is not clear from the papers available to me if any letters were sent in an amended form to local pathologists. The brain book entries show that no brains were collected from mortuaries that had not previously been involved.

Lack of progress reports to Ethics Committees and LRECs

No progress reports are contained in the records of the Prestwich and North Manchester Ethics Committees and no other reports to any Ethics Committee by the joint programme were identified during the course of this investigation, although several Committees had specifically asked for these. The NHS circular HSC(91)15 required researchers to provide these and to inform the LRECs of any changes to projects that had been approved by Ethics Committees.

Summary

To increase the number of brains retained, Dr Deakin approached consultants in seven hospitals near Manchester between 1988 and 1991.

Standard drafts were used to interest clinicians in other hospitals in providing brains for the joint programme.

The clinicians all required Ethics Committee referral and approval before agreeing to participate in brain collection for the joint programme.

When Ethics Committees were contacted, the protocol dated 17 July 1986 was offered and reference was routinely made to approval already given by Salford and North Manchester Ethics Committees.

Brain collection at Oldham and Rochdale had started before the Ethics Committees were approached.

Dr Slater was reminded in August 1991 of the importance of providing Ethics Committees with progress reports.

In December 1992 Dr Slater was reminded of the constraints of the Human Tissue Act.

In March 1995 there were further proposals by the joint team to enlarge the programme. The draft letter which would have been sent to local pathologists implied that the collection of brains from Coroners' cases was a new initiative.

Following advice that brains from Coroners' cases would require consent of the relatives, Professor Deakin requested a meeting with Mr Gorodkin.

No copies of progress reports to Ethics Committees or LRECs have been provided by the research team or can be found in the Salford and North Manchester Ethics Committees records.

References

1 Data in the joint programme brain books.
2 Extract from fax dated 28 March 1995.
3 Transcript of fax dated 4 April 1995.

CHAPTER 15

Warrington General Hospital
Application to Warrington Hospital Ethics Committee

Introduction

This chapter describes discussions in 1988 that preceded consideration of the research protocol submitted by Dr Deakin to the Warrington Ethics Committee. The findings in this chapter are based on contemporaneous documents and the recollections of staff involved.

Background

Winwick Hospital, Warrington, was a psychiatric hospital with long-stay wards but without facilities for post mortems on site. All post mortems, including "brain only" removals, were carried out at Warrington General Hospital.

Warrington General Hospital also served as a public mortuary and, like Prestwich mortuary, received the bodies of those who had died suddenly in the community.

Correspondence preceding the application to Warrington General Hospital Ethics Committee

1988

Dr Deakin wrote to Dr John, chairman of the Division of Psychiatry at Winwick Hospital, Warrington, on 6 June 1988 to ask if the Division would provide brains for the joint programme: "*I am writing to ask whether you think it may be possible to arrange for the collection of post-mortem material from patients who die in Winwick Hospital or its neighbourhood.*" Annex 68

Dr John replied on 28 June to Dr Deakin: (Your request) "*was discussed at the last meeting of the Psychiatric Services Committee ... and in principle we are agreeable to the doctors here co-operating with you in this project by asking relatives permission for academic post-mortems. However, the Committee also agreed that we should seek the permission of the Ethical Committee in the District and to this end, I will be contacting them.*" Annex 69

The Ethics Committee considered and approved the application. It appears that the application considered by the Ethics Committee was the protocol dated 17 July 1986 on the South Manchester Ethics Committee form. This does not refer to the collection of brains from Coroners' cases. The news the application had been approved was not transmitted to Dr Deakin.

1990

Dr Deakin wrote again to Dr John on 14 February 1990 to follow up the 1988 correspondence. Dr Deakin noted: "*We have Ethical Committee permission to collect post-mortem brain material from Prestwich, Manchester and Salford*", and enclosed a Annex 70 copy of the protocol dated 17 July 1986 that had been submitted to the North and South Manchester Ethics Committees.

Dr John replied on 3 May 1990 that the Warrington Ethics Committee had considered and approved the application in July 1988. Dr John also apologised for not informing Dr Deakin of the Ethics Committee's decision in 1988. Annex 71

Chronology and analysis of brains from Warrington General Hospital

Twenty-three brains were obtained from Warrington General Hospital between 1988 and 1992[(1)]. A separate Mortuary Register was maintained for bodies referred to the mortuary by the police, so Coroner's cases can be readily identified.

Twenty-two brains were obtained from patients who were, or had been, in-patients at Winwick Hospital. Two patients were on weekend leave from Winwick Hospital when they died.

The solitary "control" brain was from an in-patient at Warrington General hospital who had no previous history of neuropsychiatric illness.

The first brain was received from a hospital post mortem in June 1988.

The next 11 brains were obtained from Coroner's cases. All had been patients in Winwick Hospital. The post mortem reports show that all these deaths had been appropriately reported to the Coroner[(2)]. For example, one in-patient died following a fall in which she broke her leg shortly before death.

From June 1990 the next seven brains were all from hospital post mortems or "brain only" examinations. The reports of these post mortems are no longer available.

After October 1991 four further brains were obtained from Coroner's post mortems. The post mortem reports record two cases died at home from suicide and the others were sudden deaths in Winwick Hospital[(2)].

The last brain from a Coroner's post mortem was obtained in May 1992.

Uncertainty in the Coroner's office

In 1989, Mr Stephenson took up his duties as Coroner's Officer at Warrington. When he discovered that a brain was being retained, he questioned the legality of brains from Coroner's cases being retained for research. Mr Stephenson telephoned the Coroner's office to check. He was told that retention was allowed as the brain was going to the University. It is possible that the Coroner's office assumed the brain was destined for research that had the consent of the relatives.

Mr Stephenson did not question subsequent brain retentions, but remained uneasy as the relatives appeared to be unaware that the brain had been retained.

Summary

In 1988 the Division of Psychiatry at Winwick Hospital supported, in principle, the proposal for academic post mortems in suitable cases, but asked for Ethics Committee permission.

The protocol sent to the Warrington Ethics Committee appears to have been the protocol dated 17 July 1986. This protocol contains no reference to Coroner's cases.

Ethics Committee approval was given in July 1988 but not conveyed to the team until May 1990.

Eleven brains from Coroner's cases were obtained prior to June 1990. In all cases the referral to the Coroner was appropriate.

Between June 1990 and February 1991, seven brains were obtained from hospital or brain only examinations. No details of these cases are available.

Between October 1991 and May 1992, four further brains were obtained from Coroner's cases. All these cases were appropriately referred to the Coroner.

In three of the 15 cases referred to the Coroner a verdict of suicide was recorded. All other deaths were recorded as natural causes.

In 1989 Mr Stephenson, when newly appointed as Coroner's Officer, questioned the retention of brains from Coroner's cases. He was reassured that brain retention was in order. This could have been the result of a misunderstanding in the Coroner's office that the relatives had given consent.

References

1 Entries in the joint programme brain books.
2 Post mortem reports sent to the Coroner.

CHAPTER 16

Analysis of brains collected for the brain bank of the joint research programme 1985-1997

Introduction

This chapter summarises the information available on the 311 adult brains that were collected for the joint programme.

Sources of information

The brain books

The findings set out in this chapter derive from the entries in four brain books maintained in the Department of Physiology. These books contain a separate entry for each brain obtained for the joint programme. Summary sheets prepared by Professor Deakin supplement the entries in the books.

Mortuary Registers

At each of the main hospitals contributing to the programme it was possible to cross-check the data against the Mortuary Registers. The status of the post mortem could usually be determined from the these registers.

Coroners' post mortem reports

When post mortems were carried out on the instructions of the Coroner, further validation of the information in the brain books and Mortuary Registers was possible by cross checking with the post mortem reports and other case papers held by the Coroners. The post mortem reports were available in all but one case requested.

Hospital case records

There were some hospital cases from Prestwich and North Manchester General Hospitals where the status of the post mortem was not clear and/or it appeared that the relatives could have been asked to consent to the retention of the brain.

For these cases the hospital case notes were requested. However, 10 to 15 years after the death of a patient, very few notes were found. Most had been disposed of due to the passage of time since the death of the patient, in line with NHS time limits for retention of hospital records.

Findings

Brains collected for the joint programme

Most of the 311 adult referrals were of whole brains received directly from mortuaries in the Manchester area. The total includes 15 part brains received from the Cerebral Function Unit. The list includes a number of patients with mental handicap, such as

Down's Syndrome, and other long-stay conditions where before death the diagnosis was clear-cut.

No brains in Professor Deakin's summary lists originated from outside the Manchester area. The first brain in the brain books was collected on 1 November 1985 and the last on 29 April 1997.

Source of brains received in the programme

The table below shows the number of brains received from individual mortuaries, sub-divided into Coroners' cases, hospital deaths referred to the Coroner and hospital post mortems:

Sources of brains collected for the joint programme

By year:	85	86	87	88	89	90	91	92	93	94	95	96	97
Total	5	41	12	49	70	55	15	9	10	18	17	9	1
Coroners' cases	5	33	11	38	48	32	12	6	9	16	10	9	0
Hospital cases	0	8	1	11	22	23	3	3	1	2	7	0	1

By mortuary and status of case:

Mortuary	Coroners' Autopsies	Hospital Autopsies	Total
Prestwich	46 (11*)	7	53
NMGH	100 (60*)	32	132
Warrington	15 (7*)	8	23
Bury	27	3	30
Oldham	6	0	6
Rochdale	34	1	35
Manchester Royal Infirmary	1	6	7
Stepping Hill	1	4	5
Other Hospitals **	0	6	6
Source unknown	0	14	14

* Figures in brackets indicate the number of in-patient deaths that were referred to the Coroners.

** Withington Hospital — 3 brains
Ashton-under-Lyne Hospital)
Hope Hospital, Salford) — 1 brain each
Preston Hospital)

The mortuaries contributing to the programme provided a different balance of Coroners' and hospital post mortem cases. Overall, the number of brains from Coroners' cases was 230, including those cases where the deceased had died in hospital but the death had been reported to the Coroner.

The distinction between deaths in hospital and the other deaths reported to the Coroner is not always clear from the mortuary records because in some mortuaries, deaths before arrival in Accident and Emergency Departments are recorded as in-patient deaths.

There were 81 cases where a hospital post mortem was carried out, assuming the 14 cases where the records do not state the source were all hospital cases.

Most of the brains obtained for the programme were intact whole brains received directly from the participating mortuaries in or near Manchester. Some whole brains had been sliced by the pathologist to detect any abnormality visible to the naked eye.

Among the 311 brains recorded in the summary sheets of the joint programme are 15 part brains which were received from the Cerebral Function Unit (CFU). (There were four other part brains received from the CFU listed in the first brain book, but which are not included in the joint programme summary sheet.)

<u>Adult brains not in the programme lists</u>

There are a further 33 brains of adults recorded in the first brain book. None of these is included in the summary sheets prepared by Professor Deakin after he was first contacted by Mrs Isaacs. However, the reference numbers in the spreadsheets are in most cases the same as the contemporaneous code numbers recorded in the brain books. These brains were collected between 25 July 1984 and 19 September 1987, the majority before the joint programme began on 1 November 1985.

It is not clear from the entries in the brain books why these brains were not regarded as part of the joint programme, but the information on some is sparse. The lack of relevant data may explain why the brains were regarded as unsuitable for the joint programme.

<u>Samples of brains of babies and infants listed in the first of the brain books</u>

The first brain book also includes details of 32 children's brain samples or part brains collected between 29 October 1986 and 18 March 1988. These were all collected from Manchester Children's Hospital and other local hospitals.

The infant brain research was not part of the joint programme and did not involve Professor Deakin.

The status of the children's brain samples has been investigated by the Retained Organs Commission in a separate investigation.

Histological examination of brains recorded in the brain books

The brain books record that histology was undertaken on 37 cases, which include all 19 part brains where specimens were received from the Cerebral Function Unit. A further 13 cases are among the brains collected prior to the start of the joint programme on 1 November 1985. Of the remaining nine cases, where histology is recorded, two were of brain samples referred from hospitals outside the Manchester area and the remaining seven were from in-patients whose deaths had been reported to the Coroner and histology appears to have been carried out at the request of the consultant responsible for the patient's care. No histology appears to have been undertaken on other Coroners' cases.

Professor Deakin and Dr Slater have both commented on the matter of diagnostic histology. Professor Deakin has emphasised that histology in schizophrenia would not be informative. Dr Slater makes the same point and adds that some samples were sent by Dr Cross to the Pathology Department. *"With the dearth of neuropathologists, the delays in getting answers just took far too long and we were forced to abandon attempts".*

From the available papers it appears that histology was not requested to confirm there was no histological abnormality in brains collected as controls. Reliance was placed on the clinical history.

No reports on the research were made to the Coroners or to the doctors responsible for the care of the deceased before death. Dr Slater states that *"the fact is that we never intended to* (sic) *this and had never been asked by anyone to do so".*

Summary

Three hundred and eleven brains were obtained for the joint programme.

Two hundred and thirty brains were from Coroners' cases.

At least 78 of the Coroners' cases were in-patient deaths.

Eighty-two brains were from hospital or "brain only" examinations.

Thirty-three adult brains listed in the brain books are not categorised as part of the programme.

Thirty-two brain samples from hospital post mortems on babies and infants are recorded in the brain book but were not part of the joint programme.

The brain books record that histology was undertaken in 37 brains, of which 19 cases were specimens received from the CFU. Most of the remaining cases where histology is recorded were received in the first year of the joint programme.

CHAPTER 17

What happened to the brains obtained for the joint programme?

Introduction

This chapter describes what happened to the 311 brains obtained for the programme.

Sources of information

The chapter draws on three main sources of information:

- the brain books, which record what specifically happened to some brains;
- information provided by Dr Slater, Professor Deakin and Dr Michael Simpson, who was a member of the research team from 1985-1997;
- the list of retained organs prepared for the CMO's Census in 2000. This data was provided by Professor Freemont, and records the brains and parts of brains that were held in the Department of Physiology at the time of the Census.

Further information was found in various letters and documents and from information given by researchers in other locations.

Time intervals for collection of brains for the programme

The aim was to obtain the brain as soon as practicable after death, but the timing was dependent on the post mortem. Arrangements were made to collect the brains within hours of the post mortem examination. It was thought initially that fresh brain tissue was essential for reliable investigation of brain neurochemistry. In all mortuaries the practice was to place the brain in the mortuary refrigerator until it was collected.

The brain books record the interval between death and removal of the brain[1]. For many this was less than 24 hours. There are very few where the interval was longer than 72 hours. A prolonged interval was considered to make the brain unsuitable for neurochemical investigation. In practice, brains were not collected when the post mortem was delayed over the weekend.

Preparation of brains for research use

For transport to the laboratory the brains were placed in a cool box container packed with ice. On arrival each brain was prepared for the research programme by one of the research team. This involved separating the two halves of the brain and dividing each half (or hemisphere) into portions. Each portion was then individually packed and labelled before being rapidly frozen. The labelled portions were then placed in one of the freezers and the location carefully documented. A fuller description of the methods used in preparing the brains is included in the first of Dr Slater's applications to the Medical Research Council. Appendix 23

Validation of the suitability for research use of each brain

For use in the programme, each brain had to meet clearly defined criteria. For example, for cases of schizophrenia a firm diagnosis had had to be made during life, or validated by reference to case notes after death. The same principle applied to Alzheimer's disease and other diseases studied.

For use as a "control" the deceased must have died of an unrelated disease with no history of neuropsychiatric or other disease affecting the brain. Histology was not undertaken when "controls" were required for comparison with the brains from those who had mental disorders.

Chapter 9 referred to the system used to abstract information about the deceased's health and medication from hospital case records. In the case of "controls", this information was obtained from the general practitioner as it was important to exclude neuropsychiatric disease.

Brains used for research

Before brain samples were placed in the freezers, they were categorised so that only specimens that met the appropriate diagnostic criteria were selected for each study. Samples of diseased and "control" brains could be chosen for neurochemical analysis.

Neurochemical analyses involve the extraction of complex chemical compounds from the substance of each sample. During the process, the integrity of the sample is destroyed, so that at the end of the investigation no recognisable brain substance remains. As further samples are investigated, the volume of tissue remaining from each brain progressively diminishes.

For this reason collection of brains continued for a period of years so the newly collected brains would replace those that had been used up.

The brain tissue samples reported to the CMO's Census in 2000 were the samples that had not been used up in the neurochemical investigations. Almost all the remaining samples could still be identified, through reference numbers, and linked to a named deceased person.

Exclusion of brains that did not meet the criteria

Many "control brains" were obtained before details of the deceased's medical history became available. Among these were some that could not be used as "controls" after the deceased was found to have had a history of neuropsychiatric disease.

Some brains collected as "index cases of schizophrenia" were not used when clinical details did not satisfy the research criteria for that condition. The same criteria resulted in the exclusion of some index cases that did not satisfy the research specification. The excluded brains were not used further in the research programme.

Some brains were excluded when the medical details of the deceased's mental health could not be obtained. This was the reason why Mr Isaacs' brain was not used for research. A few brains were not used when they posed a risk of infection to the research team; for example, when the deceased was discovered to be a carrier of Hepatitis B.

The excluded brains were disposed of after their unsuitability for the programme was identified.

Other uses

Transfer to another research team

The brain books record that a small number of brains were not investigated in the joint programme, but passed on to other research teams known to be collecting brains in the same diagnostic category. These transfers were made after the deceased's medical history had been validated and found not to match a diagnosis the joint team were investigating.

The number of brains transferred to other teams was small, but this was considered a better use of scarce research material than disposal without any investigation. In the brain books such transfers were usually noted by the name of the researcher, rather than the institution where (s)he worked.

Records found in other locations suggest that not all brain samples transferred were recorded in the brain books.

Pharmaceutical company brain research

One brain book records that samples of a brain were provided to a pharmaceutical company. Further enquiries showed that during the course of the programme, brain samples were provided on three separate occasions for research by pharmaceutical companies. On each occasion a different company received the sample. On two occasions the research was a joint investigation between the company and the research team.

After the third sample had been provided, the joint team received from the company a small quantity of chemical reagents: *"As a token of our appreciation for your help in progressing our research we provided your laboratory with a set of standard radioisotopes for quantifying autoradiographic results"*. The value of the reagents was not recorded. Annex 72

This transaction goes beyond the scope of my investigation but Manchester University have been making further enquiries.

Disposal of brains and brain samples

All excluded brains and residual brain samples that were not used or needed for the programme were disposed of by incineration as "clinical waste". This method of disposal was adopted at that time by hospitals to dispose of samples and specimens of human origin that were no longer needed.

Reviews of stored brain samples

From time to time the contents of the freezers were reviewed. These reviews were prompted by shortage of space for new brains. Two members of the research team recall that in 1993 there was a more rigorous review of the brain samples then held. It is thought Mr Isaacs' brain was disposed of after this review, but this cannot be confirmed and the date of the review was not recorded.

Summary

Index and "control" brains were collected according to strict criteria.

All samples remain identifiable.

Those that did not meet the criteria were excluded.

The research process used most of the brains collected and resulted in the destruction of the brain samples used.

Brains excluded from the programme were disposed of by incineration.

The brain samples that remained in 2000 were reported for the CMO's Census.

Some brains or samples that were not suitable for the programme were transferred to other researchers.

On three occasions brain samples were provided for research undertaken jointly with pharmaceutical companies.

References

1 Data in the brain book entries.

CHAPTER 18

Approval of the joint programme by Ethics Committees and letters to general practitioners of "control" cases

Introduction

This chapter summarises the involvement of Research Ethics Committees in considering research protocols submitted by the joint programme. The chapter describes key features of the protocols considered by RECs.

Professor Deakin states that *"All Ethical Committee applications had the sole and explicit purpose of obtaining approval to approach relatives for hospital post mortems on their deceased relatives"*.

The protocols omitted any reference to the collection of brains from Coroners' cases. Professor Deakin has commented that *"reference to control brains was for information and to demonstrate the scientific design"*. However, the references to controls did not address the source or the inclusion of Coroners' cases.

The titles of the projects submitted

With the exception of the first protocol that was submitted to Salford Ethics Committee, Professor Deakin is sure that all other Ethics Committees received the same proposal. Professor Deakin states this was the protocol dated 17 July 1986 which is on a South Manchester Ethics Committee (SMEC) form.

While several Ethics Committees may have received the same protocol, the titles by which they referred to the protocol were different.

Titles of applications used in correspondence with Ethics Committees

Salford Ethics Committee, Chapter 12

The Salford EC considered and approved the protocol entitled: *"Brain research in schizophrenia and tardive dyskinesia"*. Annex 31

South Manchester Ethics Committee

The South Manchester EC received the protocol signed by Dr Deakin on behalf of Dr Slater and himself on 17 July 1986. The title was: *"Post-Mortem Brain Neurochemistry and the Major Psychoses"*. No record is available about when the protocol was considered by the Ethics Committee for the University Hospital of South Manchester. The only document available is a copy of an unsigned letter dated 26 November 1986 to Dr Brookes. Professor Deakin reports that Dr Brookes was Secretary of the Ethics Committee responsible for the South Manchester hospitals. Annex 33 Annex 73

This letter asks for comments on a draft letter which Dr Deakin planned to send to general practitioners. The draft letter itself is not attached and the terms in which the South Manchester Ethics Committee responded are not available.

However, the letter to Dr Brookes refers to *"Control samples* (of brains) *are obtained from patients who have died in the Community and who come to post mortem at Prestwich or North Manchester"*.

There is no reference to Coroner's cases and the terms *"deaths in the community"* is not synonymous with deaths reported to the Coroner.

It is also notable that the letter is addressed to South Manchester in respect of cases occurring in Salford (Prestwich) and North Manchester districts with which there was no similar correspondence.

North Manchester Ethics Committee, Chapter 13

The North Manchester EC received the same protocol as South Manchester EC. The title is to be found in the approval letter dated 11 September 1986. It appears from the date of the letter to Dr Brookes that consideration by the North Manchester EC preceded consideration by the South Manchester EC, but in the absence of other documents, this cannot be confirmed. Later correspondence with the North Manchester EC refers simply to: *"post mortem brain studies in mental illness"*.

Warrington Ethics Committee, Chapter 15

The correspondence with Warrington EC refers to: *"Post-Mortem Neurochemical Studies in Schizophrenia"*.

Oldham, Rochdale and Wigan Ethics Committees, Chapter 14

Correspondence with these three Ethics Committees refers to: *"Brain Research in Schizophrenia"*.

Macclesfield Ethics Committee

The correspondence with Macclesfield EC refers to: "*Post-mortem brain studies in Schizophrenia*".

Professor Deakin assures me that the Committees, with the exception of Salford, received the protocol dated 17 July 1986. As the Committees no longer have the protocols that were considered more than 10 years ago, I am unable to check the titles or explain the variations used by the Ethics Committees in correspondence.

Professor Deakin states that the difference in the titles probably followed the heading he used in his letters to the Committees. However, the letters available to me all have the same title *"Post-mortem brain studies in Schizophrenia"*. It is improbable that the Ethics Committees decided to change the titles of protocols submitted to them.

In view of my discussions with those who were Chairmen of Ethics Committees in the late 1980s, I am surprised that each Committee did not insist on receiving an application on its own form. One Committee Chairman has told me that the Committees in the Manchester area were very particular on this point.

References to approval by other Ethics Committees

After protocols had been approved by Salford and North and South Manchester ECs, other Committees were told of the approvals already received.

The consent of the relatives

In the protocols that survive, the team emphasise the importance of obtaining consent from relatives. This was included in the 1988 notes prepared for consultants to give to relatives of patients with schizophrenia in hospitals participating in the research. Annex 46 and 47

The protocols submitted to the Ethics Committees state clearly that the relatives would be asked to consent to the retention of brains of patients. The psychiatrist who had been looking after the patient will: *"seek permission from the nearest relative to remove brain tissue at post mortem"*.

(The need for consent was emphasised by Oldham Ethics Committee. In their approval letter dated 2 November 1990 the Committee Chairman wrote: *"It was the considered opinion of the members that a direct approach to the relative was preferable to a telephone call and that contact should be made either by you or a senior clinician"*.) Annex 56

The applications to the Ethics Committees are less specific about consent to the retention of "control" brains but state: *"We would also like to collect some brains of patients who have died from medical conditions who have not suffered from mental illness"*.

The letter to Dr Brookes refers only to *"patients who have died in the Community"*, but does not refer to consent from the relatives of these patients from whom *"control samples"* were obtained.

Access to patients' medical records

On access to the patients' medical records, the protocols to Ethics Committees include: *"We will need to look at the deceased patient's notes at some stage after collecting each patient's brain"*.

The protocols do not state how the records of "control" cases would be accessed.

Collection of brains from Coroners' cases

While the protocols to Ethics Committees (and applications for research funds) referred to collection of "control" brains, they failed to disclose that most of the control brains were obtained from Coroners' cases. There was, therefore, nothing in the protocol that would prompt an Ethics Committee to ask about the consent or collection arrangements for brains removed from Coroners' cases.

The assumption appears to be that Ethics Committees did not need to know about the collection of brains from Coroners' cases. This, in my view, did not absolve the research team from making full and complete disclosure to the Ethics Committees of their proposed activities.

Letters to general practitioners

In practice, when the team obtained a brain from a Coroner's case a letter was sent to the deceased's general practitioner. The reason for this was to establish that the patient had had no dementia and no mental illness which would exclude the use of their brain as a "control" and to identify relevant drug treatment at the time of death which might interfere with neurochemical measures.

The letter to the general practitioners in the first paragraph states: "*We are carrying out research into brain chemistry and mental illness. We collect post-mortem brain samples and these are analysed in the department of physiology in the Medical School. These studies have ethical committee approval*".

The letter sent to Dr Rosenberg, Mr Isaacs' general practitioner, is one such example. Annex 15

The second and subsequent paragraphs request particular information about the deceased's health and medication at the time of death.

At a later but unrecorded date the format of the letter to general practitioners was changed. The wording of the second letter indicates that it would have been preceded by a telephone conversation. The letter maintains the reference to *"samples of brain tissue"* but Ethics Committees are referred to at the foot of the letter: *"This research is carried out under the auspices of all local ethics committees"*. These letters, like the earlier version, were sent on behalf of Dr Deakin, but were usually signed by other members of the team. Annex 74

Professor Deakin states that the first letter had been referred in draft to Dr Brookes, Secretary of the Ethics Committee responsible for South Manchester hospitals. However, the application to the South Manchester Ethics Committee and the letter dated 21 November 1986 do not mention the collection of brains from Coroner's cases, although both refer to collection of "control" samples from patients who died in the community.

The initial letter was also sent to general practitioners in respect of Coroner's cases whose bodies had been taken to Prestwich Hospital, although the Salford EC had not been approached. The Salford EC were unaware of the collection of "control" brains from Coroner's cases or of the use of this letter.

Misleading statements

The Ethics Committees had not been told the relevant facts. They had been told about the collection of controls but not that these would be mainly brains from Coroners' cases. In particular, the Salford and North Manchester ECs were unaware of the collection of brains from Coroners' cases.

The assertion in the letters to general practitioners that *"these studies have ethical committee approval"* was regarded as misleading by at least one general practitioner.

The letter to general practitioners was also misleading in referring to "*brain samples*" when in fact the whole brain had been retained.

General practitioners would expect that, in some cases, samples of brain tissue would be retained, but would have taken issue with the University had they realised that the whole brain had been removed and retained without the knowledge of the relatives.

General Medical Council guidance

The claim of Ethics Committee approval must also be considered in the light of the General Medical Council's guidance that information for research should only be disclosed for projects that have been approved by a recognised Ethics Committee, Chapter 6.

General practitioner recipients of these letters, whose patients had been the subject of a Coroner's post mortem, would have concluded that the Ethics Committees had been informed that the research would include Coroners' cases. They could not have known that they were being asked to provide details outside the GMC guidelines. It was also not made clear that a brain from a Coroner's case had been obtained without the knowledge or consent of the relatives. Appendix 13

Professor Deakin's observations on consent – June 2001

In a letter dated 11 June 2001 to the General Medical Council, Professor Deakin notes: Annex 75
"Dr Slater initially set the system up for Alzheimer's disease but I began collaborating with him with schizophrenia sometime afterwards. The local mortuaries and coroner's offices would telephone Dr Slater's laboratory if possible cases of Alzheimer's disease or schizophrenia were undergoing post-mortem and also if non-psychiatric control subjects were.

This system continued an earlier one in which brains from all over the country were supplied to the Medical Research Council Brain Bank at Addenbrooke's Hospital. My understanding is that in Coroners' cases of non-patient deaths in the community, consent was not routinely sought in the 1970s and early 80s. In contrast, where deaths occurred in hospitals, removal of tissue could not happen without written consent of the relatives. We continued existing practise (sic) *in the NW. As far as I could see, this did not differ from practises* (sic) *in the previous research institute where I trained or from practise* (sic) *in other hospitals at that time.*

I became increasingly uncomfortable about not consulting relatives and after a discussion with Mr Gorodkin the Manchester Coroner, instigated by me in 1995; my involvement ceased.

I did obtain Ethical Committee permission as part of an attempt to set up a prospective collection. In other words, to approach patients and their relatives for brain donation in the event of subsequent death of the patient and also to approach relatives after the death. However, we had no funding to set up the ante-mortem consent scheme and nothing further came of it.

We did not have Ethics Committee permission to collect brains from Coroners' post-mortems because we did not believe it was necessary. It never entered our minds that this was required, especially as the pathologists were willing to remove tissue. We understood from our contact with other researchers and from previous experience that it was universal practice for tissue and organs to be removed for research purposes during Coroner's post-mortems".

Professor Deakin's observations in his letter of June 2001 explain why he did not seek the approval of Ethics Committees before obtaining brains from Coroners' post mortems and why he did not ask permission of the relatives.

Professor Deakin makes the same point in a letter to me dated 8 November 2001: "*It is certainly the case that Coroners' post-mortems were frequently used as a source of supply for brain and other organ material to form the control sample and indeed consent was not routinely obtained. Brains were collected from Coroners' post-mortems at Northwick Park where I trained and Professor Tim Crow would be able to tell you about that. Other collections active at the time* (were) *at Nottingham, Oxford, Institute of Psychiatry, Newcastle and Edinburgh".* Annex 76

Summary

Although the same protocol was said to have been sent to a number of Ethics Committees, the subsequent correspondence refers to different project titles. The reasons for this variation have not been satisfactorily explained.

Protocols submitted to Ethics Committees must include all the relevant facts. The joint research team did not include significant features in their protocols.

Ethics Committees who were later asked for approval may have been mistakenly reassured by references to approval given by other Ethics Committees who had not been given the full facts. The Committees could not have known that almost all control brains were obtained from Coroners' cases.

The protocols sent to Ethics Committees state clearly that the consent of relatives would be obtained when the deceased had been under the care of a psychiatrist, but are silent about whether relatives of control cases would be similarly asked for consent.

The letters to general practitioners are misleading:

- Ethics Committees had not been aware of, or approved, the inclusion of brains from Coroners' cases. The provenance of control brains was not explained;

- the statement that "*these studies have ethical committee approval*" obscured the real provenance of most of the brains collected as "controls" and the reference to "*brain samples*" hid the fact that the whole brain was retained;

- the request for medical information about the deceased's health does not appear to satisfy the GMC requirements for Ethics Committee approval.

CHAPTER 19

Pathology reports submitted to Coroners in Manchester and Cheshire

Did the report to the Coroner mention brain retention?

This chapter describes a central feature of the reports sent to the Coroners' offices in North Manchester, Central Manchester and Warrington in respect of the 230 Coroners' cases. In all these cases the brains were obtained for the joint programme.

This chapter is based on scrutiny of samples of post mortem reports provided for this investigation by the Coroners of the three districts.

The importance of full and accurate reporting of organ and/or tissue retention in post mortem reports to Coroners is discussed in Chapter 42.

Reports on post mortem examinations at Prestwich, Bury, Oldham and Rochdale mortuaries

There were 45 post mortem examinations at Prestwich mortuary undertaken for the Coroner between 1985 and 1989. A sample of 50 per cent of these reports was examined[(1)]. There is no reference to brain (or other organ) retention in any of the reports. This applies both to cases of sudden death in the community and to in-patient deaths reported to the Coroner.

There were also 67 brains retained from Coroner's cases in Bury, Oldham and Rochdale. In a sample of 25 per cent of these reports, no mention of brain retention was found.

North Manchester General Hospital

Of the 100 Coroner's post mortem examinations at North Manchester General Hospital carried out between 1986 and 1994, 60 were on in-patients. The remaining 40 were on patients who had died in the Accident and Emergency Department or had been certified dead in the ambulance on arrival at the hospital.

More than 50 of the post mortem reports were examined[(2)]. In only one report is brain retention mentioned. This report refers to retention for the research programme at Manchester University. All other reports are silent on organ and tissue retention.

Warrington General Hospital

There were 15 Coroner's autopsies at Warrington General Hospital where the brain was retained for the research programme. Of these, seven cases were in-patient deaths.

All the post mortem reports sent to the Coroner were checked. In only one report was the retention of the brain for research mentioned[(3)].

Recollections of pathologists

The pathologists undertaking Coroners' post mortems at three of these mortuaries were asked for their recollections and whether they would have recorded brain retention on the post mortem form. Their recollections were divided. One pathologist stated that he did not record organ retention on the post mortem report to avoid distress to the relatives. In this case, the pathologist believed the Coroner was aware of his practice.

The remaining pathologists all believed that they would have recorded the removal of an organ. All expressed surprise when told of the results of the examination I had made of the post mortem reports.

Coroners' procedures – Central and North Manchester and Warrington

In view of the number of post mortem reports submitted in each of these districts, it was the practice for the Coroner's office staff to check the written reports, when these arrived, and bring any unusual features to the notice of the Coroner.

Verbal reports for the release of the body

For the purpose of releasing the body, several Coroners in different parts of the country recalled that in the late 1980s they had relied on a verbal report from the pathologist to release the body. The written report would frequently arrive some days later, not always in time for the inquest.

Summary

From the post mortem reports prepared by the pathologists, the Coroners in Manchester and Cheshire could not have known that brains had been retained for research purpose.

The relatives of the deceased who asked for copies of the post mortem would have been unaware of brain (or other organ) retention.

There were only two reports found where the retention of the brain for research (as opposed to diagnostic) purposes was referred to in the 50 per cent sample of post mortem reports that were reviewed.

It was the usual practice for the staff of the Coroner's office to review post mortem reports that arrived after the inquest had been held to check that the report contained no new or significant features.

Later chapters will show that the post mortem reports in the Manchester area followed the pattern of other parts of the country. Few reports at that time referred to brain retention unless this had a bearing on the cause of death.

References

1 Post mortem reports provided by Mr Williams, Coroner for the North Manchester district.
2 Post mortem reports provided by Mr Gorodkin, Coroner for the Central Manchester district.
3 Post mortem reports provided by Mr Rheinberg, Coroner for the Cheshire district.

CHAPTER 20

Access to medical records

Introduction

This chapter describes the reasons and methods used to correlate the features of the patient's neuropsychiatric condition with post mortem brain findings.

Reasons for collection of medical details

The research team needed to obtain information from the patient's medical records. For patients with neuropsychiatric disorders, one important reason for this information was to validate the diagnosis of Alzheimer's disease, schizophrenia or another condition.

For control cases, access to patients' records was equally important as the team needed to check that the patients had not experienced any neuropsychiatric disease.

A further reason for checking the records was to document any medication the patient had been receiving prior to death, and to obtain other relevant history or lifestyle information.

Sources of data

The mortuaries contributing brains to the programme provided basic details of the patient's name, date of birth, date and time of death, date and time of post mortem examination and cause of death. The name of the patient's general practitioner was also recorded when this was known.

Retrieval of information

Hospital patients

A member of the research team would request the hospital case records some weeks after the patient's death in order to extract relevant clinical information. The abstraction of this data was not urgent and in many cases took place several months after the patient's death.

Deaths in the community

It was more complex to retrieve data about patients included in the programme who had died in the community. Many were sudden deaths reported to the Coroner so that the cause of death could be established.

In these cases, the team would try to identify the name of the general practitioner who had looked after the deceased in life. If this name was not provided at the time the brain was received, the team would make enquiries through the Coroner's office. In all cases where there was no information available from hospital records, a letter signed by, or on behalf of, Dr Deakin was sent to the general practitioner.

A copy of the standard letter was sent to Dr Rosenberg, Mr Isaacs' general practitioner. (Its discovery by Mrs Isaacs led to the setting up of this investigation.) This letter was used in the early years of the joint programme. It was later replaced by a different letter which also refers to *"post-mortem samples of brain tissue from the patient(s) for use in schizophrenia research"*; and, as a footnote, *"this research is carried out under the auspices of all local ethics committees"*. Annex 15 Annex 74

It will be seen that the format of the first form was designed to provide the research team with sufficient data to classify each brain into one of three categories:

- suitable as an index case of Alzheimer's disease/schizophrenia/other condition;

- suitable as a control (no evidence to suggest pre-existing neuropsychiatric disease);

- insufficient information available/questionable neuropsychiatric features which made the brain unsuitable as an index case or as a control.

The form used later was specifically about patients with schizophrenia. This form was only sent after an initial telephone conversation with the deceased's general practitioner.

Further enquiries

If the initial request form to the general practitioner was not returned, a further reminder form would normally be sent, followed up by a telephone call and sometimes a visit to the general practitioner.

Enquiries about Mr Isaacs

Dr Rosenberg was sent the form at Annex 15. He did not return it, Chapter 4. Annex 15

In Mr Isaacs' case, Dr Rosenberg would have known that his death had been reported to the Coroner, but this would not necessarily have been the case in other sudden deaths. The form sent to Dr Rosenberg is no different from other forms, copies of which remain in the brain books.

Further communications followed, and some general information was provided over the telephone. While this referred to *"no formal psychiatric history"*, the information was not considered to be sufficiently detailed. For this reason, Mr Isaacs' brain was not used in the programme. The relevant entry in the brain book reads: *"Notes unavailable since civil suit against GP in action"*.

Features of the letter sent to general practitioners

The misleading features of these letters were discussed in Chapter 18.

Summary

The design of the joint programme required collection of data from the deceased's medical records to establish the suitability of each brain for the research programme.

For patients who had died in hospital, the hospital records were obtained by the research team at an appropriate interval after death. These records were abstracted for information on neuropsychiatric history, medication at the time of death and any previous contact with the psychiatric services.

For deaths in the community, this information was requested by letter from the general practitioner of the deceased. Where the letter received no response, further attempts were made to obtain the medical history. The wording of the letter to general practitioners gave a misleading impression that brain samples only had been retained. In reality, the whole brain had been obtained in most cases.

The reference to Ethical Committee approval obscured the fact that the Ethics Committees consulted had not been informed of the inclusion of cases of sudden death in the community and other deaths reported to the Coroner, Chapter 18.

CHAPTER 21

Who was aware of the role of the North Manchester Coroner's office in identifying suitable brains for the joint programme?

Introduction

This chapter describes who knew about the role of the North Manchester Coroner's office in identifying brains suitable for the joint programme, who was involved, and the extent to which they might have questioned the arrangements for brain retention. It is based on the recollections of those involved and relevant contemporaneous documents.

Background

The discovery that Mr Isaacs' brain had been retained without the knowledge of his relatives poses two important questions:

- who had authorised the retention of Mr Isaacs' brain?
- why did no-one at the time take action to question the retention of Mr Isaacs' brain?

While these questions relate to Mr Isaacs' brain, they apply equally to all brains retained at Prestwich that had been identified by the Coroner's office.

Who was involved?

Three different groups of staff were privy to the arrangement - the staff of the Coroner's office, persons working in Prestwich mortuary and other mortuaries in Bury, Rochdale and Oldham, and the staff of the joint research programme.

Staff of the Coroner's office

The involvement of the Coroner's office was described in Chapter 10. Mrs Langan and other staff of the Coroner's office have stated that in the late 1980s and early 1990s cases where the brain might be suitable for research were notified to the joint programme. Mrs Langan's name and the names of other staff in the Coroner's office (Mrs Shirley Connelly, Mrs Gillian Williamson and Mrs Jean Sweat) can be found in the brain books of the joint programme.

Mrs Langan would usually telephone the Department of Physiology at Manchester University to inform Dr Slater when a suitable brain was available. However, other members of the staff of the office recall that from time to time they were asked by Mrs Langan to do so.

Mrs Langan and the other members of the Coroner's office staff are in no doubt that the Coroner, Mr North, knew of the arrangement in the late 1980s. Mrs Langan also recalls that the research programme had been mentioned during regular meetings at Birchill Hospital, Rochdale, when Mr North and Mrs Langan spoke to each new group of resident doctors about deaths that should be reported to the Coroner.

Mrs Langan and the junior members of staff all believed that the Coroner was aware of, and approved, their identifying suitable cases for research.

However, as Chapter 19 records, the post mortem reports submitted to Mr North did not mention the retention of any brains for research. The same is true for those submitted to Mr Williams after he was appointed to succeed Mr North in 1995.

The position of Coroner has always been held as one of authority. The staff of the Coroner's office in Rochdale believed they were acting on the Coroner's instructions. The staff also believed the Coroner had the authority to order retention for research. Even if one of the Coroner's staff had thought otherwise, it would have been a courageous act to question directly the Coroner's authority.

Staff working in Prestwich mortuary

The pathologists

When pathologists undertake Coroners' post mortems, they do so on the instructions of the Coroner in each case. When in the 1980s a post mortem was ordered from the Coroner's office in Rochdale, the instruction generally came from the office staff and not from the Coroner himself.

Dr Farrand, who had undertaken most of the Coroner's post mortems at Prestwich mortuary since 1975, believed that instructions coming from the Coroner's office had the authority of the Coroner. Like many pathologists, Dr Farrand believed that if the Coroner was content for brains to be retained for research then the Coroner's instruction should be followed. Dr Farrand was not the only pathologist who had undertaken Coroner's post mortems at Prestwich from which brains had been retained for the joint programme.

It has been suggested that Dr Farrand should have questioned the instruction to retain Mr Isaacs' brain because he was Jewish. Dr Farrand would have known this, as the time of the post mortem had been brought forward to 11.00am so that the burial could take place the same day.

Dr Farrand was aware that those of the Jewish faith object in principle to post mortems. This followed a previous occasion when he had arrived to undertake a post mortem at Prestwich mortuary to discover that a High Court injunction was in place to stop the examination. However, Dr Farrand also knew that the High Court injunction had been overturned on appeal.

In February 1987, Dr Farrand had not regarded the instruction that Mr Isaacs' brain be taken for the joint programme as in any way unusual. He had received the same instruction for many other deceased persons, including a few of the Jewish faith. He believed the instructions to retain the brains for the joint programme had come from the Coroner.

When asked about the Jewish faith's position on organ retention, Dr Farrand was clear that in 1987 he had believed the Jewish objection was to the post mortem procedure and not to organ retention. However, by the time of my meeting with him in

December 2001, Dr Farrand was well aware of the Jewish faith's objections to any organ retention.

<u>The mortician</u>

For his part, Mr Walkden, the mortician, was even less in a position to question the instructions given by the Coroner's office. Mr Walkden was, like Dr Farrand, also aware that the brains of other persons of the Jewish faith had been sent to the joint programme. In 1987 he did not consider that the transfer of Mr Isaacs' brain was in any way unusual.

Mr Walkden was not aware that the system was unlawful and that brains should not be retained for research unless the relatives of the deceased had given their consent. In this context, Mr Walkden had always checked the consent form for hospital post mortems when brains were to be transferred to the Cerebral Function Unit, Chapter 8.

<u>The Coroner's Officer</u>

The Coroner's Officer for Bury and Prestwich mortuaries in the late 1980s was PC Joe Cassells, who was also aware of the retention of brains for the joint programme.

> Lung retention
>
> In the late 1980s, lungs were being retained on the instructions of the Coroner for diagnostic purposes for which the lungs were sent to Nottingham. These were mainly from persons who had worked in the mines or mills and who had been in contact with coal or asbestos during their working lives and where an industrial disease might have contributed to the cause of death.
>
> Brain retention
>
> PC Cassells believed that the brains transferred to the joint programme were for a similar purpose. PC Cassells has stated that, where an organ was retained in order to identify a possible cause of death, he would inform the families and indicate that the authority for retention came from the Coroner.

In any event, PC Cassells was not in a position to challenge the instructions given him for retention of brains for research rather than diagnosis, purportedly on the authority of the Coroner.

PC Cassells was unaware of what subsequently happened to organs which had been retained.

<u>Bury mortuary</u>

The position in Bury mortuary was the same as in Prestwich. Mr Walkden, the mortician at Bury mortuary, had transferred there from Prestwich in 1988.

Dr Farrand acted as Coroner's pathologist at Bury as he had done at Prestwich.

Rochdale mortuary

Mr Paul Owen was the mortician at Rochdale. He had worked first at Oldham mortuary until 1986, when he transferred to the NMGH mortuary. At NMGH Mr Owen worked with Mr Leatherbarrow, Chapter 13.

Mr Owen recalls that no tissues or organs, except for pituitaries, were retained in the years he worked at Oldham mortuary.

During the period Mr Owen worked at NMGH he had not been involved in collecting brains for the research programme. Mr Owen moved to Rochdale in February 1990.

Mr Owen's description of the arrangement for obtaining brains corresponds in all details with the description in previous chapters. A telephone call from Mrs Langan or from Dr Slater would tell him that a brain should be retained. Later the same day Dr Slater, "or someone riding a BMW motorcycle", would arrive with a cool box to collect the brain.

The Coroner's Officer at Rochdale was PC David Rigg. He held this post from 1976 until his retirement in 1995.

Like Mr Owen and PC Cassalls at Prestwich and Bury mortuaries, Mr Rigg had never questioned the arrangement. He knew that the instruction had come from the Coroner's office, usually from Joyce Langan. He assumed that Mrs Langan was following the Coroner's instructions.

Mr Rigg recollected that the brains retained at Rochdale mortuary were usually from patients who had schizophrenia. In some cases, the fact that the deceased had suffered from schizophrenia had only come to the notice of the Coroner's office from the report that PC Rigg prepared.

In PC Rigg's view, anything that was retained after a Coroner's post mortem was held on the Coroner's instructions. He believed the Coroner had the right to authorise retention.

As the procedures at Prestwich, Bury and Rochdale were identical to all intents and purposes, the system at Oldham is not separately described.

The staff of the joint programme at Manchester University

As the arrangements with Prestwich mortuary were providing the research material needed for their work, staff of the joint programme believed the Coroner had the authority to allow them to retain brains. Some members of the staff of the joint research programme believed that Mr North, the Coroner for the North Manchester district, had authorised the retention of brains from Prestwich, Bury, Oldham and Rochdale mortuaries.

However, Professor Deakin states that he believed North Manchester General Hospital was in Mr North's district. This explanation does not take account of the fact that the arrangements for identifying brains from the NMGH mortuary were entirely different. None was identified through the Coroner's office, a feature that was clear to other members of the team.

Manchester University Administration

The contemporaneous documents show that Manchester University Administration were aware of some of the research applications submitted by the joint team as these were countersigned on behalf of the University.

However, the detailed practical arrangements, as described in previous chapters, were not made available to the University Administration. I am satisfied that Manchester University Administration were not aware of the collection of brains without the knowledge or consent of the relatives. Similarly, Manchester University Ethics Committee was not informed.

Summary

The staff of the Coroner's office believed that the Coroner, Mr North, approved of referral of suitable brains to the joint research programme.

Dr Farrand and other pathologists who had referred brains to the programme believed they were following the Coroner's instructions. They mistakenly believed the Coroner had the legal powers to allow brain and other organ retention for research unrelated to the cause of death.

The staff undertaking post mortems for Mr North in the other mortuaries were unaware that brain retention for research purposes was unlawful unless the relatives had given consent.

The staff of the joint programme at Manchester believed the Coroner had agreed to the retention of brains and for this reason they did not consider the consent of the relatives was required for brain retention from a Coroner's case.

Manchester University Administration were unaware that brains were being collected without the knowledge or consent of relatives.

CHAPTER 22

Was the retention of brains known to Coroners in Manchester and Cheshire?

Introduction

Between 1985 and 1996, 230 brains from Coroners' cases were obtained for the joint programme from three districts: North Manchester, Central Manchester and Cheshire. This chapter describes the extent to which Coroners in the three districts were aware of brain retention.

The chapter is based on contemporaneous papers and the recollections of those involved.

North Manchester

Mr North was the Coroner for the North Manchester district from 1974 to 1994. Mr North stated that he was not aware of, or had ever sanctioned, the removal of brains or other organs without the consent of the relatives unless the organ was required for diagnostic purposes.

Mr North had been asked in July 1985 by Professor Yates, Professor of Neuropathology at Manchester University, about the removal of post mortem samples of brains from Coroner's cases without any supervision of a medically qualified pathologist. Professor Yates had written: *"In all cases the families of the deceased will have known of our interest and intentions and have given their permission for the procedure before the death of the subject".* Annex 77

Mr North replied: *"I feel it difficult to agree with your request. The only way I could agree is to have my pathologist present at the time of the removal in order that he could give me a full and complete report. That would not seem to me to be a practical proposition as my pathologists are seldom able to carry out post mortem examinations as quickly as one hour after death".* Annex 78

This exchange of correspondence preceded the start of the joint programme and was about the removal of brains when the relatives had given their consent.

Mr Isaacs' brain was retained in February 1987.

In 1990 Mr North was asked about the removal of specimens for research by Dr Menon of the Department of Pathology at Birch Hill Hospital, Rochdale. Dr Menon's letter is not available, but Mr North replied on 12 June 1990: *"I am of the opinion that before any specimens or samples are taken for research purposes which do not form part of your enquiry as to establishing Coroner's cause of death that the consent of the relatives should be obtained".* Annex 79

These letters are the surviving documents that set out Mr North's position on the removal of organs and tissues for research purposes.

Four members of Mr North's staff and two Coroner's Officers from Bury police district are of the opinion that Mr North *"must have known what was going on"*.

There is no contemporaneous written evidence to resolve this divergence of opinion.

Mr Williams' views

In the mid 1980s Mr North invited Mr Barrie Williams to act as his deputy. When Mr North resigned in June 1994 on health grounds, Mr Williams continued as Deputy Coroner until he was appointed to succeed Mr North in 1995.

When asked directly if he was aware of the arrangement, Mr Williams replied ***"No"***. Mr Williams added that when he was Mr North's deputy, he had not known that the office staff were involved in identifying cases for the joint research programme. He did not find out until after Mrs Langan had retired. Mr Williams assures me that had he known at the time he would have put a stop to the practice immediately.

It is important to record that the morticians at Bury and Rochdale both commented that Mr Williams "*does everything properly*", implying that, in their view, had Mr Williams known, he would have put a stop to the practice.

The only relevant written record is a note made by Dr Farrand after an informal discussion with Mr Williams at Bury Magistrate's Court on 22 May 2000. This was a month after Mrs Isaacs had started to make enquiries about why her husband's brain had been retained. Dr Farrand's note records: *"22 May – meeting with Mr Williams before inquest at Bury Magistrate's Court. Mr Williams was aware that Joyce would arrange for brains to go for research and he said that this must have had the Coroner's approval"*. This note relates to Mr Williams' comments on events that took place at least five years previously.

Dr Farrand's note, in manuscript, is on a memo dated 14 April 2000 from Harold Howard of the Royal Bolton Hospital to Brian Senior at the same hospital. At the time Dr Farrand's note was written, Mr Williams would have recently become aware of Mrs Isaacs' enquiries.

Central Manchester

Mr Leonard Gorodkin has been the Coroner for the Central Manchester district since 1978. He was astonished when he saw the list which included 100 brains taken from Coroner's cases at North Manchester General Hospital. At least one other brain had been obtained from a death reported to him at Manchester Royal Infirmary.

Mr Gorodkin has always made it clear to the pathologists and to his staff that organs of any kind were only to be retained for diagnostic purposes and that he should be informed whenever this occurred. Mr Gorodkin would agree to organs being retained for other purposes, provided the consent of the relatives had been obtained. One such example would be for organ transplantation. However, Mr Gorodkin expected all pathologists working for him to record any organ retention in the post mortem report. As the post mortem reports did not record organ retention, the Coroner and his office staff were unaware of what was occurring in the NMGH mortuary.

Pathologists at North Manchester General Hospital and at the Manchester Royal Infirmary were well aware of Mr Gorodkin's position on organ retention, which makes it the more surprising that the pathologists did not ask questions about the intended destination and use of the brains.

In the 50 post mortem reports examined from North Manchester General Hospital, only one referred to the brain having been retained. In this case death was due to natural causes and there had been no reason to hold an inquest. In these circumstances, Mr Gorodkin had relied on his office staff to check that the cause of death in the post mortem report corresponded to the findings the pathologist had telephoned to his office and on which Mr Gorodkin released the body and notified the Registrar of the cause of death. Mr Gorodkin had required his staff to bring to his attention any discrepancies affecting the cause of death, or other significant features. He was obliged to rely on his staff in view of the very substantial number of post mortems carried out in his district.

Following advice from Professor McClure in April 1995, Chapter 14, Professor Deakin requested a meeting with Mr Gorodkin. This took place on 26 June 1995 in Mr Gorodkin's office. Professor Deakin states that his purpose was to seek Mr Gorodkin's permission to extend the brain collection system into Mr Gorodkin's Central Manchester District and to ascertain his views about retaining brains as part of the Coroner's investigation.

Mr Gorodkin was clear that the relative's consent would always be necessary. This is consistent with Mr Gorodkin's long-held position.

Mr Gorodkin's response to Professor Deakin's request was clearly a major factor in Professor Deakin's decision to end his part in the joint programme, Chapter 24. Professor Deakin states that Mr Gorodkin *"confirmed my view that the joint programme was no longer practicable"*. It is not clear what Dr Slater was told about the conversation Professor Deakin had had with Mr Gorodkin.

It appears that at the time of this meeting Professor Deakin was not aware that 100 brains already obtained by the joint programme were from Coroner's cases at North Manchester General Hospital for deaths that had been reported to Mr Gorodkin.

Mr Gorodkin's firm position on organ retention was confirmed by several staff in the North Manchester General Hospital mortuary and Manchester Royal Infirmary. One mortician who had provided brains for the joint programme even stated that he knew that this was against Mr Gorodkin's policy.

It should be noted that the programme continued to collect brains from Coroner's cases without consent until 1996.

Cheshire

Warrington General Hospital was one of the mortuaries within the district of the Coroner for Cheshire. The Coroner for Cheshire between 1988 and 1992, when brains were obtained for the programme from Warrington, was the late Mr Hibbert.

There is no doubt that the staff of the Coroner's office in Warrington were aware that brains were being sent to Manchester University. Mr Stephenson, newly appointed as Coroner's Officer in 1989, made enquiries when he first came across a brain that was being retained for the joint programme, Chapter 15.

After Mr Stephenson was reassured, he and the mortuary staff assumed that the joint programme had the Coroner's approval.

All but one of the 15 Coroner's post mortem reports are available. None makes any reference to brain retention.

There is nothing in any of the documents now available from the Cheshire Coroner's records, or from other sources, to suggest that the late Coroner, Mr Hibbert, was aware of, or agreed to, brain retention for research. There was undoubtedly confusion in the Coroner's office in 1987-88 over the referral of brains to the joint programme.

Summary

Mr North states that he was unaware that brain retention without the consent of relatives was taking place from Coroner's cases in his jurisdiction. He also assured me that he was unaware of his office's involvement in the arrangement.

Mr North's office staff and two Coroner's Officers all take the view that Mr North knew that brains were being retained.

In Central Manchester, all the evidence supports Mr Gorodkin's firmly held policy that no organs should be retained for research without the knowledge and consent of the relatives.

At Warrington, the Coroner's Officer made enquiries when he first encountered a request for brain retention. There is nothing to suggest that Mr Hibbert was himself aware that brains had been retained without consent.

The most likely explanation is confusion within the Cheshire Coroner's office where staff did not appreciate that consent had not been given by the relatives.

Changes in the procedures for Coroners' post mortems since the late 1980s are discussed in Chapter 47.

CHAPTER 23

Consent from relatives for brain retention

Introduction

This chapter first summarises the consent procedures that were planned at the start of the joint programme, and second, compares the plan with the consents that were obtained from relatives. The chapter follows from the descriptions in previous chapters, and draws on the recollections of morticians and other staff involved at the time.

The joint research team's approach to consent

The research applications submitted to the NWRHA and the Medical Research Council, Chapters 9 and 11, state that the consent of the relatives would be obtained for brain retention.

Obtaining the consent of the relatives is clearly stated in the applications to Ethics Committees, Chapters 12 to 16. For example, the protocol dated 17 July 1986: *"After a patient has died the Psychiatrists who have been looking after the patient will seek permission from the nearest relative to remove the brain tissue at post-mortem. This is already in operation at Prestwich Hospital and has been approved by the ethical committee. A standard post mortem consent form will be used".* Annex 33

Pre-mortem consent from relatives of patients in hospital

Early in the programme, Dr Deakin had discussed with consultants at Prestwich Hospital the possibility of obtaining consent from the relatives in advance of the patient's death. Annexes 45 and 46

Experience showed, however, that while pre-mortem consent may be realistic in patients with Alzheimer's disease, it was then an unsatisfactory procedure in those with schizophrenia. The patient's prognosis and life span in Alzheimer's disease is more predictable towards the end of life, whereas a patient with schizophrenia may live for many years. A premature request to the relatives about brain retention could all too easily give offence. For this reason, the idea of obtaining pre-mortem consent in schizophrenia was not pursued.

Consent to post mortem after the death of a hospital in-patient

Dr Deakin's letters and information provided to Ethics Committees written between 1986 and 1990 emphasise the importance of approaching the relatives for their agreement to brain retention: *"We should like to obtain post-mortem brains from patients in Prestwich Hospital. To lessen the distress caused by making this request of the next of kin at the time of death, we should like to discuss this with relatives before the patient's death".* Annex 31

Other contemporary letters further illustrate this approach. In a letter to the Chairman of the North Manchester Ethics Committee on 27 June 1986, Dr Deakin wrote: "*I think the only ethical difficulty is asking patients relatives routinely for permission to remove post-mortem brain material. This obviously needs to be handled tactfully and the request would be made by the doctor involved in the care of the patient who in most cases will already know the relatives. It is of course entirely at the descretion* (sic) *of the medical firm whether an approach to the relatives is made and should they feel it inappropriate such a request would not be made*". Annex 39

"*Would it be possible for you to draw the approval of this research to the attention of particularly the medical staff so that when an in patient dies a request for a post mortem examination is made of the relatives. It is of course entirely at the discresion* (sic) *of the medical firm whether they approach the relatives and no doubt some times they would feel it appropriate to make such a request*". Annex 43

"*This, at first sight, seems a difficult request to make. However, I have found that relatives are generally pleased to hear of the research effort and are only too willing to cooperate*". Annex 45

Patients with no known relatives

In the context of hospital patients who had no relatives, Dr Deakin wrote to Dr Braude on 13 February 1990, Chapter 14: "*Often chronic inpatients don't have next of kin, in which case there is no difficulty.*

There should be local consent forms, perhaps your secretary could get in touch with the pathology department or the administrator at the Victoria Road Hospital". Annex 54

There is no mention of seeking the agreement of the person designated by the hospital's manager required by HC(77)28, Chapter 5.

Coroners' cases

The arrangements described above were planned with hospital cases in mind. In the event, as Chapter 16 shows, the joint programme received many more brains from Coroners' cases than from consented hospital post mortems.

On 11 June 2001 Professor Deakin wrote retrospectively on the reasons why consent was not asked from the relatives of Coroners' cases: "*The purpose of not informing the relatives was to avoid causing distress. At the time, what went on in post mortem rooms was not felt to be a matter that public sensibilities could tolerate. The consequence – to keep things within the profession – is of course completely unacceptable by modern standards of openness and of public and religious involvement*". Annex 75

On the collection of brains of Coroners' cases as controls, Professor Deakin wrote to me on 6 March 2002: "*I have written and explained to you previously about control brains. We did not think that Ethics Committee permission was required since Coroners and Pathologists were more than willing to supply tissues of all kinds from Coroners' post mortems...We did not think that the Coroner system would yield significant numbers of brains in people with Schizophrenia and that hospital post mortems would be necessary. It seemed to me therefore essential to have Ethics* Annex 80

Committee permission to make such a difficult and possibly stressful request of a bereaved relative".

<u>Coroners' cases – lack of consent by relatives for sudden deaths in the community</u>

When a case of sudden death occurs in the community there is an important procedural objection to any approach to the relatives about organ retention between death and the post mortem. In this interval any such approach would require the Coroner's agreement. Until the post mortem examination has established the cause of death, Coroners will not sanction any such request to the relatives (except for organ donation for transplantation when the deceased had carried an organ donor card). Mr North's letter to Professor Yates in July 1985 illustrates the point. Annex 78

During the course of this investigation, a number of Coroners were asked if they would have allowed a research team to speak to the relatives about brain retention before the post mortem. All replied that they would not have agreed.

It is clear that in cases of sudden death in the community, none of the relatives was asked to consent to brain retention or whether they had any objections to retention. This applied irrespective of the mortuary to which the body had been taken.

<u>Coroners' cases – deaths in hospital</u>

For the samc reasons, Coroners would also have refused any approach to relatives about brain retention of patients whose deaths had been referred to them from Prestwich, North Manchester General or any other hospital.

Some of these in-patients with psychiatric disorders were in long-stay wards. These patients could have been assessed for the joint programme in the way set out in the research protocols, and consent forms signed by the relatives. While this may have happened for some patients with Alzheimer's disease, for the reasons already given it is much less likely that a consent form would have been requested or completed for patients with schizophrenia. If a consent form had been signed, it would have been placed in the patient's notes. None of the hospital case records of patients with schizophrenia was available for me to check.

<u>Hospital deaths not reported to the Coroner</u>

Any consent forms for post mortem and/or brain removal should have been placed with the patient's hospital notes. Very few sets of hospital case records survive. The following paragraphs summarise what was found in these notes.

<u>Prestwich Hospital</u>

There were seven deaths in this category, of which six were patients of the Cerebral Function Unit. One set of notes is available and this contains a consent form for brain removal properly signed and dated by the relatives[1].

North Manchester General Hospital

There were 32 hospital deaths. Two sets of records are available[2]. In one a consent form was found. This is the standard "post mortem declaration form" with the following wording:

"*I understand that this examination is carried out:*

a) to verify the cause of death and to study the effects of treatment which may involve the retention of tissue for laboratory study;
b) to remove amounts of tissue for the treatment of other patients and for medical education and research".

However, in the set of notes found, item *"b"* as above had not been signed by the relative but this exclusion had not been respected. The brain had still been retained for research.

Warrington General Hospital

There is little information available about the eight brains of hospital cases which include two brain-only removals. Most were, or had been, in-patients in Winwick Hospital. As these were hospital post mortems, it is likely that the standard hospital post mortem consent form was used.

Bury and Rochdale mortuaries

There is no information available on the four hospital post mortems from these mortuaries.

Brain removal from patients in the Cerebral Function Unit research programme

Chapter 8 records that all patients in the Cerebral Function Unit's programme were seen and assessed in life.

One practical feature of the CFU programme not discussed in Chapter 8 serves to confirm that the consent of the relatives was obtained before the brain was removed.

Mr Walkden explained that at Prestwich many of the brains for the CFU's programme were from "brain only" removals. These did not involve the attendance of a pathologist. In "brain only" cases the mortician removed the brain as soon as practicable after death, and in some cases in the middle of the night.

As brain removal was unsupervised, Mr Walkden would always check the consent form himself before he started the procedure. Professor Mann independently confirmed this. If the form was missing the brain removal would have to wait until the signed consent form arrived.

Similar checks were made by morticians at other hospitals from which Professor Mann had collected brains.

Summary

From contemporaneous documents it is clear that the joint research team recognised that consent by the relatives was necessary for hospital cases.

For Coroners' cases, it appears the team believed the Coroner could authorise brain retention, but at NMGH which provided the largest number of brains the Coroner was not asked, and his agreement appears to have been assumed by the pathologists who allowed the mortician to remove the brain.

As it turned out, the large majority of the brains obtained for the programme were from Coroners' cases and not from hospital post mortems.

No attempt was made to approach the relatives for consent in Coroners' cases.

Few hospital case records are now available, so it is no longer possible to check how frequently consent forms had been completed by the relatives

In one hospital case where the brain was retained at NMGH, the consent form shows that the relatives had not authorised removal of tissue for teaching or research.

In "brain only" examination, before brains were removed for the CFU programme the morticians who undertook the removal were careful to check the consent form, as they were undertaking the procedure without the supervision of a pathologist.

The comment that "*often chronic inpatients do not have a next of kin, in which case there is no difficulty*" disregards the responsibility placed on the Chief Executive or Hospital Secretary by HC(77)28.

Professor Deakin's retrospective observations that "*we did not think the Coroners system would yield significant numbers of brains with schizophrenia and that hospital post mortems would be necessary*" do not match the facts as recorded in the brain books. These show that most brains from cases of schizophrenia were obtained from Coroners' post mortems.

References

1 Case record at Prestwich Hospital.
2 Case records at NMG Hospital.

CHAPTER 24

Other features of the joint programme

Introduction

The preceding chapters have described the main features of the joint programme. This chapter covers two aspects of the programme that have not been described.

Reports to Ethics Committees and LRECs

A general principle of the operation of all Ethics Committees is that researchers whose protocols have been approved should submit progress reports to the Committees, and should inform the Committees of any major changes to the methodology of the approved project. Salford EC had this requirement in place throughout the 1980s and minuted progress reports and amendments received routinely.

The minutes and other papers of the Salford EC have been reviewed for the years from 1986 when the proposal by Dr Soni and Dr Deakin was approved. There is no further mention of this project to be found anywhere in the Salford EC's papers. This was notwithstanding the frequent reference to "*approval by Salford EC*" in submissions that were made to other ECs.

The records of the other ECs that approved protocols from the joint programme were not available for me to review to see if progress reports had been submitted.

Dr Slater should have been reminded in 1991 of the obligation on researchers to submit progress reports to Ethics Committees when the Central Manchester REC approved the application he and Dr D'Souza had submitted, Chapter 14. The records provided by the joint programme do not contain any references to progress reports having been submitted to Ethics Committees. Annex 67

Implications of HSC(IS)153 and the 1991 "Red book"

This circular was described in Chapter 6. It made clear that all research "*on the recently dead in NHS hospitals*" should be referred for consideration. The circular does not appear to have prompted any action by the joint team to inform LRECs that Coroners' post mortems in NHS hospitals were the main source of the brains that they were collecting.

Fees to morticians

Morticians in NHS hospitals were accustomed in the mid 1980s to receiving "*item of service*" fees.

Fees for Coroners' post mortems

Post mortem examinations undertaken for the Coroner were not regarded as part of a pathologist's NHS duties. The Coroner paid a fee to the pathologist for each post mortem undertaken. The Royal College of Pathologists at a meeting in

November 2001 commented that it was customary for the pathologist to pay the mortician ten per cent of the fee he received from the Coroner[1]. The post mortem fees received by the pathologist for an examination *"with specialist knowledge"* were significantly higher than the standard fee, which was set by the Home Office. The mortician could expect to receive ten per cent of the higher fee.

Payments by undertakers

In some locations, morticians also received payments from undertakers for various services. These arrangements were agreed locally.

Payments for pituitaries

Chapter 5 describes the national pituitary gland collection arrangements. Morticians in hospital and public mortuaries had become accustomed to receiving a case-by-case fee for each pituitary collected within the scheme. Morticians were aware that the scheme had the active support of the then Ministry of Health and its successor departments.

Payments for brains for medical education

Chapter 4 referred to the collection of brains from the mortuary for the Anatomy Department at the University for teaching purposes. The practice of obtaining brains from mortuaries for undergraduate teaching was at that time widespread and is described in Chapter 36.

Anatomy departments paid morticians a small sum for each brain supplied for teaching purposes. At NMGH Mr Leatherbarrow had received such payments from the University Anatomy Department until October 1985.

Payments for brains for the joint programme

When the joint programme began, morticians who provided brains were offered a fee. No record was found of the initial fee, but the letter sent to Mr Leatherbarrow at NMGH on 17 October 1986 stated: *"We can arrange payment of £10 per brain before tax, which is deducted at source".* Annex 44

A similar fee was offered to morticians in other mortuaries contributing brains to the programme. Mr Walkden, the mortician at Prestwich and later at Bury mortuary, and Mr Owen, the mortician at Rochdale mortuary, both received these fees.

By 1986 the pituitary collection programme had ceased. For comparative purposes, in 1980 the fee payable for NHS morticians for pituitary collection was consolidated into the pay scale agreed through the Whitley Council. Before this consolidation, the fee for each pituitary had been 20 pence.

Against this background, the offer of a fee to morticians for removal of each brain was not in itself remarkable, although some research teams, including the Cerebral Function Unit, did not pay any fees to the morticians. The £10 offered by the joint programme appears generous by comparison and has been interpreted as an inducement to encouraging morticians to provide as many brains as possible.

It is not clear why the letter to the mortician at NMGH was not copied to the hospital management or to any of the consultant pathologists.

Professor Deakin refutes that a fee of £10 for removal of each brain was unusual or that this level of fee would constitute a financial inducement. It should be noted, however, that the Cerebral Function Unit research programme did not offer any fee for brain removal although this, in some case, involved the morticians in extra work undertaken during unsocial hours.

Number of brains obtained from NMGH in 1994

Mr Leatherbarrow has retained all his pay advice slips from the University in respect of the brains he collected under the arrangements discussed in Chapter 13. From 1986 Mr Leatherbarrow only ever received payments from the University for brains that he had retained for the joint programme. From his payslips it can be calculated that he was paid for providing over 40 brains in 1994.

However, the brain books of the joint programme record that in 1994 only three brains were obtained from NMGH mortuary.

For earlier years the sums paid to Mr Leatherbarrow relate directly to the number of brains listed in the brain books. This highlights the discordance between payments made and the number of brains recorded in the brain books in 1994.

In this context three other points are relevant:

- when the collection of brains from NMGH ended, Mr Leatherbarrow was told that the reason was unspecified problems about the collection arrangements for brains of Coroner's cases;
- Professor McClure's advice to Professor Deakin in 1995;
- Professor Deakin's conversation with Mr Gorodkin in June 1995, Chapter 22.

Mr Leatherbarrow commented that, when the brain collection ended, he had noticed the difference it had made to his income.

The discordance between the number of brains recorded in the brain books and the number for which Mr Leatherbarrow received payment has not been explained.

Summary

There are no records that LRECs received progress reports.

The 1991 circular did not prompt any action by the team to inform LRECs of the main source of the brains they were collecting.

The payment of fees to morticians was common practice in the 1980s. A precedent had been set with the payment of fees for the collection of pituitaries within the national collection scheme.

Morticians were accustomed to receiving from pathologists a proportion of the fees paid by Coroners for each post mortem.

Fees for brains provided had been paid for many years to morticians by anatomy departments of Universities who obtained brains for teaching medical students.

The offer of a payment for each brain provided did not appear unusual, but no fee was paid for brains collected for the Cerebral Function Unit.

The fee of £10 in the late 1980s could be regarded as generous. At least one mortician considered the level provided an inducement as the extra work involved was minimal.

It is not clear why the letter to the mortician at NMGH was not copied to the hospital management or to one of the consultant pathologists.

Payments for brains were referred to in some of the grant applications made by the research team, Chapter 9.

The discordance between the sums paid for brains collected and the number of brains listed in the brain books in 1994 has not been explained.

References

1 Information provided by the Royal College of Pathologists.

CHAPTER 25

Why were brains from Coroners' post mortems retained? Unanswered questions about the joint programme

Introduction

This chapter summarises the findings from the preceding chapters and sets out a list of unanswered questions.

Sources of information

These are set out in the preceding chapters.

The central issue

The central problem in this report is the collection and retention of brains from Coroners' cases **without the knowledge and consent of the relatives.**

Why did this happen on such a large scale and continue for so long?

The short answer, in my view, is prolonged and consistent disregard of the Human Tissue Act.

The belief became established that the practice of brain retention had the approval of the Coroner, in circumstances where the Coroner had no authority to authorise retention of brains for research. The research in the joint programme had no bearing on the cause of death.

If brains were to be retained for research from Coroners' cases, the Human Tissue Act required the consent of the relatives.

The perceived authority of the Coroner to retained organs and tissues

The Coroner's powers to retain "material" that has a bearing on the cause of death is clear and unambiguous, but the Coroner's power to retain brains is limited only to those circumstances where examination of the brain has a bearing on the cause of death.

This was not the case when brains were retained for the joint programme. There was, however, a widespread and erroneous belief that the Coroner could authorise the retention of organs and tissues that had no bearing on the cause of death.

In the case of the NMGH mortuary, the Coroner was quite unaware of any brain retention.

This misunderstanding of the legal position was shared among pathologists, Coroner's Officers, morticians and researchers.

As a result, the joint programme collected brains from mortuaries in and near Manchester without the knowledge and consent of the relatives.

These misunderstandings meant the joint programme accumulated substantial numbers of brains from Coroners' cases for research, although the emphasis in the applications to research funding organisations had been on the collection of brains with consent.

Dr Deakin and Dr Slater were aware that pathologists in other locations were prepared to retain brains and other organs for research without reference to the Coroner. In the Central Manchester District Dr Deakin wrote directly to the NMGH mortician in terms that encouraged the collection of suitable brains. The letter did not distinguish between brains from hospital post mortems or those where the examination had been undertaken on the instructions of the Coroner.

Rules 9 and 12

These Rules are discussed in Chapter 31, and are mentioned here only to record that they are not once referred to in any of the papers about the joint programme. There is nothing to suggest these Rules were ever considered.

Central Manchester: collection without the Coroner's knowledge

The largest number of brains from Coroners' cases were collected from the mortuary at NMGH. The Coroner, Mr Gorodkin, and his staff were unaware that brains were being collected, Chapter 22. If Mr Gorodkin had been asked, he would have refused unless consent was first obtained from the relatives. The Coroner's authority cannot be used to explain or excuse the collection of brains from the NMGH mortuary.

North Manchester: collection of brains identified through the Coroner's office

In the North Manchester coronial district, the misunderstanding of the Coroner's authority was further influenced by the help of the Coroner's office staff who believed they had the Coroner's approval for their actions, Chapter 10. This district provided the second largest number of brains from the four mortuaries.

Warrington: misunderstandings in the Coroner's office

Only a small number of brains from Coroner's cases were collected from Warrington General Hospital. The Coroner's staff appear to have misunderstood the status of the brains collected.

How brains reached the joint programme

Prestwich, Bury, Rochdale and Oldham mortuaries

The pathologists, Coroner's Officers and mortuary staff in the four mortuaries from where brains were collected wrongly believed that the Coroner had authority to consent to brain retention and that they were following the Coroner's instructions, Chapter 10.

NMGH mortuary

The pathologists were under the impression that the brains of inpatients were collected with consent and were being collected for the Cerebral Function Unit. For Coroner's cases, the pathologists thought the Coroner had been asked and that the Coroner could agree without asking the relatives if they had objections, Chapter 13.

The Ethics Committee's approval further lulled the initial concerns that the pathologists and the mortician expressed. However, the EC had not been told about the collection of brains from Coroner's cases. The protocol reference to "controls" had not mentioned that the large majority of the brains were from Coroners' cases.

The mortician was encouraged to provide brains and was told that the research had been approved by the Ethics Committee. A fee of £10 was offered for each brain. This encouraged the collection of more brains.

Warrington General Hospital mortuary

The Coroner's Officer challenged the validity of the first case. He was mistakenly reassured.

Ethics Committees

In the applications to ECs, the protocols referred to the collection of brains with the consent of the relatives. Collection of "control" brains was mentioned in some applications, but the fact Coroners' cases were the main source of "controls" was never mentioned, Chapter 18.

As a result the Committees' approval was based on incomplete information.

The Ethics Committees approached after the programme had been in progress for two to three years were told that other Ethics Committees had already approved the programme.

The Ethics Committees never received progress reports on the research or information about where the brains had been obtained.

Research applications

The NWRHA and the MRC were in a similar position when applications were submitted to them in 1988 and 1989. The applications emphasised the consent of the relatives and referred to the collection of "control" brains but did not mention Coroners' cases as the main source of "index" and "control" brains, Chapters 9 and 11.

General practitioners

When general practitioners were asked to provide details of the deceased's medical records and medication, they were assured in writing that the studies had Ethics

Committee approval. This was not so for Coroners' cases. Ethics Committees were not told that Coroners' cases were involved, Chapter 18.

The letters to general practitioners were also misleading in referring to brain samples when the programme had received the whole brain in almost all cases.

Knowledge of brain retention

Organ retention in the mid 1980s was not the subject of discussion among pathologists. The public were unaware of what happened in mortuaries. The joint team kept the fact of brain retention from relatives of "control" cases. Professor Deakin states that this was to avoid distress. The misconceptions about the Coroner's authority meant that brains were collected without asking the relatives if they had objections, despite the fact that the applications to ECs had emphasised that consent would be obtained from the relatives of index cases.

It is difficult to reconcile these two positions. If relatives of "index" cases are to be asked for consent, why should the relatives of control cases not be given the same right?

Issues for which no explanation has been offered

Introduction

While there was in the late 1980s widespread misunderstanding of the Coroner's powers to authorise retention of organs and tissues for research, this in itself does not explain the following features and actions of the joint team.

Questions that deserve an explanation

Why, when protocols were submitted to ECs, did the references to collection of control cases not make it clear that these would mainly be obtained from Coroners' cases? The reliance on brains from Coroners' cases may not have been planned but it was, or should have been, clear to the team when the protocol dated 17 July 1986 was signed.

Why did protocols to the ECs draw attention to the importance of consent for retention of the brains of index cases, but obscure the fact that consent would not be obtained from the relatives of controls that were Coroners' cases? Did the research team consider this was not relevant to the ECs' consideration?

Why did the research team not consider Ethical Committee approval was necessary for Coroners' cases?

"Avoidance of distress" was the team's stated reason for not contacting the relatives of control cases. Why was this not revealed to the ECs?

Why were the research applications submitted to the NWRHA and the MRC in 1988 silent on the collection of control brains from Coroners' cases?

Why, when writing to general practitioners for medical details of deceased patients whose deaths were reported to the Coroner, did the joint team claim "*The studies have Ethical Committee approval*" when the ECs had no knowledge that these enquiries would be made about Coroners' cases?

Why did the same letter to general practitioners also refer to *"brain samples",* when the research team had collected the whole of the brain in the large majority of cases?

Why was the mortician at NMGH encouraged to collect the brains of normal cases when the team knew, or should have known, that most of these would be collected from Coroners' cases?

Why was the letter to the mortician at NMGH not copied to his employers or to the pathologists at the hospital?

Why was the £10 payment per brain offered to morticians in the 1980s set at this level, when other teams did not offer a fee?

Why, in 1994, when payment was made for 40 brains from the NMGH mortuary are only three brains recorded in the brain books?

Why were the Coroners not asked directly about the retention of brains from cases for which they had ordered the post mortem examination?

Why were doctors at another hospital encouraged to disregard the consent requirements for those patients who had no known relatives by the reference to "*Often chronic in-patients don't have next of kin, in which case there is no problem*"? This disregards the responsibility placed on every hospital authority to consider if a deceased person had expressed an objection.

In response to these questions, Professor Deakin and Dr Slater, during separate discussions, have claimed that they were ignorant of the legal position.

SECTION 4

Research at other locations on brains from Coroners' cases

CHAPTER 26

The Cambridge brain bank

Introduction

The third of my Terms of Reference required an examination of other centres that appeared to have collections of brains obtained from Coroners' cases.

The brain bank and research programme at Cambridge was identified as one of the centres that should be included in this investigation for the following reasons:

- brains had been transferred from mortuaries in the Manchester area to Cambridge, beginning in 1972;

- the research team at Manchester identified the Clinical Research Centre, Northwick Park, and the Cambridge systems for collecting brains as models to follow when planning the joint programme;

- the brain bank at Cambridge was one of the banks supported specifically as a *"brain tissue bank"* by the Medical Research Council (MRC) in 1985, Chapter 37;

- staff from the bank had taken part in various MRC meetings on brain banking, starting in 1974;

- the Cambridge brain bank has been widely described as the *"first brain tissue bank in this country"* and said to be one of only four worldwide at the time it was set up;

- at an early stage of the investigation, Dr Sandra Webb reported that the Cambridge brain bank had obtained the brain of her late husband, Mr David Webb, following a Coroner's post mortem at Cambridge on 26 January 1988, in circumstances similar to the retention of Mr Isaacs' brain.

Nomenclature

Since the mid 1970s the brain bank at Cambridge has been referred to by a number of different titles and has moved locations several times. Whatever the location or name at a given time, brain collection has continued as a recognisable entity. For consistency in this chapter the collection is referred to as the "Cambridge brain bank".

Sources of information

Addenbrooke's Hospital

To investigate the procedures of the Cambridge brain bank, meetings were held with present and past staff of Cambridge University and Addenbrooke's Hospital, pathologists, morticians, brain bank staff and others who had been involved in, or provided brains for, the bank from the early 1970s. The meetings began on 4 February 2002 with:

- Mr Keith Day, Administrative Director, Addenbrooke's NHS Trust;
- Professor Peter Collins, Director of Pathology;
- Mr Colin Carr, Pathology Manager.

Mr Day is in charge of the arrangements for the return of retained organs and tissues from Addenbrooke's Hospital to relatives.

Professor Collins, as Head of Pathology, has overall responsibility for the brain bank.

Mr Carr has day-to-day operational responsibility for the Pathology Department.

At this meeting full co-operation in the investigation was offered. Subsequently, Mr Carr arranged other meetings with staff of the brain bank and mortuary.

Access to staff and records

The records of the brain bank were made freely available and its filing system explained. The Mortuary Registers and reports of all post mortems at Addenbrooke's Hospital since the 1970s were made available.

At my request, lists of brains transferred to the brain bank from the Manchester area were prepared from the hospital's computerised pathology record system. This database had been set up to identify all retained organs and other specimens received from post mortems at Addenbrooke's and those referred from other hospitals. This system enabled Addenbrooke's to identify the hospital from which each organ had been referred. All referring hospitals were notified, in case the relatives should ask for the organ or tissue to be returned to them.

Further meetings about the Cambridge brain bank are listed at the end of this chapter.

Coroners for the Cambridge district

Meetings were held with Mr David Morris on 27 March 2002, and Mr John Smith, his predecessor as Coroner, on 16 April 2002.

Mr Morris has been Coroner for South and West Cambridgeshire since 1999 when the boundaries of the coronial districts were changed. From 1987 to 1999, Mr Morris had been Coroner for Huntingdon. He is also Coroner for the separate district of Bedfordshire and Luton.

Mr Smith was appointed Coroner for South and East Cambridgeshire (known together as "South Cambridgeshire" District) in 1987. At that time Cambridge City was a separate district. When Mr Sterndale Burrows, the Coroner for Cambridge City, died in post in 1990 the districts of Cambridge City and South West Cambridgeshire were combined. Mr Smith was Coroner for Cambridge City and for his first district of South Cambridgeshire until 1998. The boundaries of the districts were altered when Mr Morris was appointed.

The changes in the coronial boundaries in 1990 are significant, as Chapter 27 will show.

Source documents

The brain bank records – these start in the early 1970s and include individual records on all brains that have been retained by the brain bank; the Mortuary Registers at Addenbrooke's Hospital; and post mortem reports to Coroners.

History of the Cambridge brain bank

The brain collection at Cambridge was in 1980 the only brain tissue bank in this country[1]. At that time there were three other brain banks worldwide, two in the USA and one in Sweden. The Cambridge bank was one of the first deliberately to collect brains from other hospitals for research. Other brain collections, such as the Corsellis collection, had begun as accumulations of brains retained after diagnostic examination had been completed, Chapter 33. The value of such collections for research was later recognised.

The MRC Neurochemical Pharmacology Unit

In the 1970s the MRC provided direct funding support for the Neurochemical Pharmacology Unit (NCPU) which, as its name implies, was established to undertake research into the chemistry of the brain. The Head of the Unit was Dr, now Professor, Leslie Iverson.

Research publications by staff of the Unit show that some brains were collected specifically for research from 1970. However, the start of the Cambridge bank is given as 1974 when it was recognised by MRC within the Neurochemical Pharmacology Unit.

Operational heads of the brain bank

1974-1978 Dr E D Bird

Dr Ted Bird, a medically qualified American citizen, was a member of the Scientific Staff of the unit. In the early 1970s, Dr Bird became interested to discover if neuro-chemical factors in the brain had any significance in Huntington's disease. When the possibility of a research study on Huntington's disease was first mooted, there were doubts about the feasibility of finding enough patients for a meaningful investigation of this progressive and incurable condition.

Dr Bird was undeterred and, having explained his objectives to psychiatrists and pathologists, began to collect the brains of patients who died from this condition. Dr Bird was careful to explain his work to relatives and his research attracted the enthusiastic support of many relatives and of COMBAT, the voluntary organisation for relatives of those with Huntington's disease. Some relatives became very active in identifying for Dr Bird patients with the early symptoms of Huntington's disease. As a result Dr Bird received referrals from many parts of the country.

Dr Bird and Dr Iverson published the results of their research on Huntington's disease in 1974[2].

1978-1985

After Dr Bird left Cambridge in 1978, and in the period before the MRC awarded a programme grant for its "banking" activities in 1985, the Cambridge brain bank was headed first by Dr E Stokes in 1978, followed by Dr Martin Rosser between 1979 and 1983, followed by Dr Gavin Reynolds. During this period the bank remained within the Neurochemical Pharmacology Unit until the closure of the unit in 1985.

In the early 1980s, in addition to collecting brains of cases of Huntington's disease and control cases, the bank diversified to obtain brains of patients with a range of neuropsychiatric conditions. This was before an application for support of the "banking service" was made to the MRC.

The programme grant application to the MRC of 1985

This application was submitted by Professor Gresham, Sir Martin Roth and Dr Ian Wilkinson. The purpose of the application was to formalise the arrangements in the brain bank which had evolved to provide: Appendix 2

- a service role for tissue collection, dissection, cataloguing and storage;
- a neurochemical assay service;
- a diagnostic service;
- a major research role in the investigation of Alzheimer's, Parkinson's and Huntington's diseases.

Other topic-related proposals were submitted to the MRC at the same time. These were separate from, but dependent on, the brain banking proposals in the main programme application. Appendix 2

The brain collection procedure as described in the application to the MRC

This application refers to the bank providing a major service for tissue collection, dissection and storage. The procedures used had been: *"worked out over the last 13 years, and vary with the particular needs of the studies for which they are collected"*.

"Once a patient has died, the body should be moved to refrigerated storage, ideally within 4 hours of death. When all appropriate consent has been obtained, the post mortem dissection is performed, usually within 72 hours of death".

There is nothing in the application submitted to the MRC that implies that brains were being obtained without appropriate consent. In the context of brains from patients with psychiatric disorders the protocol records: "*Freedom to seek the help of mortuary technicians at any time and their willing co-operation in the enterprise has been a major asset ... a generous and co-operative network of support at Fulbourn Hospital* (the local mental hospital) *and Addenbrooke's Hospital has also been an important asset*".

The application included a request for funds to upgrade the mortuary at Fulbourn Hospital so that bodies did not have to be transferred to Addenbrooke's Hospital in Cambridge for brain removal.

The MRC awarded the programme grant and the research applications linked to it.

In 1985 Professor Paykel, who had recently been appointed as Professor of Psychiatry at Cambridge University, became head of the bank. While Professor Paykel was concerned with the overall direction and management of the bank as titular head, the day-to-day control was the responsibility of Dr C M Wischik, who had succeeded Dr Reynolds.

This programme grant gave the bank a firmer financial base and enabled the banking service to continue. For the next three years the bank maintained the procedures that had been used to collect brains from a widening range of diseases as well as control brains.

Application to the MRC in 1987 to change the bank's objectives

A new and different application was submitted to the MRC by Professor Paykel and Dr Wischik. This application was to change the objectives of the bank from collecting brains of many diseases to the collection of brains for particular research studies, principally on Alzheimer's disease. Thereafter the bank would have a reduced capacity to provide brain tissues for research to other investigators. It was envisaged that each research team should collect its own material.

1988

A significant redirection of the energies of the bank followed in 1988. Researchers at Cambridge and the brain bank became involved in a multi-centre epidemiological study of progressive dementias, the CFAS study(3). This is a long-term study that is still in progress. For CFAS and other studies of patients, a research nurse, Mrs Angela O'Sullivan, was appointed to work on the programme.

One of Mrs O'Sullivan's main responsibilities is to work with, support and counsel patients enrolled in the study and their families. The study has many methodological similarities to the research of the Cerebral Function Unit in Manchester, Chapter 8.

One of the objectives is to relate the progress of the patient's illness with post mortem findings. In this respect, Mrs O'Sullivan's responsibilities include discussing the possibility of examination of the brain with the family when the patient is approaching the end of life. A set of consent forms and leaflets have been in use for this purpose since 1988 which Mrs O'Sullivan uses for discussion with relatives.

With the start of the CFAS study, the balance of the bank's work moved from the provision of brain tissue to supporting this and other large-scale prospective studies.

The end of the MRC's support

In September 1998 the MRC ended its support for the "brain banking" functions of the bank but has maintained funding of the long-term prospective investigations of dementia and other similar studies.

How the Cambridge brain bank system worked

Source of brains

For the Huntington's disease study from which the brain bank evolved, brains from patients with Huntington's disease and control brains were required. In 1974 Dr Bird and Dr Iverson published details of how the brains were obtained[(2)]: "*Several consultant psychiatrists and pathologists throughout the United Kingdom provided invaluable assistance by seeking permission for post-mortem examinations of the brains of patients with Huntington's chorea and in the initial handling of the brain material".*

"Controls consisted of coroners' cases and hospital cases of various ages, on which necropsies had been performed in the University Pathology Department at Addenbrooke's Hospital, Cambridge".

The reference to collection of control brains from Addenbrooke's mortuary should be noted as throughout the 1970s and 1980s the bank continued the practice of obtaining control brains from post mortems on Coroner's cases at Addenbrooke's Hospital[(1)].

Post mortem procedures at Addenbrooke's mortuary

There was no difference in the procedure between hospital and Coroner's post mortems at Addenbrooke's mortuary. All were carried out as full post mortems and the brain was routinely removed. The procedures are described in a text book on mortuary practice published by Professor Gresham, who was in charge of the mortuary until 1990, and the Head Mortician, the late Mr Arthur Turner, entitled "*Post Mortem Procedures".*

The post mortem reports mostly did not record that a brain had been retained for the bank. Other organs retained for research or teaching were generally not mentioned, but some reports to the Coroner did record the retention of specimens that had a bearing on the cause of death.

How were suitable brains identified?

Mr Hills, the Chief Technician in the brain bank, states that after he was appointed in August 1980 he visited the mortuary each morning, on behalf of the head of the bank, to see what post mortems were scheduled. If a post mortem was from a case that would be of interest to the brain bank, he reported to the person in day-to-day charge of the brain bank who reviewed the case. If it was of interest to the bank, a request for retention would be made to the pathologist to ask that the brain be set aside at the end of the examination for the brain bank's use. Mr Hills states that this practice continued throughout the 1980s.

Mr Hills' account differs from that of the Chief Mortuary Technician, Mr Stevenson, whose recollection is that the request came directly from Mr Hills. Professor Gresham, Dr Wight and Mr Stevenson all confirm that brains were regularly retained from Coroner's cases, Chapter 27.

Brains collected

The brains collected by the Cambridge bank fall into two of the categories that were described in Chapter 7. When brains were initially retained for diagnosis a report would be sent to the Coroner or, for hospital post mortems, to the doctor who had looked after the deceased in life. Among these were brains and parts of brains referred from other hospitals for diagnosis.

The second category of brains was collected specifically for research. These include the collections of brains of suicides and the "control" brains. In the case of "controls", the brains were chosen because the deceased had no neuropsychiatric disease.

The brains received by the bank in the 1970s were referred for histology to Professor Corsellis at Runwell Hospital.

In 1985 the collection arrangements were described in the MRC application. The brain bank records show that between 1981 and 1984, a total of 367 brains had been collected of which 145 were "controls", 100 from Huntington's disease, 36 dementia, 25 schizophrenia, 19 Parkinson's disease and the remainder from patients with a variety of other conditions. Appendix 27

Coroners' cases

Two categories of brains were regularly obtained from Coroners' cases in the 1980s.

Brains of suicide victims

By definition, a death from suicide or suspected suicide must be reported to the Coroner. Among brains collected by the bank from Coroners' post mortems were those of victims of suicide. This collection started in February 1983 and continued over the next seven years. Forty-three brains were collected, including the brain of Mr David Webb, Chapter 27.

(The suicide brains were stored and, apart from a few samples from early cases which were sent to other researchers as part of the brain bank's "banking function", no research or examination of any kind was undertaken on them at Cambridge.)

Normal controls

The second category of brains frequently obtained from Coroners' post mortems were normal "controls". The first "control" brain was collected in January 1980. The total number of brains obtained in this collection was 557, not all from Coroners' cases. Collection of "control" brains is continuing but now strictly with the consent of the relatives.

The "control" brains were individually examined. This included histology to make sure each was suitable for use as a control for a particular study. The extent of the examination of a brain depended on the purpose of the study for which it was to be used. For Coroners' cases, no report on the examination was sent to the Coroner.

Mr Hills states that, when the brain of a Coroner's case was requested for the brain bank, the Coroner was asked. However, this cannot be confirmed as Mr John Smith, Coroner for South and West Cambridgeshire, was unaware of the retention of brains for the brain bank until he was appointed Coroner for the City of Cambridge in 1991, and Mr Morris, who was Coroner for Huntingdon, was similarly unaware. The question of whether Mr Sterndale Burrows, Coroner for the City of Cambridge in the late 1980s, was aware is discussed later in this chapter.

The ending of brain collection from Coroners' cases

When Mr Smith became Coroner for the City of Cambridge in 1991, the retention of brains and other organs from Coroners' post mortems, without the knowledge or consent of the relatives, was brought to his notice.

Mr Smith investigated and then gave immediate and firm instructions that no organs were to be retained for research or teaching from bodies for which he was responsible without his knowledge, and then only with the consent of the relatives.

It should be emphasised that no brains, including suicides and "controls", have been collected from Coroners' cases without the consent of the relatives since Mr Smith issued his instructions.

Ethical Committee approval for brain collection

Studies on patients

The 1985 application to the MRC does not make any reference to approval of the bank through an Ethics Committee. The MRC requirement at the time was that all studies on patients must be referred for Ethics Committee approval. In view of the MRC's conditions for grants in place at this time, it is unlikely that any studies that involved patients had not been submitted to, and approved by, an Ethics Committee. Appendix 27

Professor Paykel's clear recollection is that all new research that started after he had transferred to Cambridge received full ethical approval.

Collection of "control" brains

Whether the Ethics Committees were also informed or consulted about the collection of "control" brains by the bank is not clear in the main 1985 application for funding of the banking activities of the bank. The application does not mention EC approval. This aspect was explored with Addenbrooke's Hospital. In a letter dated 1 August 2002, Mr Carr stated: Annex 81

"You are quite correct in assuming that there is full ethical approval for research on consented brains, but this never seems to have been the case with brains collected from Coroner's cases. I am fairly certain that had ethical approval been sought for the brains, then it would not have been given on the basis of a lack of evidence of consent having been sought".

Mr Carr's statement is supported by the recollections of Mr Rick Hills, the Chief Brain Bank Technician.

It should be stressed that since Mr Smith insisted on the need for proper consent, all "control brains" have been collected with the consent of the relatives and using the same research consent procedure that is deployed for collection of index brains in the CFAS and other long-term prospective studies.

Why had brains and other organs been retained from Coroners' cases?

The pathologists at Addenbrooke's believe that before 1991 there was an understanding with the late Mr Sterndale Burrows, and that he did not object to the removal of organs and tissues for teaching and research. Other staff dispute this and have told me that Mr Sterndale Burrows would not have agreed to organ retention without the consent of the relatives. The latter view was expressed by one of the Coroner's Officers who worked for Mr Sterndale Burrows in the late 1980s.

Some of the staff of the mortuary told me that they were uneasy about the number of organs that were being retained, but did not bring their concerns to the Coroner's notice. There are no contemporaneous written documents that shed light either way. I do not have the information to reach a definitive conclusion. Mr Sterndale Burrows cannot rebut those who say they had his tacit agreement to organ retention.

Cases from other districts

The mortuary at Addenbrooke's also received bodies from other districts. In this context, when Mr John Smith was Coroner for South Cambridgeshire District, the pathologists and mortuary staff had not asked him whether organ retention had his approval. Had they done so, they would have been reminded of the legal position that nothing should be removed from the body when the relatives expressed objections except when this was necessary to discover the cause of death.

Although Mr Smith regularly visited the other mortuaries in his district, he did not visit the Addenbrooke's Hospital mortuary as frequently. This mortuary was in Mr Sterndale Burrows' district as Coroner for the City of Cambridge, and his staff had an office adjacent to the mortuary.

Until Mr Smith became Coroner for the City of Cambridge in 1991 and became aware of what was happening in the Addenbrooke's mortuary, the retention of organs from Coroners' cases continued.

Post mortem reports to the Coroner

The post mortem reports sent to the Coroner listed any tissue samples or other investigations made by the pathologist that could have a bearing on the cause of death. The reports did not mention that brains had been retained for the brain bank.

All the post mortem reports on the 43 suicide victims whose brains had been obtained for the bank were examined. The records of the brain bank confirm that these brains were retained but none of the post mortem reports mentions brain retention. These reports were made to the Coroners for Cambridge City, South Cambridgeshire and Huntingdon Districts(1).

A number of post mortem reports on cases where the brain had been retained as a control were also cross checked against the brain bank records. Again, the post mortem reports were silent about brain retention for the bank.

In this respect these post mortem reports were deficient as they did not alert the Coroners to what was going on. The reasons for this are discussed in Chapter 42.

Brains received from hospitals in the Manchester area

Between April 1973 and November 1975, 28 brains were referred by pathologists from Prestwich and other hospitals in North Manchester to the Cambridge brain bank. Ten of these were the brains of patients who had died of Huntington's disease. The remaining 18 were cases of schizophrenia. Among these were a number of Coroner's cases.

In all these cases, a report was sent back to the pathologist at Prestwich Hospital.

In keeping with the Cambridge brain bank's policy, the pathologists in Manchester who were referring brains to Cambridge were regularly informed of changes to the protocol and encouraged to send further brains. The brain bank was diligent in keeping the referring pathologists informed of the progress of research work. This practice appears to have originated with Dr Bird and followed by his successors in the bank.

Recent analysis of brains collected by the bank

The bank has provided an analysis of the brains that were collected between 1980 and 2001(1). The following table provides details.

Category	Number of Brains Received	Earliest Date	Most Recent Date
Prader-Willi syndrome (B)	3	21.01.1997	24.02.2001
Normal control (C)	557	05.01.1980	08.10.2001
Dementia: long PM delay (D)	172	10.01.1980	02.03.1993
Epilepsy (E)	39	10.05.1983	28.12.1988
Dementia: short PM delay (FD)	272	21.11.1985	23.04.2001
CC75C (L)	206	22.06.1989	29.11.2001
Huntington's disease (H)	707	17.02.1980	10.12.2001
Fronto-temporal dementia (JH)	102	20.01.1992	16.01.2002
Down's syndrome (M)	16	04.03.1981	19.10.1998
Multiple sclerosis (MS)	2	12.03.1995	22.05.1997
Parkinson's disease (P)	62	01.02.1980	02.09.1992
CFAS (RH)	86	14.05.1993	21.12.2001
Schizophrenia (S)	182	04.01.1980	22.09.1994
Spinal cord (SC)	2	Unknown	Unknown
Progressive supranuclear palsy (SR)	1	07.09.1979	-
Depression (X)	66	01.02.1983	23.12.1992
Suicide (Y)	43	18.02.1983	13.03.1989
Tissue held for Oxford CFAS	29	In one batch, sometime mid 90s	

Meetings held to discuss the Cambridge brain bank

4 February 2002	Mr Keith Day, Administrative Director, Addenbrooke's NHS Trust Professor Peter Collins, Director of Pathology Mr Colin Carr, Pathology Manager
13 February	Mr Colin Carr, Pathology Manager Mr Graham Lawrence, Records Manager Mrs Angela O'Sullivan, Research Nurse Mr Rick Hills, Chief Brain Bank Technician Mr Nick Stevenson, Chief Mortician, Addenbrooke's Hospital
1 March	Professor E S Paykel, Emeritus Professor of Psychiatry, Cambridge University Mr Colin Carr, Pathology Manager
27 March	Mr David Morris, Coroner for South and West Cambridgeshire Members of Mr Morris' staff
28 March	Professor A Gresham, Emeritus Professor of Histopathology, Cambridge University
18 April	Mr John Smith, Coroner for South West Cambridgeshire from 1984 to 1998 and for Cambridge City from 1991 to 1998
26 April	Dr Derek Wight, Consultant Histopathologist, Addenbrooke's Hospital

26 April	Mr Colin Carr Mrs Angela O'Sullivan Mr Rick Hills Mr Nick Stevenson	

Summary

The Cambridge brain bank evolved from research undertaken by Dr Bird in the Neurochemical Pharmacology Unit in the early 1970s. The first research was into Huntington's Chorea (now referred to as Huntington's disease).

The Huntington's disease study had the active support of relatives and of COMBAT (the voluntary organisation formed to support families of those with Huntington's disease). Consent was obtained for brain removal in these cases.

Further programmes developed and in 1985 the MRC received a proposal to support the brain bank as a service facility to support research teams undertaking neurochemical and other investigations that required brain tissue.

"Control" brains from "normal" subjects were collected. Consent from the relatives was not sought or obtained.

The Department of Pathology of the University provided diseased brains and "control" brains.

No distinction was made between hospital and Coroners' cases when brains were obtained.

There is no record that the collection of "control" brains was ever considered by an Ethical Committee before 1985.

The 1985 application to the MRC was ambiguous on the question of consent. One section, referring to collection of index cases, underlined the need for consent by the relatives. Elsewhere the requirement for "control" brains is set out with no linkage to consent of the relatives.

During the 1980s the brain bank technician would review the list of post mortems scheduled each day and identify brains that would be of interest to the brain bank.

In 1987 the funding basis of the bank changed. From that date it was to focus on individual projects rather than provide a "banking" facility.

In 1988 the bank became involved in a multi-centre prospective epidemiological study of dementing diseases of the elderly (the CFAS programme). This study received Ethical Committee approval.

For the CFAS programme, full consent for brain retention had been routinely obtained from the relatives.

Collection of brains from Coroners' cases as "controls" and for the suicides study continued in parallel with the large prospective dementia study.

The post mortem reports to the Coroners failed to record when brains were retained for use by the brain bank.

In 1991 Mr Smith, the Coroner for Cambridge City, discovered that brains were being removed from Coroners' cases. He ordered that no brains or other organs from Coroners' cases were to be retained for research without the consent of the relatives. Organ retention was permitted only for diagnostic purposes.

The brain bank continues to collect brains, with consent, from hospital cases.

As earlier chapters have indicated, the Cambridge brain bank was regarded as a model for other brain research routes to follow, and the methods of obtaining "controls" from Coroners' cases appear to have been copied.

References

1. Records of the Cambridge brain bank.
2. Brain 1974; Vol 97, part iii: pp 457–472.
3. CFAS – The MRC Cognitive Function and Ageing Study.

CHAPTER 27

The death of David Webb

Introduction

This chapter sets out what happened after the death of Mr David Webb in January 1988 as there are similar circumstances to events that followed the death of Mr Isaacs in February 1987. There are also parallels between the experience of Mr Webb's widow and those of Mrs Isaacs, Chapter 1.

Mrs Webb's, now Dr Webb's, experience was brought to my attention after the Terms of Reference for this investigation had been decided. (For consistency, in this chapter Mrs Webb is referred to as "Dr Webb" throughout). The third Term of Reference refers specifically to organ retention after deaths outside hospital at other locations. Dr Webb was invited to provide a detailed account of what happened following the death of her husband.

Sources of information

This chapter is based on:

- the written statements prepared for the inquest on Mr Webb;
- the post mortem report to the Coroner, Mr John Smith;
- the Cambridge brain bank records;
- correspondence between Dr Webb and Addenbrooke's NHS Trust;
- correspondence between Dr Webb and the past and present Coroners for the City of Cambridge and South and West Cambridgeshire;
- the recollections of:
  - Dr Webb;
  - Mr John Smith; and
  - Dr Wight, the pathologist who carried out the post mortem examination.

Mr Webb's health

In the last 18 months of his life Mr David Webb had suffered from depression for which he had consulted a psychiatrist and received care and medication. He had been hospitalised following a previous suicide attempt. During those months he had absented himself from his home on a number of occasions, but had later returned of his own volition, except once when he had been brought home by the police in a distressed state.

On the afternoon of 23 January 1988, Mr Webb drove away from home in an emotional state, saying that he was going for a walk and *"with luck, would not be back"*. Annex 82

As he had left in a similar manner on previous occasions, Dr Webb spoke to his general practitioner but she was not unduly concerned until 10.00pm that evening when she telephoned the police to report Mr Webb missing. As Mr Webb had gone missing before, the police noted that he had done so again.

The morning of Sunday 24 January 1988

At approximately 8.30am on Sunday 24 January Mr Webb was found in his car by a farmer who had gone to investigate as the car was well away from the road down a track. The car's engine was still running. A rubber tube led from the car's exhaust into the car. The doors had been locked, but when these were opened, Mr Webb was clearly dead and appeared to have been so for some time. The police were called and quickly attended the scene. Annex 83

A policeman called at the family home at about 10.00am to give Dr Webb the devastating news of her husband's death. The police officer was unaware that Mr Webb's disappearance had been reported by Dr Webb the previous evening.

Dr Webb's distress was made worse by the action of the attending police officer whose line of questioning left Dr Webb with the clear impression that the police considered, at that stage, she was somehow responsible for her husband's death. It was only the intervention of Mr Webb's general practitioner that changed the attitude of the police from suspicion to sympathy.

Mr Webb's body was taken to the mortuary at Addenbrooke's Hospital, Cambridge, and Dr Webb was informed that her husband's death would be reported to the Coroner and that a post mortem examination would follow. Dr Webb told the policeman, who was at this stage acting as Coroner's Officer, of Mr Webb's objections both to post mortem and tissue retention, and of her desire to follow her husband's instructions.

Mr Webb's religious beliefs

Mr Webb had been a Jehovah's Witness. He had long made it clear to Dr Webb that, in the event of his death, he did not want a post mortem and that none of his organs or tissues were to be used for transplantation because of his religious beliefs. For the same reason, Mr Webb had made it clear to Dr Webb that she should never consent to the removal of any of his organs for research purposes. Dr Webb again emphasised Mr Webb's objections to post mortem to the Coroner's Officer when she attended the mortuary at Addenbrooke's Hospital at 11.30am to identify her husband's body. Annex 82

Dr Webb felt it was important to emphasise her husband's wishes. At that time she was working for a department of Cambridge University and, through informal networks within the University, Dr Webb was aware that body parts were sometimes taken during post mortems at Addenbrooke's Hospital for research.

Mr Webb's death was reported to Mr John Smith, the Coroner for South Cambridgeshire, in whose district Mr Webb had died. In 1988 the mortuary at Addenbrooke's served as a public mortuary for the coronial districts of Cambridge City and South Cambridgeshire.

Dr Webb was told only that there would be a post mortem. While the cause of her husband's death was clear, Dr Webb understood why there would be a Coroner's post mortem. As she was her husband's executor, she particularly wished to ensure that her husband's wishes that there should be no organ retention were followed. Dr Webb was particularly concerned given her local knowledge about organ retention practices at Addenbrooke's mortuary. She was not told of her rights as in Rule 7 of the Coroners Rules. Dr Webb was only later told of her rights by a friend.

Post mortem examination

The post mortem examination was carried out two days later at 9.00am on 26 January 1988 by Dr Derek Wight. Dr Wight's report to the Coroner gives the cause of death as *"carbon monoxide poisoning"*. Dr Wight added the comment *"Death was unquestionably the result of carbon monoxide poisoning. Blood has been retained for analysis although in my view this is not strictly necessary"*. Annex 84

It is clear that a full post mortem examination was performed. The report records the brain weight and that the brain and meninges were "*normal*".

There is no reference or mention that the brain was retained.

Inquest into Mr Webb's death

The inquest into Mr Webb's death was held on 19 February 1988. Mr Smith recorded the cause of death as *(i) "carbon monoxide poisoning from vehicle exhaust fumes; (ii) took his own life while suffering from a depressive illness"*.

In the interval between Mr Webb's death and the inquest, the police were the only public agency to make contact with Dr Webb at a time of great personal distress.

Dr Webb's subsequent concerns

In the weeks after his funeral, Dr Webb continued to worry about whether any of Mr Webb's organs had been retained. In 1990 she arranged to meet Professor Gresham, Professor of Histopathology, who was in charge of the mortuary at Addenbrooke's. She asked for a copy of the post mortem report, which Professor Gresham provided. Dr Webb also telephoned Mr Smith to ask for copies of the witness statements prepared for the inquest held on her late husband.

Because of her concerns, Dr Webb's general practitioner arranged for her to attend a post mortem examination.

Looking back on the events that occurred on the day of her husband's death, Dr Webb remembers that no-one told her of her rights, in particular that she might wish to appoint someone to represent her at the post mortem, as provided in Rule 7(2) of the Coroners Rules.

April 2001

After the Redfern report of the Inquiry into the Liverpool Children's Hospital was published[1], Dr Webb's doubts re-surfaced. In April she contacted the Chief Executive of Addenbrooke's NHS Trust to ask about her unresolved anxieties that some of her husband's organs had been retained after the post mortem.

The Trust's response

The Chief Executive of Addenbrooke's NHS Trust replied by letter on 8 May 2001: *"As part of the post mortem procedure a number of organs were removed for examination. With the exception of the brain, all organs were returned to the body prior to the funeral.* ***I can confirm that your husband's brain has been retained and is still held at Addenbrooke's****.*

It is now for you to decide what happens next with regard to the organ we have retained. We will be guided by your wishes and will take things forward at your request". Annex 85

Dr Webb was devastated by this disclosure and her distress was compounded by the emphasis given to the single sentence in the letter highlighted by use of bold type.

Dr Webb was also surprised that the letter had given no indication of why her husband's brain had been retained.

Dr Webb's further questions and the Trust's answers

As the Trust's reply gave so little information, Dr Webb wrote to Dr Wight on 20 May with the specific questions numbered below to which the Chief Executive responded on 5 June: Annex 86 Annex 87

"1. Why was my husband's brain retained?

Mr Webb's brain was retained at post mortem by the Brain Bank at the request of Professor E S Paykel, Director of the Brain Bank, in order to be used for his research into depressive illness.

2. Who gave permission for this retention, and did I sign a form giving permission?

As the post mortem was a Coroner's case, performed by Dr D G D Wight, we understand that permission for retention was obtained from the Coroner. We are awaiting confirmation of this from the Coroner's Officer.

3. Is the organ still intact, or have tissue blocks been prepared from it?

The brain has been divided in two and is stored in a -80°C freezer. No histology sections or material from any other studies have been taken from it.

4. ***Has his brain been used for teaching and/or research? If so, exactly how has it been used, and what conclusions have been drawn from it's*** (sic) ***examination?***

The Brain Bank records show that the brain has not been examined or used for teaching or research.

5. ***Even if it hasn't been used for teaching and/or research, was this the original reason for it's*** **(sic)** ***retention?***

The original reason for removal was for research into depressive illness.

6. ***Where has his brain been stored since 1988? I understand that Addenbrooke's and Cambridge University's Pathology Department operate a Brain Bank. Was his brain retained as part of this resource?***

The brain is currently stored in a freezer in the Brain Bank laboratory, which recently moved to the Division of Molecular Histopathology.

7. ***The letter that I received from Addenbrooke's Trust stated that, with the exception of my husband's brain, all the other organs were returned to the body prior to the funeral. Further down the letter, however, it stated that organs and/or tissue samples may have been sent to other centres. These are two contradictory statements. How can I be sure that all the other organs were returned with the body? Is there a positive record that this actually happened?***

The brain was retained as stated above, otherwise according to the post mortem report by Dr Wight, no material for histopathology or for any other investigation was taken from the body at post mortem. As the post mortem was carried out at the request of the Coroner, I am afraid that we are not at liberty to provide you with a copy. However, the Coroner will be able to, he can be contacted on ……

8. ***Will the continued retention of my late husband's brain be of any use to anyone in the future?***

This is difficult to foresee. Presently, there are no projects on depressive illness but such may start up in the future. The brain has been kept at -80°C and thus could be used for a wide spectrum of analytical techniques in a research project studying depressive illness."

Approach to the Coroner

As Addenbrooke's letter of 5 June stated that *"we understand that permission for retention was obtained from the Coroner",* Dr Webb wrote to the Coroner, Mr David Morris, who having retrieved the archived file, replied to Dr Webb on 4 July. He indicated that the inquest had been held by his predecessor, Mr Smith, and added: *"Except with the consent of the next of kin, no organ should be removed and retained unless, in the opinion of the Coroner on the advice of his Pathologist, this*

Annex 88

was necessary to ascertain the full cause of death. This requirement has not changed although the procedure has been refined and is now fully documented.

In the particular circumstances of your husband's suicide whilst suffering from a depressive illness the medical cause of death was given by the Pathologist to my predecessor on 26 January 1988 and I cannot immediately see why his brain, properly removed for examination in the autopsy process, should have been retained and not returned to the body before its release to the Funeral Director. Indeed, I was surprised to learn that his brain had been retained as it was not required for Coroner's purposes. The Post Mortem report sent to the Coroner did not indicate this but did specifically state that no specimens or sections (other than blood) were retained for toxicology or further examination".

Dr Webb's subsequent correspondence with Addenbrooke's

Following the Chief Executive's reply dated 5 June, Dr Webb attempted, through the Addenbrooke's Helpline, to request a meeting. She wished to ask further questions about the circumstances in which her husband's brain had been retained for the brain bank without her knowledge or consent. She was asked to write in again.

As her contacts with Addenbrooke's Helpline were not addressing Dr Webb's concerns or giving her the further details she was seeking, Dr Webb made an approach to Professor Paykel through a colleague whom she knew personally.

Following this approach, the Chief Executive arranged for Dr Webb to meet Professor Paykel and others. This took place on 12 November.

Dr Webb's meeting with Professor Paykel

At this meeting Dr Webb met Professor Paykel, Professor Collins, Professor of Histopathology, and Mr Day, Administrative Director. Professor Paykel explained the background to the bank and of the plans to collect the brains of suicide victims. This research had not been developed as no funding had been obtained.

The Chief Executive's letter of 5 June had indicated that Mr Webb's brain was retained *"at the request of Professor E S Paykel, Director of the Brain Bank, in order to be used for his research into depressive illness".*

During the course of these meetings Dr Webb was informed that her husband's brain was still held intact by the brain bank and that no investigations or studies had been undertaken.

The reason for retention of Mr Webb's brain

Professor Paykel in a recent reply to me has stated that the Chief Executive's reply to question 1 in his letter of 5 June implied that he, Professor Paykel, had specifically requested that Mr Webb's brain should be retained for the brain bank. This was incorrect. Professor Paykel's request was a general request to the pathologists working at Addenbrooke's for retention of the brains of all victims of suicide. Professor Paykel had made this on behalf of the brain bank. There had been no specific request for the retention of Mr Webb's brain.

However, this point was not made clear to Dr Webb at the meeting on 12 November.

Dr Webb's continuing concerns

Following from her correspondence with Addenbrooke's and the meeting on 12 November, Dr Webb remains concerned about a number of points:

- first, as her husband's brain remained intact, why had it not been further examinedduring or after the post mortem examination?

- second, had other of her husband's organs had been retained? No satisfactoryinformation on this point had been provided. (The post mortem report was not sufficient evidence as this did not mention retention of the brain);

- third, Dr Webb asked at the meeting if she could also meet Dr Wight who had carried out the post mortem examination, but no meeting was arranged or offered.

On these points Dr Webb remains unsatisfied.

Dr Webb's meeting with Mr John Smith

As Addenbrooke's Hospital had stated in the Chief Executive's letter of 5 June that *"permission for retention was obtained from the Coroner"*, Dr Webb wished to ask Mr John Smith, the Coroner who had held the inquest into her late husband's death, if this was so.

Dr Webb arranged to meet Mr Smith in May 2002. Mr Smith told Dr Webb that he had certainly not agreed to the retention of her husband's brain. This had happened without his knowledge or consent.

While Mr Smith was Coroner for South Cambridgeshire District he had been unaware of the organ retention practices that had been a regular feature of Coroners' post mortems at Addenbrooke's mortuary.

When Mr Smith succeeded Mr Sterndale Burrows as Coroner for the City of Cambridge in 1991, the organ retention practices of the mortuary had been brought to his attention. He had immediately confronted the pathologists and told them that organ retention without the consent of the relatives must stop. Mr Smith was aware that his instruction was not welcomed by some of the pathologists, who had believed they were practising with the tacit agreement of Mr Smith's predecessor.

Dr Webb appreciated this opportunity of speaking directly to Mr Smith and for the assistance he gave her.

Collection of brains of suicide cases

The records of the brain bank show that no brains of Coroners' cases have been retained since Mr Smith was appointed Coroner for the City of Cambridge in 1991(2).

Summary

There are several similarities in the way the police approached Dr Webb and Mrs Isaacs in the immediate period following the deaths of their husbands.

Both Mrs Isaacs and Dr Webb, on looking back, consider the police could and should have given them more information about their rights as next of kin and on what was to happen next.

The Coroner's Officer failed to inform Dr Webb of her right to send a representative to the post mortem.

Mr Webb's brain was retained for research despite Dr Webb's emphasis on her husband's and her own objections.

The post mortem report, while describing Mr Webb's brain, does not mention that it had been retained for research by the Cambridge brain bank.

Dr Webb only discovered that Addenbrooke's had retained her late husband's brain as a result of an enquiry prompted by the revelations of the Redfern Report.

The research study of suicide brains for which Mr Webb's brain had been retained never took place.

The circumstances in which Mr Webb's brain was retained, and the initial explanation given to Dr Webb, serve to illustrate the misunderstanding by many NHS personnel that the Coroner has the absolute right to retain organs, including brains. The Coroners Rules are clear that retention is only lawful when the organ or tissue is needed for diagnostic reasons. Any other retention requires the consent of the relatives.

In Mr Webb's case Mr Smith, the Coroner, was not asked about the retention of Mr Webb's brain. Had Mr Smith been asked, he would have insisted that Dr Webb's consent should be sought.

References

1. The Royal Liverpool Children's Inquiry Report, 2001.
2. Records of the Cambridge brain bank.

CHAPTER 28

Queen's Medical Centre, Nottingham
Department of Neuropathology

Introduction

This chapter describes a brain collection that resulted from different procedures to those used to collect brains at Manchester and Cambridge. The collection at Queen's Medical Centre (QMC) includes brains from Coroners' cases retained for diagnosis, but **no brain was retained specifically for research.** Brains from Coroners' cases were only used for research after the diagnostic process was complete.

The circumstances in which brains were retained from Coroners' post mortems came to light from enquiries made into the retention in 1991 of the brain of Mr Stuart Fayle. The investigation of Mr Fayle's death is described in Chapter 29.

This chapter describes the retention procedures, the policy of "a full post mortem examination", and reporting arrangements for Coroners' post mortems.

The only reason brains were retained from Coroners' cases was the pathologist's intention to carry out a histological examination.

There were, however, other similarities with the brain collections at Manchester and Cambridge in that retention of the brains was not always reported to the Coroners. However, the relatives were not told about brain retention.

For hospital post mortems the position was different. The relatives of some hospital patients gave specific consent for brain retention. In other cases the post mortem consent form was considered in the early 1990s to include consent for organ retention, although this was not mentioned on the form.

Sources of information

This chapter is based on:

- what happened to the brain of Mr Stuart Fayle;
- post mortem reports provided to the Coroner;
- the record books of brains investigated in the Department of Neuropathology;
- the recollections of:
  - Dr Chapman, Coroner for Nottinghamshire since 1993;
  - Professor J Lowe, Professor of Neuropathology at Nottingham since 1985;
  - Dr K Robson, Consultant Neuropathologist at Nottingham since 1990;
  - Mr Mulligan, Chief Mortician since 1974;
  - Mrs Lianne Ward, Head Neuropathology Technician since 1989.

The mortuary at Queen's Medical Centre

This mortuary serves a dual purpose as hospital mortuary for the Queen's Medical Centre and as the main public mortuary for the City and surrounding area. The bodies of those who had died suddenly in the community and those whose deaths were reported to the Coroner for other reasons were brought to the mortuary to await a decision by the Coroner on whether a post mortem should be carried out.

The collection of brains at Queen's Medical Centre

This brain archive is located in the Section of Neuropathology. This is a specialist centre that, in addition to examining the brains from post mortems carried out by many different pathologists at the hospital, also receives brains and brain samples from other hospitals in the region for specialist histological examination.

The Section of Neuropathology moved to Nottingham from Derby in 1985. At the time of the move a brain archive at Derby was transferred to the new department in Nottingham.

Brain books

The number and identification of all brains and brain samples referred for diagnostic examination and held by the department are all recorded in the brain books. The books list all brains or samples received since the opening of the department in 1985. The oldest brain transferred dates from 1967.

Numbers of brains retained at the Queen's Medical Centre

The brain archive at the Queen's Medical Centre in 2000, as reported to the Chief Medical Officer's Census, included 1,700 brains from Coroners' cases. These had been obtained over the previous 20 years. Approximately 100 brains from Coroners' cases had been retained annually in recent years for diagnostic review, a procedure described later in this chapter, and for other purposes.

Examination procedure

Every brain was examined histologically after fixation, Chapter 7. As fixation takes four to six weeks, the brain was not returned to the body before the funeral or cremation.

Prioritisation of histology examinations

In the years 1985 to 1995 there was a very substantial backlog of brains awaiting histological examination. The backlog was inherited when the neuropathology service transferred from Derby. As a consequence, a prioritisation policy was put in place.

Surgical specimens and brains from Coroners' and hospital post mortems where there was a possibility of unexpected findings were given priority.

The histology of brains from post mortems which were considered to have a low probability of showing anything unusual or unexpected were examined when time permitted. Priority was given to examination of samples from patients over post mortem specimens. In some cases there was a delay of months before the histology on low priority post mortem samples became available.

Disposal procedure at QMC

For each brain or sample retained for histological examination, a "processing sheet" was raised. This would record the number of tissue blocks kept and the different stages of the laboratory procedure. When the pathologist had completed the histological examination he would decide to retain or dispose of the brain by incineration.

When there were no new or unexpected histological findings the pathologist would generally decide to dispose of the brain and would write this on the processing sheet. Brains were disposed of in batches by one of the laboratory staff when sufficient numbers had accumulated.

After each brain had been disposed of, the brain book would be marked with a "T" to show that the disposal instruction had been carried out. The "T" was entered by the head laboratory technician. However, the date of disposal of each brain was not recorded.

Brains that were not to be disposed of were differently marked, such as "UC". This would indicate where the brain was held and that it had been retained. When a brain was later disposed of, the "UC" was crossed out and replaced by "T".

The decision to dispose of or retain a brain was applied without regard to the status of the post mortem from which it had been retained. All brains were considered on the same basis.

In some cases criminal or civil proceedings might follow the Coroner's inquest and in these cases the pathologist might decide to continue to retain the brain or brain samples in case they were needed in evidence.

Some pathologists at the QMC never retained brains after diagnostic procedures were completed.

The policy of conducting a full post mortem

The Pathology Department at Nottingham has always followed the policy of carrying out a full post mortem. This includes examination of the brain in all cases. The policy was adopted to ensure that no significant pathological findings were missed, and had the endorsement of the Royal College of Pathologists, Chapter 44. The College's guidance on the scope of a post mortem was first made explicit in recommendations issued in 1993, but its view that a full post mortem should be routinely carried had been well known for years before the guidance was issued. Appendix 29

At Nottingham no distinction was made between hospital and Coroners' post mortems. The policy was that all post mortems should be conducted to the highest standards.

Coroners' cases

In implementing the "full post mortem" policy, the brains of all Coroners' cases were routinely examined. In most cases the brain was returned to the body at the end of the post mortem.

In a minority of Coroners' cases, for example when death had followed an injury to the head, the brain would be routinely retained for histological examination. In cases of sudden death where the cause was thought to be a stroke or other disease process affecting the brain, it would be retained for histological examination.

The brain would also be retained in Coroners' cases where for medico-legal purposes it was important to exclude any disease or injury to the brain that could be relevant to the cause of death.

The reason that reports to the Coroner did not routinely mention organ retention

The late Mr Jenkin Jones, the Coroner for Nottinghamshire until 1993, told a newly appointed pathologist that the post mortem reports should provide the Coroner with the pathologist's interpretation of his findings. If the pathologist considered it was necessary to retain the brain for histological examination, Mr Jenkin Jones was content. He had not expected to be asked about organ retention on a case by case basis.

In practice, the pathologists differed in the recording of brain retention. Some reports did not refer to retention unless the pathologist expected the results of brain histology to alter the cause of death. For the same reason Mr Jenkin Jones did not expect to receive the histology reports that revealed nothing new.

There are no contemporaneous papers that document Mr Jenkin Jones' instructions, but from reading the reports sent to him the Coroner could not have known of the frequency or number of brains that were being retained.

Cases where brain histology is relevant to the cause of death

In a small proportion of cases, the pathologist considered that brain histology was essential to determine, or might alter, the provisional cause of death. Histology was given priority in these cases as the inquest verdict might depend on the findings.

The pathologist would also inform the Coroner, so that the date of the inquest would be delayed until the histology results were available. The relatives would be informed of the reason for the delay. The initial post mortem report to the Coroner would indicate that investigations were in progress.

Cases where brain histology is unlikely to affect the cause of death

In cases where, following visual examination, the pathologist considered that it was possible, but unlikely, that histology would alter his conclusion about the cause of death, the brain would be fixed. The full histological examination was not, however, given priority and in many cases was not available until after the inquest had been held.

In such cases the pathologist would not usually mention the fact that the brain had been retained in the post mortem report. The Coroner would only be informed of unexpected findings that affected the cause of death.

The pathologists working for Mr Jenkin Jones believed he was well aware of their procedures.

The backlog of brain histology reports referred to above was another reason why there was a delay of months in non-urgent cases before brain histology became available.

When did the practice of brain retention in Coroners' cases change?

When Dr Chapman succeeded Mr Jenkin Jones as Coroner in 1993, he was unaware of the extent and frequency of brain retention. Few of the post mortem reports sent to him recorded the fact of brain retention.

Dr Chapman is clear that this practice continued until 1994. He then discovered that brain retention was being widely practised without his knowledge. This had come to his attention as the result of a particular, well-remembered, case. Dr Chapman gave instructions that brains and other organs must only be retained for diagnostic purposes and with his knowledge and agreement. Dr Chapman insisted that once the diagnostic process was completed, the brain could not be further retained unless the relatives gave their consent to the purpose for which further retention was requested. Some pathologists report that Dr Chapman's instructions were conveyed verbally and that the date was later than 1994.

Practices for brain and tissue retention were eventually unified and formalised in 1999 after further discussion between the Coroner and the pathologists. These included instructions regarding disposal of retained brains and other tissues once the diagnosis was complete.

Who was aware that brains were being retained from Coroners' cases?

The pathologists, mortuary staff, and neuropathology technicians were all aware that brains from Coroners' cases were being retained. Until 1994 they believed the Coroner was aware of the practice and was content, although retention was not routinely mentioned in the post mortem report. This changed when Dr Chapman gave instructions that he should be informed and agree to all organ retention.

For their part, the pathologists believed that once a brain was retained for diagnosis it could be held after diagnosis was complete without informing the Coroner or the relatives, for the reasons set out in Chapter 42. This mistaken belief was based on the fact that the brain had been originally held under the authority of the Coroner.

As in Manchester and Cambridge, the relatives did not know as the post mortem report did not mention retention. At QMC, unless the relatives asked specifically, there was no mechanism through which they could have discovered that the brain had been retained.

As Mr Stuart Fayle's case demonstrates, when relatives did ask they were not always given comprehensive information, Chapter 29.

Reasons for prolonged brain retention after the diagnosis was completed

There were a number of reasons why brains were retained at QMC:

- some were retained for teaching as they exhibited unusual or important features, and would be valuable for teaching and training. Prolonged retention of these brains provided an archive that could be used in future research. The value and importance of brain archives is discussed in Chapter 46;

- in some cases the diagnosis was not certain and the significance of some histological features was not clear. In these the initial diagnosis was, in effect, provisional. The brain and/or slides were retained to enable the diagnosis to be reconsidered at a later date. Retention in these cases was an extension of the diagnostic process;

- brains were also retained at QMC for "*diagnostic review*". This term is generally used to refer to the reexamination of the slides to confirm or amplify the original diagnosis. That use of diagnostic review is directly relevant to the disease that affected the deceased;

- following diagnosis, some brains retained for the purposes stated above have also been used for research into the classification of neuropsychiatric diseases, including dementia.

In summary, the reasons for prolonged brain retention were for teaching, "diagnostic review", audit and research. Brains from Coroners' and hospital cases were retained for all three purposes.

The purpose of "diagnostic review"

At QMC the term "diagnostic review" was also used to describe a different procedure where groups of brains from patients who had died of similar neuropsychiatric diseases were reexamined to identify new and previously unrecognised diagnostic sub-categories. Brain archives and collections are essential for this work and the future of neuropathology would be seriously hampered without such reviews. The Neuropathology Department at QMC did not regard this type of "diagnostic review" as research for the reasons set out in Annex 89. Annex 89

It is argued that this form of "diagnostic review" should not be regarded as research as no specific hypothesis is being tested. Also, with rare exceptions, the knowledge gained will not alter or affect the cause of death as reported to the Coroner.

However, in my view, when "diagnostic review" is used in this way it is unquestionably a form of research. When brains are re-examined for previously unidentified features, the outcome of the process is unknown. The purpose of the re-examination is the enhancement of knowledge. This is a research process to improve diagnostic accuracy. It is a valuable procedure that has the potential to identify previously unrecognised conditions. One recent example was the identification in 1996 of variant CJD as a new condition.

However, the argument that diagnostic review is not research misses the central point of this investigation. The Human Tissue Act requires that relatives should be informed of brain retention when the purpose has nothing to do with the Coroner's investigation, as provided by the Coroners Rules. Diagnostic review, however, plays no part in the Coroner's proceedings as the cause of death has been given to the Coroner long before any review process begins.

At QMC the relatives were not asked for their consent to diagnostic review until 2000.

In Coroners' cases, should the views of the relatives influence the decision to undertake a full post mortem and/or brain retention?

This issue will be considered in Chapter 45, which discusses the purposes of a Coroner's post mortem and the extent to which the objections of relatives should influence the extent of the post mortem.

Were brains retained from Coroners' cases ever transferred elsewhere for research?

Some brains were referred to other specialist centres for purely diagnostic reasons and there is an audit trail of referred material held by the QMC laboratory. Importantly, all material referred away for such investigation has been returned to QMC where it is archived.

Apart from these diagnostic referrals, the only brains sent to other centres were some from patients with schizophrenia that were referred to the Neuropathology Department at Charing Cross Hospital in the early 1990s. These brains were all returned to QMC in 2000[(1)].

Apart from these cases, Professor Gavin Reynolds took some brain specimens for neurochemistry examinations when he transferred from Nottingham University to Sheffield University in 1989. He continues to retain the brain samples originally referred to him. Samples held are carefully documented.

No other brains had been sent or referred to other centres since 1989 except for particular diagnostic purposes, for example, the referral of a suspected brain to the CJD Surveillance Centre in Edinburgh.

Appointment of nurse advisers

The QMC responded promptly to public concerns and emerging guidance about retained organs and appointed three specialist nurse advisers to help, counsel and assist relatives who made enquiries about retained organs. The nurse specialists remain in post and are available to discuss organ and tissue questions with relatives of those who have died in the hospital and in cases reported to the Coroner. The nurse specialists also assist relatives who have made enquiries about retained organs and work closely with the QMC's bereavement services.

Summary

Approximately 1,700 brains from Coroners' cases are retained in the collection at Queen's Medical Centre, Nottingham. These have been accumulated mostly since 1970 but the oldest brain was retained in 1967.

All the brains were obtained or referred from other hospitals for diagnosis. None was collected solely for research.

Brains from Coroners' cases were retained as part of the routine of a "full post mortem", with brain retention in all head injuries and other cases where brain pathology was considered likely, or needed to be excluded, from the cause of death.

Post mortem examinations at QMC were carried out to the "highest standards" as widely practised in the late 1980s and early 1990s.

The large majority of brains were disposed of after the diagnostic process was completed.

No distinction was made between the way brains from hospital and Coroners' cases were investigated.

Some pathologists at the Queen's Medical Centre never retained brains for research, teaching or for "diagnostic review".

The fact of brain retention was, until 1994 with some exceptions, not reported to the Coroner or recorded on the post mortem report.

The relatives, with a few exceptions, had no way of knowing that the brain had been retained after a Coroner's post mortem.

When the diagnostic process was complete, the pathologist would decide whether to dispose of or retain each brain.

The relatives were not informed when brains were to be disposed of.

Brains retained for prolonged periods were kept for teaching, research and diagnostic review.

For Coroners' cases the purpose of the post mortem is to establish the cause of death. Diagnostic review has no part in establishing the cause of death in a Coroner's case.

Whatever the status of diagnostic review, the relatives should have been informed when a brain from a Coroner's case was retained for review purposes.

The nurse advisers at QMC provide a most valuable source of advice and counselling to bereaved relatives in Nottingham.

References

1. Records of the Neuropathology Department at QMC.

CHAPTER 29

The death of Stuart Fayle

Introduction

The retention of the brain of the late Mr Stuart Fayle was brought to my attention by Mr Robert Fayle, Stuart's father, during a meeting of the Retained Organs Commission on 30 May 2002. Mr Robert Fayle described the circumstances by which he had discovered that his son's brain had been retained after the Coroner's post mortem carried out at the Queen's Medical Centre, Nottingham, on 15 May 1991.

Mr Robert Fayle asked me to investigate these circumstances under the third of my Terms of Reference.

Sources of information

This chapter is based on:

- examination of the contemporary hospital medical records;
- the post mortem report to the Coroner, Mr Jenkin Jones;
- correspondence between Mr Fayle and the Queen's Medical Centre;
- the recollections of:
  Dr Robson, Consultant Neuropathologist who carried out the post mortem;
  Mrs Lianne Ward, Head Neuropathology Technician at QMC.

The chapter describes what happened, and the reasons why Mr Fayle's brain was retained in line with the post mortem practices and the policies at the Queen's Medical Centre, Nottingham, in 1991.

Mr Stuart Fayle's accident

Mr Fayle was riding his motorcycle when he was involved in a road traffic accident on 14 May 1991[(1)]. He was severely injured and taken to the Queen's Medical Centre where he was found to have suffered major abdominal and pelvic injuries as well as a head injury. An emergency operation to control internal bleeding was undertaken but Stuart died despite all efforts to save his life.

In view of the accident which precipitated Mr Stuart Fayle's death, the Coroner, Mr Jenkin Jones, ordered a post mortem examination. This was carried out by Dr Robson, a consultant neuropathologist at the QMC, on 15 May 1991.

Post mortem findings

Dr Robson's report to the Coroner identifies the cause of death as multiple injuries, adding that: *"This man died as a result of extensive pelvic injuries which caused surgically uncontrollable bleeding, death occurring shortly after admission* (to the Queen's Medical Centre). *In addition there is a severe head injury which may well have proved fatal had he survived the other injuries. His management has been appropriate, but death was inevitable due to the severity of the injuries. Death is not due to natural causes. The injuries are entirely compatible with a history of a motorcyclist who has been involved in a road traffic accident".* Annex 9(

Dr Robson's report also notes the weight of the brain and its naked eye appearance but does not mention that Mr Fayle's brain was retained for further examination.

The retention of Mr Fayle's brain was not referred to during the inquest and the Coroner did not refer to detailed examination or ask Mr Fayle's relatives about their wishes regarding eventual disposal. As a result, Mr Fayle's family had no reason to believe Stuart's body was not complete when the hospital gave the body to the undertakers.

Had the family been aware that Stuart's brain had been retained, they would have wished to know the results of the histological examination and would have expressed their wishes about disposal.

Mr Fayle's enquiries in February 2001

Mr Fayle senior did not give further thought to the possibility of organ retention until February 2001 when he was prompted to write to the Chief Executive of the Queen's Medical Centre by an article in the Nottingham Evening Post. This article reported that the Centre had 2,700 stored organs. Mr Fayle wanted to be sure that none of his son's organs had been retained after the post mortem carried out ten years previously. Annex 9

Mr Fayle received a letter dated 3 July 2001 from one of the QMC's specialist pathology nurses to say that the results of the hospital's search of its documentation had been completed and that Mr Fayle should telephone the Help Line. When Mr Fayle did so, he learned for the first time that his son's brain had been retained at the post mortem, but the brain had since been disposed of. Annex 9

Mr Fayle and his family were greatly distressed, as they had believed they had buried Stuart's body complete. Had they known otherwise at the time, because of their religious beliefs, the funeral would have been delayed until Stuart's brain could be re-united with his body. The family's distress was further increased when they learned that Stuart's brain had been disposed of as clinical waste.

Since learning of the retention of his son's brain, Mr Robert Fayle has endeavoured to obtain answers about why it had been thought necessary for his son's brain to be retained, why he had not been informed and why his son's brain had been disposed of without his knowledge or consent. Mr Fayle has also questioned the timing of the neuropathology investigation in relation to the date of the inquest into his son's death. Annex 9

Meeting with Dr Robson on 13 August 2002

This meeting was arranged to clarify the reasons why Mr Stuart Fayle's brain had been retained. In discussion with Dr Robson it became clear that Mr Fayle's brain had been retained for the reasons set out in Chapter 28.

The QMC policy of "full post mortem" was in place for Coroner's cases in 1991, and was carried out in all accident deaths. In all cases of head injury the brain was retained and examined histologically. What happened to Mr Fayle's brain was the routine at that time. The brains from Coroners' cases had been similarly retained at the QMC in the years before 1995. The "full post mortem policy" and brain retention has been described in the previous chapter.

<u>Was the Coroner aware that Mr Fayle's brain had been retained?</u>

There are no papers or other records that set out the late Mr Jenkin Jones' views on organ retention. What follows is based on the recollections of Dr Robson, who undertook many post mortems for Mr Jenkin Jones, and other pathologists and staff of the Neuropathology Department.

Dr Robson clearly remembers that in 1990, when he started undertaking post mortems for Mr Jenkin Jones, he was informed that he should provide a pathological interpretation of his post mortem findings. Mr Jenkin Jones was content for Dr Robson to retain the brain, or other organ, if he considered detailed histological examination was necessary. Dr Robson believed Mr Jenkin Jones did not wish to be informed about organ retention in each case. However, this would inevitably mean that Mr Jenkin Jones was not in a position to ask the relatives about their wishes for disposal of any brain or other organ retained from a Coroner's post mortem.

These practices had been well established when Dr Robson began working at the QMC.

<u>Why was the retention not mentioned on the post mortem report?</u>

The reasons why retention of the brain was not mentioned on the pathology form were described in the previous chapter. In Mr Fayle's case, Dr Robson did not expect the histological findings would change his opinion about the cause of death. The naked eye findings suggested strongly that the cause of death was "multiple injuries".

There was, however, a small possibility that at the time of the accident, or possibly later, there could have been a period of anoxia (deprivation of oxygen), recognisable only by microscopic changes in the brain that were not visible to the naked eye.

Dr Robson did not expect to find such changes but until he had examined the brain histologically he could not be absolutely sure. In deciding to retain Mr Fayle's brain, Dr Robson had been influenced by this possibility as well as the policy that histology should be routinely performed.

Had Dr Robson considered that the microscopic findings were likely to influence the Coroner's verdict, he would have alerted Mr Jenkin Jones and advised that the inquest should be delayed.

Why was there a delay in the histological report on Mr Fayle's brain?

The histological examination was certainly delayed and was not carried out until after the inquest had taken place. The reasons for prioritisation have been discussed already. Mr Fayle's death occurred when there was a major backlog awaiting histology and his brain was not considered an urgent case. Like many other non-urgent cases in 1991, the examination was delayed for some months.

Why was no histological report sent to the Coroner?

No report was sent to Mr Jenkin Jones for the reasons described in the previous chapter.

Has Mr Fayle's brain been disposed of?

The entries in the brain book clearly indicate that Mr Fayle's brain was disposed of after the histological examination was finished, although the date is not recorded.

Why was Mr Robert Fayle not informed when the decision was taken to dispose of his son's brain?

In the early 1990s it was not the policy to inform relatives, for the same reasons that the relatives were not informed that the brains or other organs had been retained after the post mortem.

Was there a possibility that Mr Fayle's brain was retained because of possible further legal proceedings?

There is no record of the time for which Mr Fayle's brain was retained. It is known there was a possibility of legal proceedings. Whether this had any bearing on the length of time for which Mr Fayle's brain was retained can now only be speculation.

Was Mr Fayle's brain retained or transferred elsewhere for research?

Dr Robson is clear that he has never retained a brain for research without the consent of the relatives. The brains he has retained are all from hospital post mortems. Dr Robson assured me he has never retained a brain from a Coroner's case for research, and Mrs Ward independently confirms this.

The previous chapter described the occasions when brains were referred from QMC to other centres for diagnosis or research. The brains referred in this way did not include Mr Fayle's brain.

I am satisfied that there has never been a programme of research into head injury at QMC and that brains from patients who died from head injury have not been transferred to other centres for research.

I am also satisfied Mr Fayle's brain was not used at Nottingham for any other research.

Summary

A full post mortem was carried out on the late Mr Stuart Fayle in accordance with the policy and practice at QMC in 1991.

Mr Fayle's brain was retained for two reasons, as part of the policy to undertake histology in all fatal head injuries and to exclude the possibility of anoxic damage. The relatives were not informed.

In keeping with practice in many other places, the post mortem report did not mention brain retention which the pathologists believed had the late Coroner's agreement.

Similarly, the fact of histology being available at a later date had not been recorded in the report as it was not expected that the histology would alter the diagnosis.

The histology examination was, in fact, carried out after the inquest. There were no unexpected findings and a copy of the report was not sent to the Coroner.

Mr Fayle's brain was disposed of on the instructions of the pathologist on an unrecorded date. The relatives were not informed.

The circumstances in which Mr Fayle's brain had been retained for a limited period of time were no different from those of many other brains that had been held for diagnostic purposes.

Mr Fayle's brain was not referred elsewhere for research, or used in research at Nottingham.

When Mr Robert Fayle began making enquiries of QMC, he did not feel he was being fully informed. It was for this reason that he asked that his experience should be considered under my Terms of Reference.

References

1. Evidence given at the inquest into Mr Fayle's death.

CHAPTER 30

The Radcliffe Infirmary, Oxford
Department of Neuropathology

Introduction

This chapter describes an established and well-documented research archive of long standing. Coroners' cases make up a small proportion of the collection. All brains and brain samples in the archive were referred for diagnosis. Apart from a very small number recently archived with the consent of relatives for research on schizophrenia, no brains were collected specifically for research.

The prospective investigations now in progress involve study of the patients in life and retention of brains only with consent of the relatives.

The collection was included in this investigation for two reasons:

- to exclude the possibility that Mr Isaacs' brain had been transferred to the brain collection; and
- to obtain details of the large-scale prospective studies that are ongoing.

Sources of information

The information on the collection, which is held in the Department of Neuropathology at the Radcliffe Infirmary, was obtained from the registers that were available during a meeting with Professor Margaret Esiri on 9 April 2002 and from her recollections of the studies that had been undertaken.

In addition, reports published from the Department of Neuropathology and the protocols of ongoing studies indicate the wide range of investigations that have been undertaken.

The brain collection at the Radcliffe Infirmary

There are over 4,500 brains and samples in the archive. The oldest brain dates from the 1940s but, as a result of a fire in 1971, many other historic specimens were destroyed.

The archive is so extensive that from time to time older specimens, that do not have unique features, are disposed of to make space.

Documentation of the archive

Every specimen has a unique number. The comprehensive documentation of brain and brain sample includes all clinically relevant information about the origin of the brain and the pathological findings. Manual registers are now in use to supplement an earlier card index system. This enables a rapid search to be made by name and date of death of every individual. A computerised register is in the process of being compiled.

The registers for the years after February 1987 were carefully reviewed. There are no entries referring to Mr Isaacs.

Regional referrals

As the main neurological, neurosurgical and psychiatric centre for the Oxford region, the Neuropathology Department receives brains and brain samples from hospitals and Coroners' cases from a wide geographical area.

Coroners' cases

When the Chief Medical Officer's Census was carried out in 2000, it was found that fewer than 5 per cent of the cases in the Oxford brain archive were from Coroners' cases. Prior to 1970, very few Coroners' cases had been retained. With the reduction in the number of hospital post mortems, the proportion of Coroners' cases in the archive has increased. All were referred for diagnosis.

Mortuary arrangements

There is no separate public mortuary in Oxford. The bodies of those who die suddenly in the community and other deaths reported to the Coroner are taken to the hospital mortuary at the John Radcliffe.

The Oxford Coroner usually asks one of the neuropathologists to carry out the post mortem examination on any case where a neuropathological cause of death is suspected. Other histopathologists sometimes carry out post mortems on traumatic deaths that involve a head injury. In these cases, when the brain is retained it is referred to the Department of Neuropathology for further examination.

In recent years the number of Coroner's post mortems undertaken by the neuropathologists has been relatively small, but the Coroner is aware that the neuropathologist will retain the brain for investigation in those cases.

The Coroner has also arranged for the Coroner's Officers, who in Oxford are police officers, to ask the relatives for consent for brain retention in certain cases, such as schizophrenia, where the Coroner is aware of ongoing research.

Consent in hospital cases

The consent form previously in regular use at Oxford hospitals includes a specific reference: *"To remove limited amounts of tissue for further study and research"*. Annex 94

This part of the form could be deleted by relatives if they so wished.

The consent form currently in use is more detailed and follows the recommendations made by the Royal College of Pathologists in 2000.

Ongoing studies

A research study that has been in progress at Oxford for more than a decade is the OPTIMA Study (Oxford Project to Investigate Memory and Ageing). This study has collected brains from over 200 patients with dementia and 150 "control" brains. All patients are assessed in life and a consented post mortem rate of 96 per cent achieved.

One of the responsibilities of the research nurse, who is a member of the research team, is to maintain contact with relatives of the patients.

Oxford is also one of the participating centres in the CFAS (Cognitive Function and Ageing Study), Chapter 26. The organisation of this study is identical to that of other centres involved in this investigation.

Schizophrenia study

Strenuous efforts have been made to obtain consent from the relatives for the retention of brains of patients with schizophrenia, but the number of brains obtained has been small. In this study it has proved very difficult to obtain consent for "control" brains.

Consent from relatives

The OPTIMA and CFAS studies involve contact with the patient and relatives prior to death and full consent to brain retention. This is obtained in principle during the life of the patient and confirmed with the relatives after death.

In other cases (schizophrenia and other "medical interest" cases) the consent is obtained from relatives after death, using the consent form mentioned above.

Ethics Committee involvement

In the 1980s, EC approval for purely post mortem studies had not been routinely sought. However, with the start of the OPTIMA and other prospective studies, LREC approval has always been obtained, even for very small scale case studies.

Benefits of research on post mortem brains

Professor Esiri provided references to studies that conclusively demonstrate the benefits of post mortem research on the brain. She and her colleagues at the Radcliffe Infirmary believe that the benefits of consented post mortem studies of the brain are at risk of being disregarded. Experience at Oxford has shown that consent can be obtained for prospective studies, but there is greater difficulty in obtaining consent for "control" brains.

Summary

The Oxford brain archive is the second largest in England, second only to the Corsellis collection.

All brains referred to the collection were for diagnosis. While some "control" brains were obtained, diagnostic histology was always carried out for confirmatory purposes.

The records of the Oxford brain archive are exemplary in the detail held about all brains and brain samples referred.

There are some Coroners' cases in the archive, but these comprise a small proportion of the total.

Until recently, where brains were retained from Coroners' cases for diagnostic purposes, the brains would have been held without the knowledge of the relatives.

The brains retained and used in research studies in the last decade have all been consented, as for example in the OPTIMA and CFAS studies.

CHAPTER 31

Brain collections used for research under Coroners Rules 9 and 12

Introduction

This chapter describes the principal procedures that were followed for research on retained brains and brain samples that was carried out under Coroners Rules 9 and 12 with the knowledge and agreement of Coroners.

Chapter 32 describes some research programmes carried out under Rules 9 and 12 in the 1980s and in subsequent years.

Sources of information

The Coroners Rules and the recollections of Dr D R Chambers, Coroner for Inner North London District, and contemporaneous correspondence of other Coroners who agreed to research under these rules.

The purpose of Rules 9 and 12

The stated purpose of both rules is to ensure the preservation of "material" (tissues and organs) that after further examination may provide the Coroner with additional information about the cause of death.

Rule 9 - *"Preservation of material"*

"A person making a post-mortem examination shall make provisions, so far as possible, for the preservation of material which in his opinion bears upon the cause of death for such period as the coroner thinks fit".

Rule 12 - Special examination

"Preservation of material" - "A person making a special examination shall make provision, so far as possible, for the preservation of the material submitted to him for examination for such period as the Coroner thinks fit".

At first sight, these two rules appear as a duplication. The term "special examination" derives from Section 20 (4) of the Coroners Act 1988: *"In this section 'special examination', in relation to a body, means a special examination by way of analysis, test or otherwise of such parts or contents of the body or such other substances or things as ought in the opinion of the coroner to be submitted to analyses, test or other examination with a view to ascertaining how the deceased came by his death".*

Research studies undertaken as "special examination"

Rule 12 has greater potential than Rule 9 to permit new forms of research on post mortem brains. In a number of districts researchers have, with the agreement and support of Coroners, carried out innovative research on brains obtained from post mortems. For example, studies planned to investigate whether there were common neurochemical findings in the brains of those who had died from suicide or some other behavioural disorder were authorised by Coroners and successfully carried out.

Investigations were permitted under Rule 9 when the Coroner was satisfied these could be carried out on ordinary post mortem brain tissue samples.

Origins of research under Rules 9 and 12

Dr D R Chambers was appointed Coroner for St Pancras in 1970. Dr Chambers' district later became Inner North London District and he continued as Coroner for the district until 1994. He was also appointed Coroner for the City of London from 1994 until he retired in 2002. Dr Chambers was contacted in the late 1970s by a researcher working for the Medical Research Council's Institute at Mill Hill. The MRC research team wished to investigate whether levels of serotonin in the brains of those who had committed suicide were different from the levels in normal and diseased brains. As all deaths by suicide must be reported to the Coroner, the research could only be carried out if a Coroner was willing to authorise access under Rule 9 or 12.

Dr Chambers agreed to the retention of brains from suicide victims under the "special examination" provisions of Rule 12, as he considered that the findings could have a bearing on the cause of death.

Over a period of five years, the brains of 17 persons who were suspected of having committed suicide were collected from public mortuaries in North London with Dr Chambers' agreement. These brains were compared with those of patients who had died from other conditions, including Alzheimer-type dementia. This research was published in 1984 and 1986[1 and 2]. Appendix 30

Use of the methodology in other places

When other research teams learned that Rules 9 and 12 could, if a Coroner agreed, provide access to brains from Coroners' cases, the same methodology was adopted in other locations with the agreement of a number of Coroners. The Coroner had first to be satisfied that the research would have a bearing on the cause of death.

There is, however, a second condition that applies to Rules 9 and 12. A report on the examination must be made to the Coroner in all such cases.

There were a number of Coroners who, like Dr Chambers, were willing to authorise the removal of brains or brain samples for research purposes provided they were satisfied with the purpose of the research and the researcher agreed to provide them with reports on their results, Chapter 32.

As some of these investigations also required samples from "normal" brains for comparison, some Coroners were content for specimens to be obtained from the brains of other deceased persons (usually sudden deaths) who had no history of neuropsychiatric disease. However, not all Coroners who authorised the removal of brains or brain samples under Rule 9 or 12 were willing to authorise the removal of control samples.

Some Coroners who agreed to research under Rules 9 and 12 also allowed each index brain to be matched for age and gender with the next suitable "control" that became available from the same public mortuary.

Reports to the Coroner

Chapter 42 describes the reasons why post mortem reports to Coroners did not record that a brain sample or the whole brain had been retained. However, Coroners who authorised research under Rules 9 and 12 expected to receive a report of the outcome.

Summary

Coroners Rules 9 and 12 enable the Coroner to order the retention of material, including brain samples, if an examination may have a bearing on the cause of death.

Dr Chambers, the Coroner for Inner North London, agreed to a proposal for research on the brains of suicide victims under Rules 9 and 12.

Other research teams followed suit and adopted the same methodology which satisfied other Coroners that the research proposed would have a bearing on the cause of death.

Some Coroners permitted collection of brain samples from normal brains as "controls".

The Coroners expected reports to be provided, as these are required for Rules 9 and 12.

References

1 Neurotransmitter Receptors and Monoamine Metabolites in the Brains of Patients with Alzheimer's type Dementia and Depression and Suicides. Neuropharmacology 1984; Vol. 23 (12B): pp 1561-1569.

2 Serotonergic Mechanisms in Brains of Suicide Victims: Brain Research 1986; Vol 362: pp 185-188.

CHAPTER 32

Centres that carried out research under Coroners Rules 9 and 12

Introduction

The previous chapter set out the principles by which research was authorised by Coroners in a number of locations under Rules 9 and 12 of the Coroners Rules. This chapter describes work at two centres that carried out research permitted under these rules.

Sources of information

This chapter is based on documents, correspondence and the recollections of Coroners and members of the research teams at the locations described.

The Clinical Research Centre, Northwick Park Hospital

The Clinical Research Centre (CRC) was established in 1974 as one of the Medical Research Council's major research institutions. It was located next to the newly built Northwick Park Hospital in Harrow. The CRC included a Division of Psychiatry which was headed by Dr (now Professor) Tim Crow. Other staff in the Division were Dr (now Professor) Eve Johnstone and Dr (now Professor) David Owens[(1)].

The programme at the CRC was one of the models on which Professor Deakin and Dr Cross based the methodology of the joint programme in Manchester, Chapters 9 and 10.

CRC records

It has not been possible to access the CRC records as these were not retained centrally when the centre closed in the early 1990s. Details of the research programme can be found in publications by those who worked in the Division of Psychiatry, and from contemporaneous correspondence with Dr Chambers, Coroner for the Inner North London District.

Information about the CRC's policy on Ethics Committee referral was provided by the Medical Research Council Headquarters[(2)], and further details were provided through the recollections of Professor Tim Crow and Professor Eve Johnstone.

Research on schizophrenia and suicides

The study of the brains of suicides referred to in the previous chapter began in November 1978. This study was undertaken with the help and agreement of Dr Chambers. A letter from the Division of Psychiatry shows that when the study was planned there were discussions about the number of suicide brains that might be collected. Another subject considered was the need for Ethics Committee clearance before collection of brains from hospital patients with schizophrenia began.

A letter from Dr Johnstone to Dr Chambers, dated 2 November 1978, states: *"Dr Crow and I are both very pleased that you anticipate being able to provide us with so many brains. Dr Crow does not think that we should approach the hospitals for ethical permission at this stage. As he says there will be no particular hurry, the brains will be in the freezer and the case notes will not change after the patients have died. It is probable that we are more likely to get agreement in terms of specific cases than in terms of general collaboration".*

The letter continues: *"It would seem to us that the best arrangement would be if you let us know the names of any suicides whose brains you obtain together with the names of the doctors and hospitals concerned with them and we will write to them at that point".* Annex 9

Dr Chambers received a letter from Dr Crow, dated 14 November 1980 reporting progress: *"I am enclosing a list of the names and dates of death of 19 brains we have received so far. We are uncertain about three of the dates of death ...".* Annex 9

Dr Crow wrote on 7 April 1983 to Dr Chambers: *"Finally we have got round to studying the brains of the suicide cases that you sent us. Some of the results look quite interesting, although so far we have not detected any systematic differences between patients and controls".* Annex 9

Brains of hospital patients collected by the CRC Division of Psychiatry

The brains of suicides were one part of this research programme. Brains from patients with schizophrenia were obtained from patients who died in Shenley hospital.

Documentation of the mental health of patients with schizophrenia

All the patients in long-stay wards at Shenley and other hospitals were carefully assessed several times during life by staff of the CRC Division of Psychiatry. The clinical features of their condition and the treatment they received were fully documented.

Consent procedure

The initial plan had been to approach the relatives for consent to brain removal before the patient died. This was tried and abandoned as impractical. Instead, an index of all patients who had been fully assessed by the CRC research team was set up. This identified the name and address of the patient's next of kin. When a patient who fulfilled the research criteria died, one of the CRC research team would immediately try to make contact with the patient's next of kin and would visit to explain the purpose of the research and ask the relatives for consent for the brain to be removed. While these interviews were undertaken at a difficult time for the relatives, they were largely successful, and most relatives agreed once the purpose of the study had been explained to them.

Where a patient had no known relatives, the NHS hospital manager was approached under the guidance issued in HC(77)28.

Publication of the CRC research

The results of the research were published in 1984. Appendix 30

St George's Hospital, London

In the early 1980s Dr, now Professor, Horton, Professor Paykel, and others had carried out clinical research on patients with depression at St George's Hospital, Tooting, London. These investigations had full Ethical Committee approval.

Using a similar methodology under Rules 9 and 12, Dr Horton collected brain samples for research on suicide and depression in a programme which followed from his previous collaboration with Professor Paykel on clinical studies. Professor Paykel was, however, appointed Professor of Psychiatry in Cambridge before the research on brain samples began, Chapter 26. Professor Paykel and Dr Horton continued to collaborate on clinical studies after Professor Paykel had moved to Cambridge.

In 1984 Dr Horton and Ms Cheetham, a PhD research student, planned to extend the work on chemical receptors to post mortem investigation of the brains of suicides. He discussed his plans with Dr Crompton, a forensic pathologist who carried out post mortems for Coroners in South London.

Dr Crompton advised Dr Horton to explain the purpose of his proposals to Coroners in London. Dr Horton wrote to Dr Knapman, Coroner for the Inner West District of London, on 16 October 1984. Annex 98

Starting in October 1984, brain samples were first obtained from victims of suicide whose bodies were taken to the mortuary at St George's Hospital.

To increase the number of samples available, Dr Horton wrote again to Dr Knapman in the early months of 1986 and to a number of Coroners in South, West and Central London to explain the purposes of the suicide study. The Coroners all agreed to the collection of brain samples, subject to conditions in the replies set out below and providing the pathologists were prepared to collect the brain samples.

Dr Horton first wrote to Dr Burton, Coroner for the Western District of Greater London, on 6 February 1986. Annex 99

Dr Burton replied on 10 February: "*If you are examining the material as a special examination, then you would have access to the other information about the cases that you need.....*". Dr Burton emphasised that a report must be made to the Coroner in such cases. Annex 100

Dr Horton wrote a further letter to Dr Knapman on 21 April 1986: "*... to seek your permission for us to receive suitable brain samples from Dr West and to study these as a 'special investigation from the Coroner'*". Annex 101

Letters from Dr Horton to Dr Gordon Davies and Mr Paul Rose followed similar wording to the letter to Dr Burton.

Dr Gordon Davies, Coroner for Inner South District, replied on 2 May: *"I have no objections to your requests for brain samples from suspected suicides ... I would also allow access to the case histories as long as the confidentiality was observed".* Annex 102

Mr Paul Rose, Coroner for the Southern District, replied to a later letter from Dr Horton: *"I do consider that the research which you are carrying out into the biological basis of depressive illness is most valuable ... It seems to me that Dr Knapman's approach permitting a "special examination" for the Coroner commends itself".* Annex 103

Brain samples from victims of suicide were obtained from the public mortuary at Thornton Heath from December 1989.

It should be emphasised that all the correspondence about the study consistently refers to provision of samples under Rule 12.

The Coroners permitted Dr Horton confidential access to records to abstract clinical information that was relevant to the study.

In order to compare the brains of suicides with the brains of "normal" individuals, the Coroners in South London and Croydon districts also allowed samples from the brains of "normal" people who had met with sudden death, matched by gender and age to cases of suicide to be collected.

The study of suicides and depression at St George's continued until the mid 1990s and over 100 brains were collected. The first report from the study was published in Brain Research in 1988. The paper described the methodology of the study. Later, the results of the study were published in the same journal in 1997. Appendix 31 Appendix 32

On 10 December 1992 Dr Knapman sent a circular letter to pathologists undertaking post mortems for him. This letter was entitled *"REMOVAL OF TISSUE AT AUTOPSIES".* Dr Knapman emphasised *"I have previously indicated that my staff are not necessarily expected to enquire about donor cards, and consent from relatives must be obtained from pathologists undertaking research projects themselves".* Annex 104

Ethics Committee involvement

All the studies involving patients at St George's Hospital had been referred to and approved by the relevant Ethics Committee.

For the study of the brains of suicides, Dr Horton in 1984 asked the then Chair of the Ethics Committee if the suicides study should be submitted for Ethics Committee clearance. He was advised that there was no need to do so, as patients were not involved.

Summary

The investigations carried out at the Clinical Research Centre and at St George's Hospital were undertaken specifically under Coroners Rules 9 and/or 12.

All the Coroners had authorised the removal of brains or brain samples from cases of suicide, after they had considered the research protocols and agreed that these investigations satisfied the Coroners Rules.

Some Coroners permitted the collection of brain samples from the bodies of the deceased who had no history of neuropsychiatric disease. These samples were matched for gender and age with the brain samples obtained from suicide cases.

In respect of post mortem reports, practice varied. Few reports recorded the fact that a sample or, in some cases, the whole brain had been removed.

Some Coroners insisted that a report be made to them on every "special investigation" sample that was removed.

The CRC study

In the CRC investigation, consent of the relatives was obtained before the retention of the brains of patients who had schizophrenia.

Ethics Committees were consulted about this study, but only after some brains of patients had been retained.

The relatives of the suicide cases were not aware that the brains had been removed for a special examination.

Research at St George's Hospital

In 1984 the Chairman of the Ethics Committee was approached about whether the protocol of the suicide investigation should be referred to the Ethics Committee, and indicated that this was not necessary.

The relatives of the suicide cases and "controls" were not aware that brain samples or, in some cases, the whole brain had been retained for a special examination.

References

1. Derived from publications by members of the CRC Division of Psychiatry.
2. Information provided by MRC headquarters staff.

CHAPTER 33

The Corsellis collection

Introduction

This chapter provides a short account of the work of Professor Corsellis who began to collect brains at Runwell Hospital in 1950. The Corsellis (or Runwell) collection is now held by the West London Mental Health NHS Trust.

The Corsellis brain collection was the first in this country. It began as an accumulation of brains that had all been referred for diagnostic reasons. Although every brain was well documented there is uncertainty about the extent to which brains from Coroner's post mortems were collected in the early years, and of any agreements with Coroners.

Purpose of the Corsellis (or Runwell Hospital) collection

In 1950 Dr Corsellis was Consultant Pathologist at Runwell Hospital in Essex. Runwell was a long-stay mental hospital with a large population of institutionalised patients with neuropsychiatric conditions. At that time there was no effective treatment for many of these conditions. Very little was known about the causes of mental diseases. Many patients had been in hospital for years.

When a patient in Runwell Hospital died, a post mortem was almost always carried out for diagnostic reasons. The original brains in the collection were examined by Dr Corsellis as an integral part of the post mortem. Instead of disposing of the brains after he had examined them, Dr Corsellis retained those that were of diagnostic interest.

No brains in the collection were obtained solely for research. To be of any value, the medical history of the deceased was always obtained and each brain was fully examined histologically. This applied irrespective of whether the brain was from a hospital or Coroner's post mortem. Brains showing features of significance were retained. "Control" brains were also collected when neither the patient's history nor the post mortem findings indicated any neuro-psychiatric disease.

From diagnostic collection to research archive

As early as 1953, the Medical Research Council awarded Dr Corsellis a grant for his research on the collection.

Later, as the number of brains increased, the value of the collection for further research and teaching was recognised. In this way an accumulation of brains referred for diagnosis evolved over the following decades to become an invaluable research archive.

A paper written in 1994 summarises the early history of the collection:

"Brain collection began slowly; for several years almost all specimens were from Runwell patients, although a few neurological cases were received from nearby Southend General Hospital. Later Dr Corsellis' research interest in epilepsy brought referral brains from Epileptic Colonies and over three hundred epilepsy surgery specimens from the Maudsley Hospital. By the mid 1960s the workload increased as the department flourished; neuropathological support was provided for the neurosurgical unit from Oldchurch Hospital. From 1969 Runwell also provided a post mortem service for South Ockenden Subnormality Hospital. Brains from patients with all types of mental deficiency were received until that Unit closed in 1985.

A long-term collaboration with Dr Ted Bird at Cambridge beginning in the early 1970s resulted in the world's largest collection of Huntington's brains... Large numbers of normal control brains, including over 500 nonagenarian and more than 20 centenarian specimens, were collected for investigations of normal human ageing".

Dr Corsellis' skills as a neuropathologist

Dr Corsellis devoted his life work to research on the collection. As the importance of his research was recognised so his reputation as a neuropathologist grew. The result was that an increasing number of brains were referred to him for his expert opinion. To begin with, the referrals came mainly from the South East but later from all parts of the country. Brains that exhibited unusual features were referred for his opinion. Often these, with the agreement of the referring doctor, were added to the collection.

Dr Corsellis' then unique experience was recognised by his appointment as Professor of Neuropathology at the Institute of Psychiatry and his reputation as an international authority on neuropathology became widely recognised.

When Professor Corsellis retired from his academic post at the Institute, he continued to develop the collection and his research based on it.

The collection under Dr Clive Bruton

After Professor Corsellis died in 1994, the collection continued under the leadership of his colleague, Dr Clive Bruton, who had joined the research team in 1968. Under Dr Bruton's influence the collection diversified, collecting brains of cases of Parkinson's disease, depression, and Creutzfeldt Jacob disease. When Dr Bruton died in 1996 the collection was closed. It was subsequently transferred to the West London Mental Health NHS Trust in 1997.

The significance of the Corsellis collection

Other brain collections and banks were set up following the basic pattern pioneered by Professor Corsellis in the Runwell collection. Some banks are condition-specific, others collect brains from patients with many different neuropsychiatric diseases. Some collect control brains from those who have died without any of these disorders.

Some banks act as repositories from which established research teams can request brain samples of the conditions they are investigating.

Professor Corsellis was both a pioneer and a successful researcher. To give one example, his work identified the damage to the brains of boxers from repeated blows to the head. This finding has had important consequences for the safety of both professional and amateur boxing. In amateur boxing head protection is now obligatory and the length of professional fights has been limited. This was just one of the practical benefits from Professor Corsellis' research.

Professor Corsellis' most enduring contribution was that he drew attention to the knowledge that can be acquired through painstaking investigation of the post mortem brain.

Historical features

In this short description of the origins of the Corsellis collection, two points must be emphasised:

- the collection started 11 years before the Human Tissue Act (1961), and the procedures for collecting brains 50 years ago were entirely consistent with medical and legal requirements of that time;

- discoveries of major clinical importance have only been possible through research based on the number and diversity of the Corsellis collection.

The importance and value of brain archives and brain collections is discussed in Chapter 46.

Summary

The first brain collection in England was started in 1950 by Professor Corsellis in the pathology department of a long stay mental hospital.

The bank began as an accumulation of brains referred for diagnosis but the potential value for research was soon realised.

Professor Corsellis pioneered the concept of research based on brain archives and collections.

Other brain banks have since been set up and brain bank archives have become an essential research resource.

CHAPTER 34

Questionnaire to NHS Trusts

Introduction

This chapter reports on the results of the questionnaire sent to NHS Trusts that were not visited during this Investigation but which at the time of the Chief Medical Officer's Census in 2000 held substantial numbers of brains retained from Coroners' cases.

Background

A review of the Census returns showed there were 17 Trusts in England that reported holding substantial numbers of brains from Coroners' cases. These Trusts were asked to provide details of the arrangements that had been in place when brains from Coroners' cases had been retained, and in particular the consent procedures. Most of the collections were held in pathology departments but some collections were in other hospital departments. Some Trusts referred to the collections as research or teaching "archives".

Questionnaire

The questionnaire at Annex 105 was sent to the 17 Trusts with collections of more than 50 brains from Coroners' cases. Trusts were asked if brains of Coroners' cases had been retained solely for research or for teaching and if any brains had been collected specifically to serve as "controls" for research studies. Other questions concerned the use in research of brains initially referred for diagnosis. Further questions explored the arrangements for any consents given by Coroners or relatives. Annex 105

A modified questionnaire was sent to Trusts that reported holding more than 100 brains in an archive, as all the archives contained brains from both Coroners' and hospital post mortems. The replies from archives were collated and analysed separately from the collections. Annex 106

It should be noted that the Trusts responded on the basis that the data provided would be collated with no Trust individually identifiable. Every Trust completed the questionnaire.

Number of Trusts and brains held

In all there were 17 collections and nine archives held in 25 hospitals, with a total of 23,190 retained brains. Over a 20-year period, the collections had retained 14,670 brains, all reportedly from Coroners' cases. In the nine archive collections there were 8,520 brains but the number of these from Coroners' cases is unknown.

Trusts were specifically not asked to report on the collections of brains from hospital post mortems that had been separately reported to the Chief Medical Officer's Census. Trusts that only held brains from hospital post mortems were not sent the questionnaire. It is clear that brains from hospital post mortems had **not** been included in the responses received.

The largest of the 17 collections held over 4,000 brains from Coroners' cases, while the two smallest collections held more than 70 brains each.

The largest archive holds over 3,000 brains and the smallest in this survey 125 brains.

Responses to questionnaire on 17 collections and nine archives

Introduction

All 17 collections responded to questions 1 to 3, but only 14 needed to respond to questions 4 to 7. No brains from the remaining three collections had been used for research or teaching. The nine archives were expected to answer all the questions.

Results

1. *Were any brains from the Coroner's autopsies retained solely for research and/or teaching purposes?*

	Collections		Archives
	1970-1989	1990-1999	1970-1999
"Yes"	6	5	3
"No"	11	12	5
Unknown	-	-	1

2 Were any brains from Coroner's autopsies retained specifically for use in research as "controls" for studies unrelated to any illness or to the cause of death of the deceased?

"Yes"	3	3	3
"No"	14	14	5
Unknown	-	-	1

3 Were any brains from Coroner's cases initially retained for diagnostic purposes, later used for teaching or for research, either as index cases or as "controls"?

"Yes"	14	14	6
"No"	3	3	1
Unknown	-	-	2

4 *If the reply to either question 1, 2 or 3 is "yes", was the Coroner aware of the retention of brains for teaching or to research use?*

(Three collections did not need to respond to this or subsequent questions.)

"Yes"	6	4	3
"No"	4	5	4
No answer	4	5	2

5 *If the reply to question 4 was "yes", was the Coroner's consent given in writing or orally?*

Orally	6	5	3
In writing	0	0	1*
Unknown	8	9	3
No answer	0	0	2

* written consent was introduced in the late 1990s

6 *Was consent also requested from the relatives of the deceased? Routinely/Sometimes/Rarely/Never*

Routinely	0	2	2*
Sometimes	1	1	1
Rarely	3	1	1
Never	6	5	4
No answer	4	5	2

* routine consent introduced in late 1990s.

7 *Are any brains from Coroner's autopsies now retained for future research or teaching use without the knowledge of the relatives?*

"Yes"	3	1	0
"No"	11	13	8**
No answer	0	0	1

** One reply qualified by "after 2000".

<u>**Features of the replies**</u>

Six collections and three archives include some brains collected solely for research. These collections have similarities of purpose to the joint collection in Manchester and the Cambridge brain bank.

Only three collections and three archives collected brains of Coroners' cases as controls.

Of the 26 collections and archives, all but three had been used for research and/or teaching.

No explanation was offered about why brains had been retained in the three collections which had not been used either for research or teaching. As each of these collections reported holding more than 100 brains, the purpose for which they were retained is unclear.

Six collections and three archives reported that the Coroner was aware of retention, and had given oral approval. In these collections it was reported that consent from relatives was mostly "never sought" before 1990. Consent from relatives became routine in only two collections during the last decade.

Written consent from Coroners was noticeably not reported until the late 1990s.

The majority of brains in these collections, accounting for some 80 per cent in total, were originally retained after the diagnostic process had been completed.

Archive collections

Trusts that had archive collections reported that brains from Coroners' post mortems had been retained specifically for teaching or research. Almost 80 per cent of the sample had originally obtained the collection of Coroners' brains for diagnostic purposes but later used it for teaching or research.

Almost all collections reported they had never asked relatives for consent to brain retention in their archives. In only one case was it reported that relatives' consent had been sought *"sometimes until 1993 and then routinely"*.

Summary

Of the brains held in pathology departments, the great majority are accumulations of brains not disposed of after the completion of the diagnostic process. Some of these were later used for teaching or research. Less than half of the sample reported that Coroners were aware of the arrangements. Where Coroners had given consent, this was only on an oral basis.

These results demonstrate that the practice of retaining brains from Coroners' cases for research and teaching was well-established between 1980 and 2000. In this manner, over 21,000 brains had been collected.

The consent of relatives was almost never sought.

CHAPTER 35

The importance of openness where brains from Coroners' cases are retained for diagnostic purposes

Introduction

This chapter illustrates the distress to relatives that can follow brain retention without their knowledge in circumstances where the brain is properly retained for diagnostic reasons. This distress is compounded when relatives only discover at the inquest or later that brain retention has been hidden from them.

Chapter 29 described the distress of Mr Fayle's relatives when they discovered, ten years later, that Stuart's brain had been retained. Many relatives with similar experiences feel deeply deceived and betrayed. In this chapter the deceased is not named at the request of his relatives in view of the profound distress that the events described have already caused for his relatives.

For identification purposes, the deceased is referred to as *"CP"*.

Sources of information

This chapter is based on the correspondence between CP's parents, the Coroner, the hospital where CP died and the pathologist who carried out the post mortem examination.

Background

CP was aged 24 at the time of his death. He suffered from Asperger's syndrome and lived in a residential home.

On 20 February 1999 CP was a passenger in a minibus which was travelling at speed when he fell on to the hard shoulder of a motorway. His injuries were further compounded by a second vehicle that ran over him.

CP was transferred unconscious to the Neurosurgical Department of the hospital where he died six days later without regaining consciousness.

In view of the accident which had led to CP's death, the circumstances were reported to the Coroner who ordered a post mortem.

CP's parents were with him when he died. They were told that they would be able to visit his body in the mortuary. When they tried to make the necessary arrangements they were informed that their son's body had been transferred to another hospital for the post mortem examination. This took place on 1 March.

CP's body was released to his parents on 5 March 1999.

Investigations

During the interval between CP's fall from the minibus and the release of his body, the police and the Health and Safety Executive were carrying out the appropriate investigations. The Crown Prosecution Service decided not to begin criminal proceedings, thus enabling the Coroner's inquest to resume on 19 August.

The inquest

At the inquest there was no reference to the fact that CP's brain had been retained. After the inquest CP's parents requested copies of the notes of evidence on which the Coroner had reached an open verdict. On receiving the reports they discovered for the first time that his brain had been retained for further tests. This caused them great distress. They had no idea they had buried their son with a major organ missing.

The histology report

CP's parents were further distressed to discover that the histology report was not available to the Coroner at the time of the inquest. The date of the report is 26 August, a week after the end of the inquest.

The immediate impact on the family

Had CP's parents been informed from the outset of the reasons for retention of his brain, much unnecessary distress could have been avoided. His parents, following their discovery, immediately wanted to know: Annex 107

Whose decision was it to retain the brain?

Who gave authority to retain the brain, for what period and purpose?

What documentary evidence was such authority included within?

Who gave authority to carry out tests further to those carried out as part of the post mortem?

Why were those further tests not forwarded to the Coroner until after the date of the inquest?

Why were tests still being carried out on the brain after the inquest had closed?

CP's parents also wanted to know:

Why had they not been told in advance that their son's body would be transferred to another hospital when they had been assured that they could see CP in the mortuary?

Why had no one informed them of their right to have a medical representative attend the post mortem examination? Urgency could not have been the reason, as there was a delay of three days between CP's death and the post mortem.

Why did no one ask for their views on what should happen to their son's brain, until they started asking questions?

The lack of an explanation

The discovery that CP's brain had been retained deeply shocked his parents. At first they could not believe the report was accurate. Their initial enquiries did not resolve their anxieties. When they later discovered that the histology report was not written until after the inquest, this reinforced their belief that CP's brain need not have been retained in the first place. The histology could not have had any influence on the inquest verdict, so *"why was it necessary to retain the brain?"*

Further correspondence did not answer their questions but served to undermine their confidence that they were being given full information.

The position of CP's parents is best described in their own words:

"... we feel that the lack of information and the resulting feelings of abuse do parallel (in Coroner's cases) *the now widely-recognised situation with hospital post mortems.*

We feel the apparently needless retention of this organ (CP's brain) *does parallel the widely-recognised situation with hospitals where organs appear to have been retained casually and needlessly and where the whole issue has been approached with less sensitivity and seriousness than proper".* Annex 107

The reasons for retention of CP's brain

The decision to retain CP's brain in these circumstances was certainly justified. CP had suffered a grievous head injury when he fell from the minibus. This undoubtedly contributed to his death from other major injuries. The Coroner would have expected the pathologist to investigate the extent to which the head injury and brain damage had contributed to CP's death.

As police and HSE investigations were continuing, there was also the real possibility that these could lead to criminal prosecution. In such cases, the extent of the brain injury would have been a central factor. Any defendant would have had the right to an independent assessment of the injury to the brain.

While the retention of CP's brain at the post mortem was justified, it is difficult to understand why this was not explained to his parents. They had been informed only that a Coroner's post mortem would be carried out.

It is also difficult to understand why the histological examination of the brain was delayed until after the inquest, unless the naked eye appearances of damage to the brain were so grave that his histology was not relevant.

No research or teaching was ever undertaken or intended on CP's brain.

As no one explained these matters to CP's parents, their questions are fully understandable.

Long-term consequences

CP's brain is still held in the hospital pathology department. It is not there for research or teaching purposes, but solely because his parents have been so distressed by what has happened since CP's death three years ago that they have difficulty accepting that the brain is indeed that of their son. Such is the breakdown of trust that they have even considered requesting a DNA test to make certain before they are prepared to ask for the brain to be buried with CP's body.

Summary

The case of CP graphically illustrates the distress and confusion of relatives that can follow when an inadequate explanation is given of the need for organ retention in a Coroner's case. This is particularly important when retention is necessary for medico legal purposes.

CP's parents' discovery after the inquest that his brain had been retained has caused an enduring sense of loss and betrayal that they were kept in the dark.

The end result has, for CP's parents, been a complete loss of trust and a belief that the truth is being withheld from them.

These feelings are shared by many relatives who initially believe they have buried or cremated their loved one's body complete.

For relatives whose religious beliefs have been disregarded, hidden organ retention compounds these feelings.

This chapter demonstrates the importance of a proper explanation to relatives at the time when decisions are taken about organ retention. Enquiries by relatives should be fully and sensitively answered so that they are aware of any organs or tissues that are retained, and of the reasons for retention.

SECTION 5

The collection and use of brains for teaching

CHAPTER 36

The retention of brains for teaching

Introduction

This investigation is primarily concerned with the retention of brains for research after post mortems ordered by the Coroner, but brains were also retained for teaching purposes.

Sources of information

This chapter is based on contemporaneous records from Sheffield and Manchester Universities and the recollections of those involved.

History

In the 1950s most medical students dissected the brain as part of their anatomy course. For these courses large numbers of brains were obtained from both hospital and Coroners' post mortems.

Human Tissue Act 1961

Following the enactment of the Human Tissue Act in 1961 it should have been routine for relatives to be asked if they had objections before any brain was retained for medical education. In order to continue brain dissection, some medical schools introduced post mortem consent forms that referred specifically to retention of tissues for medical education.

The Medico Legal Centre and the Anatomy Department of Sheffield University

An incident at Sheffield Medico Legal Centre in December 1986 brought the retention of brains for medical education to public notice. The following paragraphs describe this incident which was widely reported in the local and national media at the time. A full investigation was carried out by Sheffield City Council, and a debate in the Council chamber followed. This closed the incident.

December 1986

Just before Christmas 1986, a telephone call was received by the manager of the Medico Legal Centre from the Department of Anatomy at Sheffield University.

The manager, who had recently been appointed, was surprised to receive a request for a further supply of brains for teaching medical undergraduates.

The caller from the Anatomy Department was put through to the Coroner's Officer, who then informed the Coroner, Dr Popper, who was concerned to know whether consent had been given.

The manager of the Medico Legal Centre also informed Sheffield City Council headquarters as the Council had responsibility for the Centre which serves as the public mortuary for the whole city.

The Coroner's investigation

Dr Popper made immediate enquiries. These revealed that in 1983 his predecessor as Coroner, the late Dr Pilling, had agreed to the removal of heart valves for transplantation from bodies under his jurisdiction but only with the written consent of the relatives of the deceased.

Dr Pilling had also agreed that the Department of Anatomy could receive blocks of tissue to make slides for teaching purposes, but only from those bodies for which the relatives had given consent for heart valves to be removed.

At some stage between 1983 and December 1986 the terms of Dr Pilling's agreement had been extended from the supply of blocks and tissue for slides to include whole brains. This had not been Dr Pilling's intention.

January 1987

Staff of Sheffield City Council arranged a meeting on 9 January to investigate "*the apparent unauthorised removal of organs during post mortems and organs being sent to the University*". The City Council were particularly concerned by the suggestion that mortuary staff were receiving payments for brains transferred to the Anatomy Department. This was in clear breach of the Council's policy.

At that meeting Dr Popper reminded those present that "*removal of human tissue may only be done under the provisions of the Human Tissue Act*".

Dr Popper stated that, as Coroner, he was "*not aware of the removal of any organs or tissues, except the heart valves which his predecessor had allowed to be removed with the consent of the relatives. The only other tissue or organs that could be removed were those required for the purpose of establishing the cause of death*"(1).

Professor Usher, Professor of Forensic Pathology at Sheffield, is recorded as saying: "*All practices are traditional and the inherited situation, which had been long-standing between the Chief Technician of Anatomy at Sheffield University and the Senior Technician in the Public Mortuary ...*"(1).

Action taken

Dr Popper gave immediate instructions that: "*He would not agree to the removal of organs without consents, but would approve of any agreed system, which could be devised within the law*"(2).

He ordered that all transfers of brains should cease and wrote to all pathologists to say that: "*No tissue was to be taken without consent*".

20 January 1987

The Sheffield Star reported the brain transfers on the front page. There was further publicity in the national media.

The City Council's investigation proceeded. A full report was prepared which was submitted to and debated by the City Council.

Since January 1987, Dr Popper and Mr Dorries, who succeeded him as Coroner for Sheffield in 1991, have followed a policy that no organs or tissues should be retained without the consent of relatives. The only exception to this rule is the retention of those organs or tissues that are needed for diagnostic purposes and the examination of which will bear on the cause of death.

Further investigations were started to discover how many brains from Coroners' autopsies had been transferred from the Medico Legal Centre to the Anatomy Department at the University, and over what period of time, but this information was not forthcoming.

Wider implications

When the irregular and unconsented transfer of brains from the Medico Legal Centre to the Department of Anatomy was discovered, the late Dr Paul Mason, who was then HM Inspector of Anatomy, was informed. On 27 January 1987 Dr Mason wrote to anatomy departments to tell them to review the arrangements through which they obtained brains for teaching and to ensure that these arrangements complied with the Human Tissue Act. Annex 108

Anatomy Department of Manchester Medical School

In reply to Dr Mason's letter, Professor P F Harris, Professor of Anatomy, drew attention to the arrangements he had introduced in the 1970s. All brains obtained by his department for medical education were collected with the consent of the relatives.

Professor Harris' letter, which by coincidence was written on 27 February 1987 (the day after Mr Isaacs' death), states: *"We have two sources of supply to the Manchester Medical School and in both instances the position is very clearly covered by the wording on the postmortem declaration form which is signed by a relative. Our established practice has worked well over many years".* Annex 22

In fact, the practice had been in operation for the previous 12 years.

The post mortem declaration form includes the words: *"I understand that this examination is carried out (a) to verify the cause of death ..."* and *"(b) to remove amounts of tissue for the treatment of other patients and for medical education and research".* Annex 22

The consent form clearly states that the relative could, if they so wished, delete paragraph (a) or (b). The relative's signature on the form was required to be witnessed.

The form includes a further note: *"A relative of the deceased should not be invited to sign this form if the hospital is itself aware of objections on the part of other relatives".*

Brains collected by anatomy departments

I have made enquires in other anatomy departments to see if any records remain available of brains collected for medical education. I have not been able to identify any extant records.

A significant factor in the ending of brain dissection by medical students was the recognition in 1992 that Creutzfeldt Jacob disease could be transmitted by contact with brain tissue. A direct result of this discovery was the removal of brain dissection from the curriculum by those medical schools that had maintained brain dissection up to that time.

Summary

Before the Human Tissue Act 1961 it was common practice for medical schools to obtain brains for teaching purposes from hospital and Coroners' post mortems.

The use of brains in medical education continued largely unchanged through the 1960s but thereafter diminished, although in some locations brain dissection continued until the early 1990s.

In the 1970s Manchester University Medical School introduced a consent form for tissue retention for research and education, for relatives to sign. Though not explicit, the form was considered as providing consent for brain retention. No brains were accepted for teaching purposes in Manchester unless this consent form had been signed.

The incident at the Medico Legal Centre in Sheffield in December 1986 showed that brain retention for medical education was continuing without the knowledge or consent of the relatives and outwith the requirements of the law.

Steps were taken by HM Inspector of Anatomy in 1987 to remind all anatomy departments that brains (and other organs) must not be used for teaching purposes without the consent of the relatives.

Anatomy departments are required by the Anatomy Regulations 1988 to keep records of the body parts they hold. The records of individual brains now held in anatomy departments in England do not identify the deceased or when and where the brain was retained.

References

1. Records of the Medico Legal Centre.
2. Records provided by Dr Popper.

SECTION 6

Brain retention and the Special Hospitals

CHAPTER 37

Brain retention from post mortems after deaths in the Special Hospitals

Introduction

This chapter describes the procedures in place at the Special Hospitals following the *"Report of the Committee of Inquiry into Complaints About Ashworth Hospital"*, published in 1992. During this investigation my attention was drawn to this report as it contains a number of recommendations that are relevant to this investigation.

The report of the Committee of Inquiry was presented to Parliament in August 1992 and subsequently accepted by the Government.

Sources of information

The chapter is based on:

- the report of the Committee of Inquiry and the subsequent legal advice obtained by the Special Hospitals Service Authority (SHSA), and other guidance documents prepared by the Special Hospitals;

- the recollections of the Coroners, medical staff, pathologists, Coroner's Officers, morticians and other staff involved in the preparation for, and procedures during, post mortem examinations on the bodies of patients who have died while detained in the Special Hospitals.

The recommendations of the Committee of Inquiry

The following recommendations made by the Committee are relevant to the retention of brains for histological examination after post mortems carried out on the instructions of Coroners.

Recommendation 8

"We recommend that if a brain-damaged patient dies in a Special Hospital, the brain should be preserved for further examination". Annex 109

Recommendation 62

"We recommend that the Home Office should send a reminder to the Coroner's Society of the value of using Home Office pathologists in all suspicious deaths (and not simply those where there is a suspicion of homicide) which would include deaths in Special Hospitals". Annex 109

The Committee also commented that *"every death of a person in custody should be treated with suspicion, even if it rarely turns out that suspicion is justified".*

Basis of the Committee's recommendations

The Committee had heard evidence about the death and subsequent post mortem on a patient who was known to have pre-existing brain damage and who had died suddenly.

Dr Cocker, the Responsible Medical Officer (RMO) for this patient, had drawn the Committee's attention to the limitations of the post mortem examination. To Dr Cocker's surprise, the examination had not included any histological examination of the brain. Dr Cocker had expected the deceased's brain would be examined histologically, as the diagnostic findings could have been relevant to the cause of the patient's sudden death.

The Committee in their report state *"We commend the attitude of Dr Cocker, who told us that in future if a brain-damaged patient for whom he was the RMO, died in hospital, he would immediately contact the pathologist with a request to have the brain preserved for further examination".*

In making this recommendation the Committee had also heard evidence from Professor Michael Green, Professor of Forensic Pathology in the University of Sheffield. Professor Green had emphasised that when a post mortem was ordered following a death in an institution for the mentally disordered, the post mortem should be *"altogether more thorough, than if a death occurred in normal surroundings".*

Professor Green had emphasised that, whenever there was a history of previous head injury, the brain should be histologically examined after fixation. The Committee of Inquiry stated *"we endorse all that Professor Green states as a requirement for the proper post mortem examination of a patient who has died in a Special Hospital".*

It should be noted that the recommendation is intended to ensure a proper post mortem is carried out for diagnostic purposes in cases of previous head injury.

The Coroner's jurisdiction and procedures followed

All deaths in the Special Hospitals are reported to the Coroner, whether or not there are any suspicious circumstances, as all these patients are "in custody". This applies not only to patients who die in the Special Hospitals but also to those patients normally resident in the Special Hospitals but who die from natural causes in other hospitals to which they have been transferred for their medical care.

Specific procedures have been agreed with the Coroners of the three districts in which the Special Hospitals are located. These procedures require a full investigation to be made of all deaths, including those where the death was expected due to known and well-documented disease such as cancer.

To ensure that each death is fully investigated, the police and Coroner's Officers are routinely involved in the preparation of reports that are made available to the pathologist before the post mortem, in addition to the documents prepared by the staff of the Special Hospital concerned.

A Home Office pathologist appointed by the Coroner will carry out the post mortem examination. A Home Office circular requires that deaths in these institutions should be treated in the same way as if deaths were in prisons.

In addition to the Home Office pathologist and the mortician, the post mortem examination is attended by other official observers. While the persons in attendance vary between the three coronial districts, in each the police and/or Coroner's officer and other officials are present for the whole of the post mortem examination until the body is closed.

A very detailed post mortem report is available to the Coroner in every case.

An inquest in which the Coroner sits with a jury is held into all deaths in Special Hospitals.

The adoption of these procedures fulfils the recommendations made by the Committee of Inquiry.

Advice from the Special Hospitals Services Authority (SHSA)

Following the recommendation of the Committee of Inquiry, and having taken legal advice, the SHSA in March 1993 agreed to revised death procedures in the Special Hospitals.

This advice is significant as it emphasised that the approval of the next of kin should be obtained before the brain of a patient in a Special Hospital could be preserved for further examination, unless the examination was relevant to determining the cause of death. In doing so, the SHSA recognised the requirement for consent by the relatives that is an integral part of the Human Tissue Act.

What happened at each Special Hospital

I have investigated whether any brains were retained specifically as a result of this recommendation made by the Committee of Inquiry after their report was published in August 1992.

Ashworth Hospital

My enquiries show that there have been on average three deaths per year in the last six years with a maximum of six deaths in any one year. These figures include patients who were transferred for medical care to nearby NHS hospitals before their death. Almost all of these deaths were due to natural causes.

Coroners to whom deaths in Ashworth were reported

Mr Christopher Sumner succeeded Mr Gordon Glasgow as Coroner for the Sefton district of Liverpool in August 1998. Since that date, all deaths of Ashworth patients, including those who die in other Liverpool hospitals, have been reported to Mr Sumner.

Prior to August 1998, deaths in Ashworth Hospital itself were reported to Mr Glasgow, while deaths in NHS hospitals were reported to the Coroner responsible for the hospital in which the patient died.

All deaths have been followed by post mortem examinations at the Liverpool University Hospital (Aintree). The examinations have been carried by a Home Office pathologist appointed by the Coroner. Since 1996, most of the post mortem examinations on patients from Ashworth Hospital have been undertaken by Dr C P Johnson.

Policy at Ashworth

Following the advice of the SHSA in March 1993, Mr E A Jones, then the Director of Planning and Administration at Ashworth, issued a letter to all Responsible Medical Officers on 9 July 1993. This letter states:

"The purpose of this letter is to inform you of the legal advice the SHSA has received in relation to this (brain preservation), *which is as follows:*

1. *If the patient has expressed the wish, then it is easier but unfortunately likely to be rare. The hospital would contact the patient's relative asking for written permission for the brain to be used for research purposes and the relatives confirm that there is no reason to believe that the wish was withdrawn later. The next of kin cannot prevent removal where the patient has authorised but need to be consulted as to whether the patient had changed his or her mind.*

2. *If the patient did not express a wish it is much harder (and also more likely to be the more usual case). The Hospital would contact the patient's relative asking for written permission and confirmation that neither of the following has happened:*

    a) *The deceased actively expressed an objection to removal which was never withdrawn.*

    b) *The surviving spouse or* <u>*any*</u> *surviving relative objects.*

It should be noted that action needs to be taken within 4 days to be of any use.

It is usual after a special hospital death for there to be a Coroners Inquest and the Coroners consent for research is needed (though that is not expected to be a problem). The Coroners use of brain is confined to determining cause of death and so should return to the body when extracted for these purposes only.

The essence of the above advice is that the necessary checks have been made and authority has been received from the family in writing."[1]

This policy was implemented at Ashworth from July 1993.

Officials attending post mortems on patients in Ashworth Hospital

The post mortem examinations on patients from Ashworth Hospital have, in addition to staff assisting the pathologist, been attended by the police who had investigated the death, the Coroner's Officer and a representative of Ashworth Hospital who had collated the documentation available to the pathologist. The latter was on most occasions Mrs Elizabeth Greenley, who has undertaken this responsibility since 1986.

Discussions with those involved in arranging or carrying out post mortems on patients from Ashworth Hospital

I have discussed the recommendation made by the Committee of Inquiry with:

Mr Sumner, Coroner for Sefton district;
Dr Di James, Medical Director of Mersey Health Care (which includes Ashworth Hospital);
Dr Johnson, Home Office pathologist;
Mrs Greenley, the member of Ashworth staff who collates the documents on each death;
Dr Cocker, whose observations led to the 1991 recommendation.

In addition, Dr James, on my behalf, has checked the documents of patients who have died in Ashworth Hospital.

None of those with whom I have spoken has any recollection of any brain being retained for diagnostic purposes from a post mortem examination on a patient in Ashworth Hospital since 1992, when the report was published. There had certainly been no occasion on which a brain has been retained for research.

Further reassurance that no brains had been retained is provided by the attendance at each post mortem of the police and other independent observers. Had brain retention occurred, this would have been observed and reported.

Broadmoor Hospital

All deaths in Broadmoor are reported to the East Berkshire Coroner and since 1991 had been followed by post mortem examinations at East Hampstead public mortuary until this mortuary closed in 1992. Since closure, post mortems have been carried out in NHS mortuaries. Where patients from Broadmoor died in nearby NHS hospitals, the post mortem examination was undertaken in the NHS hospital mortuary.

The number of deaths in Broadmoor was variable, but there had not been more than eight deaths in any recent year. Many of these deaths are from natural causes.

Coroners to whom deaths at Broadmoor were reported

Mr Peter Bedford has been Coroner for the East Berkshire district since 1998. Mr Bedford succeeded Mr Robert Wilson.

Mr Bedford had been unaware of the recommendation of the Committee of Inquiry and had no knowledge of any brain retention from patients who had died in Broadmoor Hospital, except where further examination was necessary for diagnostic purposes.

Following my letter to him, Mr Bedford had discussed the recommendation with his predecessor Mr Wilson, the pathologists who had carried out post mortems for him and for Mr Wilson, and with Mr Thomas, the Coroner's Officer with responsibility for investigating the deaths of patients who had died in Broadmoor Hospital.

Brain retention at Broadmoor Hospital

There are two separate aspects to the retention of brains of patients who have died in Broadmoor Hospital since 1991. These are separately described. The first relates to a research project in 1992 and 1993 under which four brains were collected, with consent of the relatives of the patient. This project had received Ethical Committee approval[(2)].

The second aspect is the development of the hospital policy in the light of the recommendation of the Committee of Inquiry[(2)].

Research project entitled *"Post-mortem Study of Special Hospital Patients"*

The details of the project described below are set out in the Broadmoor Hospital archived records that were made available to me for the purpose of my Investigation[(2)].

In 1991 there were discussions between Dr Crow in the Division of Psychiatry at the Clinical Research Centre, Northwick Park, see Chapter 32, Dr Bruton at Runwell Hospital, see Chapter 34, and Dr Tidmarsh, Chairman of the Research Committee at Broadmoor Hospital.

These discussions led to the development of a research proposal for the study of brains of patients who die in the hospital. It was agreed at the outset that the study would require the consent of the patient's relatives.

In August 1991 the Coroner, Mr Robert Wilson, was approached. Dr Hemsted, the pathologist who undertook the post mortems, was also asked about the practical arrangements for the study if it proceeded.

In November 1991 the Broadmoor Ethics Committee considered the proposal. The Committee emphasised the importance of consent being obtained from the relatives of the deceased.

Further discussion of the proposal followed at the next meeting of the Committee in January 1992.

The project was formally approved at the meeting of the Ethics Committee held on 1 April 1992. This was before publication of the report of the Committee of Inquiry, see below.

The study was undertaken with the knowledge of the then Coroner, Mr Robert Wilson, who had agreed to the project on the basis that consent would be obtained from the relatives. The pathologist involved was the late Dr E H Hemsted.

It is clear from subsequent correspondence between Dr Tidmarsh, Director of Research, and the Coroner that few relatives were willing to give consent. By November 1993 after four brains had been collected, the project was discontinued.

On the information available to me it is clear that few relatives had been willing to consent to the retention of brains, which may explain why the project lasted less than 18 months.

It is also clear that the development of a new policy for Broadmoor Hospital, in the light of the recommendation of the Committee of Inquiry, had begun towards the end of the research project.

Development of a new hospital policy

Following the advice of the SHSA in March 1993, the hospital reviewed its policies. On 21 July 1994 Mr Alan Franey, the General Manager, circulated a new policy document entitled *"Hospital Policy on the Death of a Patient"* to *"all Designated Hospital Policies/Procedures Manual Holders"* at Broadmoor Hospital[(2)].

This policy in its opening paragraph states that *"the death of any patient in the Special Hospital must be reported to HM Coroner".* The policy continues to set out in detail many of the practical arrangements that should follow every death in Broadmoor Hospital.

A section headed *"Communication with Relatives"* states:

"Consideration should be given to making a sensitive approach to relatives concerning the preservation of the brain, primarily in the case of brain-damaged patients".

In a separate section on post mortems the policy states:

"Post Mortems

The RMO should contact the Pathologist before the post mortem takes place and advise, in particular, of any unusual circumstances ..."

This part of the policy did not specifically refer to the retention of the patient's organs or brain.

Communication with relatives and the pathologist

However, detailed procedure sheets attached to the policy include the following:

"If appropriate, liaise with relatives and the Coroner's pathologist about neuropathological investigations".

It is clear from these references that those responsible for the development of the policy had not only taken account of the advice of the Committee of the Inquiry and the SHSA but also recognised that brain retention for research unrelated to the cause of death was only lawful with the consent of the relatives.

1996 revision of the policy

The hospital's policy was next updated in 1996. The reference to *"preservation of the brain"* was removed from the policy as staff who had been asked to discuss brain retention with relatives had become reluctant to do so and the practice had ended.

Pathologists

Three pathologists carried out post mortem examinations on patients from Broadmoor for Mr Bedford and Mr Wilson between 1991 and 2002. Dr Robert Chapman had carried out post mortems since 1994, the late Dr Hemsted, who retired in 1999, and Dr Fegan-Earle who had succeeded Dr Hemsted. Dr Hemsted was the pathologist involved in the research study already described.

Neither Dr Chapman nor Dr Fegan-Earle was aware of the recommendation of the Committee of Inquiry. Neither had retained brains from any patients who died in Broadmoor, except where further examination of the brain was relevant to the cause of death.

Coroner's Officer

Mr Brian Thomas has been Coroner's Officer since 1991. He has the responsibility for investigating all deaths of patients in Broadmoor Hospital. Mr Thomas has made it his practice to attend all post mortems on patients from Broadmoor Hospital. He has always remained in the mortuary until the post mortem is complete. In the context of the recommendation of the Committee of Inquiry, Mr Thomas has confirmed to me that to the best of his knowledge he does not recall any brains being retained after post mortem.

As Mr Brian Thomas has attended the post mortems on all patients who have died in Broadmoor Hospital since he became Coroner's Officer, he would have observed if brains had been retained in the circumstances recommended by the Committee of Inquiry.

Deaths in other hospitals of patients from Broadmoor

There have, however, been two occasions since 1991 when patients from Broadmoor died in other hospitals and the brains were retained for diagnostic reasons. Both died in nearby NHS hospitals where they were under care for medical conditions. In both cases, the papers available to me show that the pathologist considered that further examination and histology of the brain would contribute to determination of the cause of death.

The retention of the brain in these cases was for entirely proper purposes and agreed by Mr Wilson. On both occasions the relatives were aware that the brain had been retained. After histological examination, the brains were returned to the relatives of the deceased.

Summary of brain retention from patients who died at Broadmoor

There were two occasions when the brains of patients from Broadmoor Hospital were retained following post mortems carried out on the instructions of the Coroner. In both these cases histological examination of the brain was relevant to determining the cause of death. Both patients had died in nearby NHS hospitals to which they had been transferred for medical care.

Four brains were retained with the consent of the relatives for a research study undertaken in 1992 and 1993. This study had been approved by the Coroner and the Broadmoor Hospital Ethical Committee.

I am satisfied that, apart from these retentions which were authorised by the Coroner or with the consent of the relatives, no other brains were obtained from patients from Broadmoor Hospital.

Rampton Hospital

The SHSA's advice would have been available to the managers of Rampton Hospital, but no consequential policy statement has been made available to me and there is no recollection of any such policy being developed. There is no reference to the procedures recommended in the 1991 report in the current Rampton policy documents.

My enquiries confirm that all deaths of patients from Rampton are reported to the Nottinghamshire Coroner and that the post mortems are carried out by a Home Office pathologist at the mortuary at Bassetlaw Hospital. This mortuary serves as a public mortuary as well as providing mortuary services for the NHS.

The Coroners to whom deaths at Rampton Hospital were reported

Dr Nigel Chapman has been Coroner for the Nottinghamshire district since 1993. This district includes responsibility for Rampton Hospital. Dr Chapman's predecessor as Coroner was Mr Jenkin Jones. Dr Chapman was unaware of the recommendation prior to my enquiry.

The number of deaths in Rampton Hospital is similar to that at Ashworth. There have been between three and five deaths each year in recent years. The majority of deaths are due to natural causes.

Pathologists

Professor Rutty, Home Office pathologist, who is now based at Leicester University, has carried out the majority of post mortems on patients who have died in Rampton

Hospital since 1996. Professor Rutty initially carried out these examinations when he worked in the Department of Forensic Pathology at Sheffield. He has continued to undertake the examinations at Dr Chapman's request since he took up his appointment at Leicester in 2001.

Professor Rutty was unaware of the recommendation of the Committee of Inquiry. However, he and his predecessors acting for Dr Chapman had retained brain tissue samples, but not whole brains, as a matter of routine during post mortems on patients from Rampton. This procedure follows Home Office advice when an inquest will follow.

Professor Rutty states that the only circumstance in which he would retain the brain would be for fixation prior to histological examination. In his experience, this was rarely necessary. He did not recall any occasion when a brain had been retained except for diagnostic reasons, which he had always reported to Dr Chapman.

Mortician at Bassetlaw Mortuary

At Dr Chapman's suggestion, I made further enquiries of the mortuary staff at Bassetlaw General Hospital. The post mortem examinations on patients who die in Rampton Hospital are attended by a number of officials. (This follows a similar pattern to attendance of officials at post mortems on patients who die in the other Special Hospitals.)

Mrs Patricia Dady is the senior technician at the Bassetlaw mortuary and has worked there since August 1993. Mrs Dady confirmed that the bodies of all patients who die in Rampton are transferred to the Bassetlaw mortuary where a post mortem examination is always undertaken by a Home Office pathologist.

Mrs Dady confirmed that the brain is examined in all post mortems undertaken by Home Office pathologists and tissue samples taken. The brains are returned to the body before closure.

Mrs Dady could remember only two occasions when the whole brain of a patient from Rampton Hospital had been retained at the end of the examination. On both occasions, retention had been for histological examination relevant to the cause of death. The retention of these brains had been reported to Dr Chapman. In one case, disposal of the body had been delayed so that the brain could be returned to the body.

Brain retention from patients at Rampton

I am satisfied, on the basis of the recollections of Professor Rutty, Mrs Dady, Dr Chapman and others who they have consulted, that brains have not been retained from patients in Rampton Hospital except when histological examination was required for diagnostic purposes and this was discussed with the families.

Summary

In 1991 the Committee of Inquiry into Complaints about Ashworth Hospital recommended that *"if a brain damaged patient dies in a Special Hospital, the brain should be retained for further examination"*.

The Special Hospitals Services Authority provided legal advice to the three Special Hospitals in England in 1993. This emphasised that the consent of the relatives was a necessary pre-condition for further examination of the brain when this was not required to determine the cause of death.

A new hospital policy was issued to staff in Ashworth Hospital in 1993, and at Broadmoor in 1994. The Broadmoor policy was further changed in 1996.

At Ashworth and Rampton Hospitals no brains have been retained as a consequence of the Committee of Inquiry's recommendation.

At Broadmoor Hospital brains were retained on two occasions to determine the cause of death and four brains were retained in 1992/1993 for research. The retention was with the consent of the relatives.

At Rampton, brain samples were routinely retained. On two occasions whole brains were retained for diagnostic reasons. On both occasions the Coroner informed the relatives that retention was required for his purposes.

References

1. Ashworth Hospital archived papers.
2. Broadmoor Hospital archived papers.

SECTION 7

Research funding organisations and Royal Colleges

CHAPTER 38

The Medical Research Council and post mortem brain banks for research

Introduction

This chapter sets out the Medical Research Council's (MRC) involvement in post mortem brain research from the beginning of the Council's support in the 1950s. The chapter describes the MRC's early research support for the Corsellis (Runwell) and Cambridge brain collections, the Council's relevant ethical policies and research grant conditions, and the grants the MRC awarded to the joint research team in Manchester in 1988/89.

The role of the Medical Research Council

The MRC is the Government's main agency for fostering and funding biomedical research. In keeping with this important role, the MRC has made a pivotal contribution to the development of clinical and basic research on the brain in this country. This has been achieved in two ways.

First, the MRC has a distinguished record of supporting world class neuropsychiatric research in its designated research units, and by awarding programme and project grants to other research teams through the Council's competitive research funding systems.

Second, and of equal importance, have been the Council's thematic reviews of different research fields to identify the most promising future lines of research. The subjects identified through these reviews then become priority areas for future Council funding.

Through these mechanisms the MRC has kept this country's basic and clinical research competitive with the best in the world in many fields including the neurosciences.

Sources of information

For this investigation the MRC has provided a written response about the policies and procedures for brain research and brain banking which have been developed over the last four decades. Annex 110

The chapter also draws on contemporaneous notes of workshops and other MRC meetings, and programme and grant applications to the Council. The minutes of MRC meetings on brain research, brain banking and related subjects have been particularly informative, and have provided a contemporary insight to the thoughts of the research community in the 1970s and 1980s.

The MRC's Topic Review issued in December 1995 entitled *"The MRC's Role and Guidelines for MRC-funded Brain Banks"* provides a clear statement of the Council's policies in the mid 1990s[(1)]. This followed from the work of the Brain Bank Review Committee set up in 1991. The review includes principles that all researchers funded by the Council were required to follow.

Why did the MRC decide to support research on the brain?

The importance of studying the brain and of investigating the causes and effects on the brain of neuropsychiatric disorders such as Alzheimer's disease and schizophrenia, has long been recognised. The MRC's reasons for supporting post mortem research on the brain are set out in the 1995 Topic Review:

"Systematic brain banking has added a new dimension to neuroscience, contributing to major advances in research into human neuroimmunological and neurodegenerative diseases. New treatments of Parkinson's disease and Alzheimer's disease were originally based on discovery of neurotransmitter abnormalities (in the 1960s and 1970s) in post mortem tissue obtained from clinically and neuropathologically diagnosed cases".

The section later continues: *"All pathological studies of the human brain depend on fundamental knowledge of the distribution of key components (receptors, transmitters, peptides, cytoskeletal proteins). These have been mapped over the last two or three decades using normal, banked tissue".*

Historical perspective of the MRC support for brain research

Starting in the 1950s, the MRC funded brain research though programme and project grants, and from the 1970s supported this field of research in its own units. The brain related programmes and projects that MRC has supported are far too numerous to list, but collectively the results achieved have made, and continue to make, a substantial contribution to new knowledge and to improve the care of patients with neuropsychiatric diseases.

MRC support for brain banks

The Corsellis (Runwell) Collection

For consistency in this report this collection has been referred to as the "Corsellis collection" although in earlier years it was referred to as the Runwell collection.

Research on brains from hospital post mortems was a novel development in 1950 when Dr Corsellis began to collect and study brains in the Pathology Department at Runwell Hospital. The MRC soon recognised the importance of this new field of research and in 1953 awarded Dr Corsellis a research grant, Chapter 33.

MRC support for research on the Corsellis collection continued for the next four decades. In 1985 the MRC provided support through staff attached to the Division of Psychiatry at the Clinical Research Centre. The research programme of the Division was linked to studies based on the Corsellis collection, Chapters 31 and 32.

The research at CRC was led by Dr Tim Crow and Dr Eve Johnstone. Dr Crow was subsequently appointed Professor of Psychiatry at Oxford University and Dr Johnstone was appointed Professor of Psychiatry at Edinburgh University.

When the Clinical Research Centre closed in 1994, project grant support for research on the Corsellis collection was maintained by MRC. In 1995 Professor Crow received MRC support to use Magnetic Resonance Imaging on fixed brains to study: *"Developmental anomalies of cerebral asymmetry and corpus callosum in schizophrenia and psychoses"*.

The Cambridge brain bank

The MRC recognised the importance of chemical mechanisms within the brain when it set up the Neuro Chemical Pharmacology Unit (NCPU) at Cambridge in 1971. As its name implies, the Unit was established to research the chemistry of the brain. The origins of the Cambridge brain bank were described in Chapter 26.

The Huntington's disease project, also described in Chapter 26, began in 1970. This project came about because of the freedom MRC gives to senior scientific staff in all its units to undertake research projects of their own choosing in the context of the proposed programme of work approved by the Council.

In 1975 the MRC awarded a grant specifically for investigation of Huntington's disease. From this beginning MRC support for the Cambridge brain bank evolved. The banking functions were formally recognised by the MRC in 1980.

The MRC decided to close the NCPU in 1985, but awarded a five year programme grant to maintain the brain banking facility. This was administered through the Department of Psychiatry, which was headed by Professor Paykel. Other research applications were submitted in parallel, Chapter 26.

In 1987 the MRC decided in principle to refocus the bank's activities on collecting brains for specific projects. This was a reflection of the Council's view that MRC brain banking activity should focus on systematic collection and distribution to underpin high-quality and peer reviewed research relevant to the Council's strategy. Research teams were expected to make their own arrangements for collection of brain samples relevant to their work rather than to rely on brain banks.

Prospective studies at Cambridge and elsewhere

The MRC approved the *"Cognitive Function and Ageing Study (CFAS)"* in 1988. As its name implies, this is a long-term investigation of the ageing process. Cambridge was one of the six participating centres. The MRC changed the direction and emphasis of its support for brain research with the funding it provided for this and other prospective studies. For these studies a research nurse was appointed to the programme.

The MRC carried out a further review in 1992 as a result of which the Council funding for the banking function at Cambridge came to an end in September 1998, but support for CFAS and other long-term prospective investigations is ongoing.

Other brain banks the MRC had supported prior to 1991

The MRC brain metabolism unit in Edinburgh

The brain bank in this unit was funded by the MRC from 1978 until 1989 when post mortem studies in the unit ended. The brain collection was later transferred to the Department of Pathology in Edinburgh where it was no longer dependent on MRC support.

The Department of Neuropathology at Oxford

The brain bank in this Department had received MRC support since 1980 for research on Alzheimer's disease, other dementias and schizophrenia, which included brain tissue collection, Chapter 30.

Newcastle brain tissue bank

This bank had been funded by the MRC since 1980. It was located within the Council's Neuro Chemical Pathology Unit.

Institute of Psychiatry, London

The London brain bank on Alzheimer's disease at the Institute of Psychiatry has been funded by MRC since 1988.

UK HIV brain banks

Three banks to study the neurological effects of HIV were funded by the MRC in 1990. These are located at the Institute of Psychiatry, London, the Department of Neuropathology, Oxford, and the Western General Hospital in Edinburgh.

Further details of all these banks can be found in the MRC 1995 Guidelines on Brain Banks(1) and Annex 110. Annex 110

MRC ethical guidelines

The MRC's 1962/63 annual report was the starting point for the ethical structures that are now in place in this country. It reflected a signal change to the way that research on patients was to be conducted and the MRC was the first organisation in this country to formulate ethical principles to be observed by those undertaking medical research. Appendix

Since that first statement in 1963 the MRC has progressively developed and strengthened its policies on the ethics of medical research. The MRC's statement provides full details and indicates the ethical requirements the Council place on all researchers who received MRC funding. Annex 110

At all times since 1962/63, the MRC has expected all researchers it supports to follow current ethical guidelines issued by the MRC and other organisations as appropriate and to comply with the MRC's conditions and grant rules.

There are, however, five dates in the subsequent MRC chronology that are particularly relevant to this report.

In 1972 the MRC issued a new statement on "*Responsibility in the use of medical information for research*". This provided guidance on investigations involving the transfer of medical information of identifiable patients. It made no reference to research on post mortem material. Appendix 33

In 1985 the earlier statement was updated: "*Responsibility in the use of personal medical information for research; principles and guide to practice: a statement by the Medical Research Council*". Although this updated statement did not mention the use of human material, the role of Ethical Committees was referred to. Appendix 34

In 1992 a further update was issued: "*Responsibility in investigations on human participants and material and on personal information: guidance by the Medical Research Council*". This refers to human tissue although post mortem material was not specifically mentioned:

"*Where the approval of the appropriate local ethical body is appropriate, evidence of such approval must be forwarded with the application. In some cases this may lead to a dialogue ...about whether a particular proposal needs such approval, and the Council may require a letter from the relevant ethical committee chairman confirming that it does not*". Appendix 35

In 1995 the "*Guidelines for MRC-funded Brain Banks*" contained a section devoted to "*Consent for Removal and Retention of Tissue*"[1].

On Coroners' post mortems the guidelines state: "*While HM Coroners do not require relatives' consent to authorise medico-legal autopsies and retention of tissue to establish the cause of death, the constraints on retention of tissue for other purposes such as research still apply*".

On ethical aspects, the guidelines include: "*The requirements for decency and respect for the dignity of human remains are important ethical considerations*".

"*Health Departments' guidance makes it clear that Local Research Ethics Committees should be consulted about proposals involving the recently dead*".

In April 2001 the Council updated its guidance in its Ethics Series in: "*Human tissue and biological samples for use in research*"[2].

This guidance emphasises:

- *"Informed consent is required from the donor (or the next of kin, if the donor has died) whenever a new sample is taken wholly or partly for use in research";*
- *"All research using samples of human biological material must be approved by an appropriately constituted research ethics committee*";
- *"Researchers should treat all personal and medical information relating to research participants as confidential".*

Project grant regulations

The MRC's regulations issued in 1979 state: Annex 110

"(1) If the proposals involve procedures for the removal of human tissue at post-mortem examination applicants are required to confirm they will conform with the relevant Code of Practice.

(2) Any procedures undertaken during the course of a project that involves the removal of human tissue at post-mortem examination (Human Tissue Act 1961) must be carried out in accordance with the guidance issued by the Health Departments/Local Authority".

The first of these regulations was amended in 1983 so that the applicants had to confirm "*at the time of their application that they will conform with the relevant Code of Practice".*

MRC discussions on brain banking

The MRC considered collection of brains for research and banking procedures on a number of occasions. Ethical aspects of brain research, taking account of the policies described above, were discussed several times starting in the 1970s.

1976 Workshop on brain banking

The MRC hosted a workshop chaired by Professor Corsellis on 5 July 1976. This was attended by many of the UK leaders of brain researchers at that time. Appendix 3

At the start of the workshop the MRC made clear "*that although the Workshop was held under the auspices of the MRC, it was not intended that the Council should monopolise brain banking in the UK or be responsible for all of its support financially*".

It was also agreed that "*discussion should be restricted to the banking of human post-mortem tissue, except for biopsy specimens in the case of Creutzfeldt-Jacob disease".*

The section of the workshop report headed *"Collection of brains"* records *"The meeting noted that the major source of supply was the Hospital Pathology Department. Mortuary technicians generally appreciated some payment for their efforts to provide specimens."*

"Coroners courts provided a further source of supply of post-mortem brains. In law the Coroner has the absolute right of disposal of any part of the body, but in practice there were frequently ethical and religious objections to this. These could sometimes be circumvented by the Coroner requesting the further examination of brain material as an extension of his own investigations. There were certain advantages inherent in suicide cases."

It is clear from the record of that meeting that those present believed that Coroners had authority to allow the retention for research of any organs and tissues, although Coroners would take account of the objections of the relatives.

National pituitary collection programme

Chapter 5 outlined the national pituitary collection programme. This began as an MRC-funded research project before the enactment of the Human Tissue Act in 1961. No documents were available about collection arrangements that took place in the early years of the research project.

1977 MRC Steering Committee for Human Pituitary Collection

The legality of retention of tissues on the authority of the Coroner was questioned eighteen months later at a meeting of the MRC Human Pituitary Collection Committee held on 16 December 1977. Appendix 37

A member of the Committee reported that he *"had been approached by a number of pathologists supplying pituitaries who were disturbed by the difference in procedure between hospital post-mortems and Coroner's post-mortems regarding the permission of relatives for the removal of tissues. Some pathologists were uneasy about the situation and were concerned about possible adverse publicity."*

"After discussion the Steering Committee agreed that interpretation of the Human Tissues (sic) *Act was quite clear and the spirit of the act was not being broken by present procedures because as Coroners were in legal possession of the bodies of those whose deaths were reported to them, they were legally entitled to say whether human tissues (i.e. pituitaries) could be taken from the bodies and used for medical education and research.....DHSS would discuss and clarify with the Home Office the whole situation. For its own part, the Steering Committee agreed that the Chairman should write to the Coroner's Association making them aware of the various points which had been raised".*

In this connection Circular HC(77)28 had been issued to the NHS in August 1977. Appendix 5
This addressed directly the question of the removal of pituitaries for the national collection programme. Referring to the Human Tissue Act, it stated: "*specific consent is not required by the Act"*.

At a meeting between MRC and DHSS officials on 17 January 1978, discussion about the prospects for collecting more pituitaries referred to the need for "*Reassurance that pathologists and mortuary technicians were legally safeguarded"*... "*the Council had always understood that the method of collecting pituitaries for the MRC Collection conformed with the necessary requirements".* Appendix 3

On 17 April 1978 the MRC wrote to the DHSS about an approach to the Coroners Society to encourage the collection of pituitaries from Coroners' cases, but it is not clear if the letter to Coroners was ever sent. Appendix 3

At the next meeting of the Steering Committee on 23 May 1978, the Committee was informed that the DHSS "*had drafted a letter to pathologists advising them of the legal position regarding the removal of glands".* Appendix 4

Further correspondence followed and on 15 December 1978 the MRC was informed that the Regional Medical Officers had considered the matter. "*Their opinion was that the problem had generally settled down and they did not wish to draw attention to it again unless the need should arise".* Appendix 4

The correspondence between the MRC and the DHSS apparently ends at this point but further advice about pituitary collection was sent to the NHS on 25 April 1980. This letter was issued after the DHSS had taken over responsibility from the MRC and encouraged an increase in pituitary collection. Annex 23

Review of MRC brain tissue banks, 22 October 1991

The first meeting of this Committee reviewed the operation and procedures of nine brain tissue banks supported by the MRC, and for comparative reasons, information about three other banks in the UK and three in Europe. In their comments to the Committee, one bank noted: "*Although always in short supply, normal tissues were obtainable through a network of links with coroners and London hospitals".* Appendix 4

At the same meeting another bank referred to the need to obtain "*the confidence and consent of patients and their families".*

The Committee "*recognised that Banks would wish to refuse to supply material for uses which did not have appropriate ethical approval",* but made no specific comment about ethical approval for the collection of brains or brain samples.

The Committee recommended that an expert working party should help the MRC set up *"a national register of stored and available brain-tissues".*

The MRC Brain Bank Review Users Conference, 3 June 1994

The Council convened a conference on 3 June 1994 at the Clinical Research Centre. This was planned to discuss the guidelines which the Council intended to publish following the work of the review committee set up in 1991. The conference was attended by the leading MRC-supported research teams and considered all aspects of post mortem brain research. For each condition discussed, the papers referred specifically to ethical considerations. There were also many references to the involvement of families in decisions affecting brain donation. Appendix 4

A paper prepared for the meeting by Professor Eve Johnstone considered in detail the ethical requirements and emphasised that consent was as essential as approval by LRECs.

The difficulty of obtaining control material was stressed at this Conference.

MRC funding of brain research at Manchester University

In 1988 and 1989 the MRC awarded grants to three brain-related projects in the Department of Physiology at Manchester University. These did not involve the MRC in supporting the general activities of the joint programme's brain bank.

Dr Paul Slater was the applicant in all three projects. These involved investigation of the neurochemistry of the brain and were planned to compare the results obtained in diseased brains with those taken from neurologically normal people.

These applications were described in Chapter 11 and were supported by the MRC. Appendices 23-25

In 1993 a small project grant of one year's duration was also awarded to the Department of Psychiatry, the details of which are not available.

Summary

MRC policies, ethical principles and regulations

In 1962-63 the MRC led the way in developing the first set of principles for ethical evaluation of research in human beings. These were published in 1964.

The MRC's approach to, and involvement in, brain banks and brain banking can be seen to follow the general evolution of professional practice over the four decades since the enactment of Human Tissue Act in 1961.

To ensure that ethical principles were observed, the Council imposed a requirement that all grant holders must obtain clearance from Ethics Committees. This was made explicit in the 1979 regulations.

Despite the clarity of the MRC's regulations, this investigation has identified two research teams that received support from the Council but disregarded the Council's requirements.

While the Council regularly updated its guidance on the ethical responsibilities of researchers, it was not until 1995 that specific guidance on brain banks was given. This drew attention to the need for Ethics Committees to be routinely consulted on research relating to the recently dead.

Following the publication of the Redfern Report(3) in 2001, the MRC published further guidelines on "*Human tissue and biological samples for use in research*". This provides a comprehensive and clear set of principles for the lawful and ethical use of human tissues.

All researchers supported by the Council are expected to follow the policies, regulations and procedures that the MRC has developed. Through these the Council has sought fully to comply with all legal, ethical and administrative requirements.

Support for brain banks and research

The Medical Research Council recognised the importance of post mortem research on the brain as early as 1953 when the Council provided support for Dr Corsellis.

In 1970 research into Huntington's disease was undertaken at the MRC's Neuro Chemical Pharmacology Unit at Cambridge.

In 1979 the MRC formally supported the Cambridge brain bank, and some MRC support continued until September 1998.

In 1987 the main focus of the brain collection at Cambridge changed to the prospective collection for a long-term study of Cognitive Function and Ageing (CFAS).

The MRC funded two other brain banks before 1980 and five more between 1980 and 1990.

The MRC was also active in supporting research projects and programmes in other centres.

In 1991 the MRC set up a Brain Bank Review Committee. Following the Committee's deliberations, the Council published *"Guidelines for MRC-funded Brain Banks"* in 1995.

In 1988 and 1989 the MRC supported three project grants in the joint programme at Manchester University.

Brains from Coroners' cases

The use in research of brains obtained from Coroners' post mortems was brought to the MRC's notice and discussed at a number of meetings convened by the Council starting in 1974.

When the legality of collecting brains was discussed in the 1970s, the view was taken that the collection of brains, pituitaries and other tissues from Coroners' cases was lawful. It was believed that Coroners had authority and discretion to agree to the retention of tissues for research and teaching.

On the collection of pituitaries, legal advice was specifically obtained about the National Collection Programme and the DHSS was consulted after legal doubts had resurfaced in 1977. The DHSS Circular issued earlier that year gave reassurance that specific consent was not required.

The MRC's 1995 guidance drew attention to the limitations to the authority of the Coroner to order the retention of organs and tissues unrelated to the cause of death.

Applications submitted to the MRC on behalf of the Cambridge brain bank in 1985 and by the joint team at Manchester in 1988 did not mention that brains had been collected from Coroners' cases. There may have been other applications that similarly slipped through the net.

Future priorities

Research applications to the MRC or to other funding organisations should contain all the relevant information. However, when research involves ethically sensitive matters, it may in future be necessary for the Council to check key features, as envisaged in the 1992 Statement of Responsibility.

The restoration of public confidence must be given high priority. This is discussed in Chapter 46. As part of the process it may be necessary for the MRC to check more frequently on the terms of ethical approval and to make direct enquires about the source of human organs and tissues and the consents that have been given by the patient and/or relatives.

References

1 The MRC's Role and Guidelines for MRC-funded Brain Banks, 1995.
2 Human Tissue and Biological Samples for Use in Research, 2001.
3 The Royal Liverpool Children's Inquiry Report, 2001.

CHAPTER 39

The Wellcome Trust: funding of brain research

Introduction

The Wellcome Trust has been a major supporter of research on the brain for the last two decades. This chapter is included as two research grants, among the many funded by the Trust, were awarded to the joint programme in Manchester, Chapter 11.

Sources of information

This chapter is based on:

- a meeting with Dr Michael Dexter, Director of the Trust, on 14 May 2002 when the Trust's conditions for its grants and awards were discussed;

- the Trust's awards to the joint programme that are recorded in contemporaneous papers.

Development of the Trust's policy on ethical approval

Since Ethics Committees were first established, all researchers receiving support from the Trust have been expected to obtain Ethics Committee approval when necessary, complying with the requirements of the Circulars issued to the NHS in 1963 and 1975 (Chapter 6) without the necessity for the Trust to remind them of their obligations.

From the early 1980s, applications to the Trust were routinely checked to ensure that these included reference to approval by an Ethics Committee.

At that time the Trust did not have any special requirements for research on organs and tissues from post mortems, and it did not provide advice on ethical questions for applicants who intended to work on post mortems specimens. In this regard the Trust's procedures were no different from those of other research funding bodies.

A specific question was added to the Trust's grant application form in 1987 to confirm that LREC permission had been obtained, and the Committee which gave it. This requirement was further strengthened in 1990 when the head of the institution applying to the Trust was required to confirm in writing that *"all necessary licences and approvals have been obtained or are being sought"*.

Policy statement

In 1994 the Trust issued a policy statement on the conditions that applied to all its grants and awards which, among other matters, stated *"The Trustees will consider applications before the consent of the relevant ethics committee is obtained, but no award will be made until it is satisfied about the ethical aspects of the proposal*". The Annex 111
1994 statement remains in force as does the application form.

The Trust recently updated its guidelines and in January 2002 issued *"Guidelines on Good Research Practice"*.

Ethical practice is one of the subjects covered by the guidelines which also address the specific question of access to confidential personal information about research subjects. The guidelines have been widely distributed. Appendix 44

Research awards to the joint programme

In 1988 a three year project grant was awarded to the joint team in Manchester and a second grant was awarded in 1991, Chapter 11. Both these awards were made after 1987, so the Trust would have required written confirmation that ethical clearance had been or would be obtained.

Other brain research

The Trust has made grants to other researchers who planned to study post mortem brains, but has not issued any guidance about access to post mortem material from Coroners' cases.

The statement the Trust issued in 1992 referred specifically to the Human Tissue Act. In doing so the Trust drew researchers' attention to the Act before post mortem retention of organs became a matter of public concern.

The Wellcome Trust Standing Advisory Group on ethical aspects of Trust-funded research

While it has been firm policy since 1987 to ask about LREC approval for all applications, the Trust has its own Ethics Committee. The Committee can be asked to consider any applications about which the Trust has ethical concerns.

Summary

Since the first circulars on Ethics Committees were issued to the NHS, the Trust has expected researchers to comply with the guidance and obtain appropriate consents from Ethics Committees.

In 1987 the Trust introduced an additional check to ensure that ethical aspects of all research applications submitted to it had been properly considered.

The two applications from the joint programme that were funded by the Trust would have required written confirmation of ethical clearance.

The Trust has its own Ethics Committee to which applications of concern can be referred.

In guidelines issued in January 2002, the Trust has further strengthened the ethical principles and requirements for all research that it supports.

CHAPTER 40

The Royal College of Pathologists: guidance

Introduction

This chapter describes the guidance provided by the Royal College of Pathologists to Fellows and Members of the College in 1991, 1993 and 2000 that set out the College's policies on post mortem procedures and reports.

Sources of information

The chapter is based on:

- a report issued jointly by the College and the Royal College of Physicians of London and the Royal College of Surgeons of England in 1991;

- guidance documents issued by the College in 1993, 2000 and 2002;

- discussion with Professor Sir John Lilleyman, then President of the College, and Professor Sebastian Lucas at the College on 23 November 2001.

1991 recommendations by the Royal Colleges

In August 1991 a report was issued entitled *"The Autopsy and Audit"*. This report had been prepared by a joint working party of the Royal College of Pathologists, the Royal College of Physicians of London and the Royal College of Surgeons of England. The report included a number of recommendations that are directly relevant to this investigation.

Recommendations *"concerning the performance of autopsies"* included:

"6.1 i) responsibility for obtaining permission for an autopsy should lie with the consultant in charge of the case. The task may be delegated to junior medical staff in individual cases. Specially trained bereavement officers could approach relatives for consent at the request of the consultant in charge;

viii) the final complete report should normally be issued within 3 weeks of the autopsy, except in cases where the report may be further delayed by special investigations ...;

ix) diagnostic or confirmatory paraffin section histopathology should be done in every case. Retention of tissue for purposes other than to establish the cause of death is subject to the requirements of the Human Tissue Act, 1961;

x) Coroner's autopsies should be performed with the same thoroughness demanded by autopsies prompted by clinical requests."

It is notable that the report of the joint working group emphasised that any retention of tissue for purposes other than establishing cause of death should comply with the Human Tissue Act.

In a separate set of recommendations the report included:

"6.2 vi) the value of the autopsy in medical audit should be emphasised in the undergraduate medical curriculum".

The report of the joint working party is at Appendix 45. Appendix 45

1993 guidelines on post mortem

In April 1993 the College issued guidelines on the content of post mortem reports. This document recommends the information that should be included in all post mortem reports. Appendix 29

At the time these guidelines were issued, they reflected *"best practice"* in the way post mortems should be carried out *"whether funded by the National Health Service, Coroner or Procurator's Fiscal"* and the content of the reports subsequently provided by pathologists.

This document is relevant to this investigation as no distinction is made between reports on hospital and Coroners' post mortems.

A single standard for all post mortems

The introduction to the guidelines recommends that all post mortems should be carried out to a single standard: *"The Royal College of Pathologists emphasises that a single standard should be applicable to all post mortem examinations, whether funded by the National Health Service, Coroner, or Procurator's Fiscal. The major difference between these types is in the frequency of histological examination. Recent publications indicate the desirability of retention of tissues for histological examination in most cases. The extent to which Coroners will support and finance this is limited, but the principle is clear".*

On histology the guidelines imply that tissue retention should be routine:

"5. Histology report and other investigations

(a) Indicate whether material has been taken for histology.
(b) Indicate what other material has been saved, ie toxicology, microbiology, etc.
(c) Record tissues sent to any third party for further investigation, such as genetic analysis, tissue culture, etc".

Neuropathology

The guidelines include an appendix on neuropathology that describes the extent of the examination and advises: *"The brain should not be sliced before fixation. Careful macroscopic examination will often provide information for a preliminary cause of death".*

A list of blocks that should normally be taken for histological sampling is included.

Other appendices

There are separate appendices that do not concern this investigation on deaths in babies and infants, maternal deaths and the National Confidential Enquiry into Perioperative Deaths (NCEPOD). However, the guidelines do not mention consent.

The scope of a routine post mortem examination

In discussion Sir John Lilleyman and Professor Lucas emphasised that the 1993 guidelines were *"best practice"* when they were issued. The recommended procedures had been developed over time. In the years preceding publication the College would have expected histopathologists to work to similar standards although no formal guidance had been issued by the College.

The College had always advocated a single high standard for post mortems that made no distinction between hospital and Coroners' post mortems.

Influence of the College on post mortem practice in the 1990s

The guidelines issued by the College in 1993 reflected professional opinion and practice. The advice was then that all post mortems should be carried out to a uniform high standard. While laudable in the context of encouraging high class professional standards and practice, this advice obscured the different purposes of hospital and Coroners' post mortems.

The 1993 guidelines did not refer to the fact that a proportion of Coroners' post mortems were ordered against the objections of relatives. Similarly, the Human Tissue Act requirement for consent of the relatives was not mentioned. Appendix 29

The College's review of policy in the light of the retention of organs of children reported from Liverpool and Bristol

Before the first of these reports[1,2] the College had recognised the 1993 guidelines required revision. Many histopathologists had been concerned about the legal and ethical aspects of organ and tissue retention. This prompted the College to start work on revising the guidelines in the mid-1990s and, after full consultation, new guidance was issued in March 2000.

2000 guidance

These guidelines are entitled *"Guidelines for the retention of tissues and organs at post mortem examination"*. Appendix 46

These guidelines provide a clear statement of the legal position of organ and tissue retention in Coroners' post mortems. The requirement for consent by the relatives for organ retention is clearly stated.

The guidance includes separate sections on *"post-mortem examinations required by law"* and *"post-mortem examinations performed with relatives' agreement"*. The different purposes of Coroners' and hospital post mortems are the root cause of the objections of those relatives who would refuse consent for a post mortem if they had a choice. The different purposes are discussed further in Chapter 44.

Principal features of the new guidelines

Respect for the concerns of relatives:

The emphasis in the introduction recognises the concerns that many relatives had expressed: *"The Royal College of Pathologists promotes and maintains high standards of post-mortem examinations, and this includes a requirement to ensure that the bereaved are treated with respect".*

Retention of tissue:

Under the heading *"Legal and ethical principles"* the retention of tissues is described:

"The following principles apply to the retention of tissues:

- *Retention of tissue must be lawful, i.e. must not contravene statute or breach a common law tenet (e.g. obscene display).*
- *Reasons for the retention of tissue must be defensible, open, and justifiable in law and in clinical practice.*
- *Unless the post-mortem examination is directed by law, the procedures must be sufficiently flexible to reflect the wishes of relatives, while maintaining standards of diagnostic accuracy.*
- *If the post-mortem examination is directed by law, where possible and practicable the relatives should be fully informed before the examination of what is to be done and its purpose.*

Taking into consideration these principles, these guidelines seek to ensure that the retention of tissues and organs at post-mortem examination complies with the relevant legislation and is professionally regulated to high ethical standards".

Organ retention in Coroner's cases:

"Coroner's autopsy reports should state when whole organs have been retained, and the reasons given in the report. However, disclosure arrangements will need to be discussed with local Coroners who may themselves wish to review their approach in the light of these guidelines. Coroners should inform relatives and advise them of the date when the organ(s) may be released. However, if the relatives declare that they wish to have the organ(s) cremated or reunited with the body after burial, Coroners should make it clear that this would be the relatives' responsibility".

The consent of relatives to retention that goes beyond the Coroner's requirements:

"If retention of tissues or organs not within the remit of the Coroner's post-mortem examination appears desirable, the agreement of relatives should be obtained in accordance with the HTA 1961. The Coroner's authorisation must also be sought; it is only where there are good grounds for refusal that the Coroner's authorisation is likely to be withheld. Coroners may forbid such extra samples to be taken even when the relatives agree, but cannot authorise them without their agreement".

Advice of the Crown Prosecution Service

The guidelines recorded that the Crown Prosecution Service had given advice about retention of *"relevant material"* when criminal procedures might follow.

In these guidelines the College implicitly acknowledged the shortcomings of the earlier document. These guidelines recognise that, while post mortems are a legal safeguard and essential in many cases of sudden death, the extent of procedure can be modified when there are objections from relatives, although not in all cases.

2002 guidelines

In September 2002 the College issued further guidelines entitled *"Guidelines on autopsy practice".* Following from this document, the College will be publishing evidence-based guidance on what should be done in, and retained from, post mortems in different categories of death.

Summary

In August 1991 the report of a joint working party of the Royal College of Pathologists, the Royal College of Physicians of London and the Royal College of Surgeons of England on *"The Autopsy and Audit"* emphasised that *"retention of tissue for purposes other than to establish the cause of death is subject to the requirements of the Human Tissue Act".*

"*Guidelines for Post Mortem Reports*" was published in August 1993 by the Royal College of Pathologists.

This guidance reflected best practice at the time.

The 1991 and 1993 guidance documents advocated a single standard for both hospital and Coroners' post mortems.

The Royal College of Pathologists issued revised guidance in March 2000 after wide consultation. This emphasised the legal and ethical requirements for tissue and organ retention while at the same time maintaining the principle that high standards should apply to all post mortem examinations.

The Royal College's forthcoming guidance on what should be done in and retained from post mortems in different categories of death will be welcome. For relatives who object in principle to post mortems, there will be further benefit if this advice includes recommendations about limiting the extent of Coroners' post mortems once an obvious cause of death has been identified.

References

1. Royal Liverpool Children's Inquiry Report, 2001.
2. The Bristol Royal Infirmary Inquiry Report, 2000.

CHAPTER 41

The Royal College of Psychiatrists: guidance

Introduction

This chapter is included for three reasons.

First, to follow up the advice from the College, which is referred to in the guidelines on Local Research Ethics Committees (the Red Book), distributed to the National Health Service in 1991.

Second, to discover if the College has issued guidance on post mortem research on the brains of patients with mental disorders.

Third, to obtain the College's views on benefits to patient care that have resulted from post mortem research on the brain.

Sources of information

- Documents provided by the College.

- Discussion on 23 May 2002 with Dr Michael Shooter, then Registrar, now President of the College.

Guidance to Fellows and Members of the College

The College has issued guidance on a wide range of subjects and has well-established mechanisms to develop new policies.

Ethics Committee approval of research involving patients with mental health problems

The College has always supported the LREC system from the inception of these committees. The committees have a particularly important role to fulfil in considering research on patients with mental health problems whose ability to consent for themselves is, or may be, impaired by mental illness or learning difficulties.

Although the College had not issued guidance in the 1980s, it had expected Members and Fellows to seek Ethics Committee approval for any research on patients with mental health problems without the need for specific prompting from the College.

1990 guidance from the College

In 1990 the College issued guidance on research in the Psychiatric Bulletin. This contains sections on confidentiality and consent. A section on special problems includes paragraphs on "*incompetent patients*". The guidance emphasised the importance of referral to an Ethics Committee. Annex 112

"Proposals for research where capacity to consent is impaired will need particularly careful consideration by the LREC, with regard to its acceptability in terms of the balance of benefits, discomforts and risks for the individual patient and the need to advance knowledge so that people with mental disorder may benefit".

"The LREC and researchers will find the guidelines issued by the Royal College of Psychiatrists particularly useful in considering these issues".

The same guidance required that: *"An LREC must be consulted about any research ...involving the recently dead in NHS premises".*

Post mortem research on the brain

The College's 1990 guidance had not addressed pre mortem consent for examination of the brain of patients who were no longer mentally competent. However, the principles in the NHS guidance on the responsibilities of Ethics Committees had the support of the College.

June 2000 updated guidelines

The College in June 2000 issued new *"Guidelines for researchers and research ethics committees on psychiatric research involving human participants".*

This report refers to "*archived samples*" and states that all research on such samples must be referred to an Ethics Committee:

"As with any other type of research involving human subjects, approval of research using records and archived samples must be sought from the appropriate ethics committee, which will need to consider the usual ethical issues with respect to purposes, reputability of researchers, lack of inappropriate constraints on publication, source of funding and other matters outlined in this document".

Archived brain specimens are clearly included, although not specifically mentioned.

April 2002

In responding to the Department of Health's draft interim statement on the "*Use of Human Organs and Tissue*", the College emphasised the importance of obtaining valid consent from the patient and/or relative after the death of the patient. The College advice is that there are occasions when consent should be sought before death from the individual himself rather than from relatives: *"in which case, we feel this is best practice".*

What has been learned from research on the brain?

The College is firmly convinced of the value of brain collections and archives, not only for reference purposes but also as a resource essential for the future progress of research in neuropsychiatric diseases.

Another part of the College's response to the Department of Health's draft interim statement draws attention to the advances in understanding of neurological diseases that have been entirely dependent on the use of donated organs:

"Perhaps the first, and to date most successful treatment for a neurological condition is the use of Levodopa in Parkinson's disease. This treatment was developed directly as a result of the early work by Arvid Carlsson (winner of the 2000 Nobel Prize in Physiology or Medicine) and was dependent upon the brains donated to the University of Lund in Sweden. Organ research has been essential to an understanding of the dementias and today, when patients are assessed by clinicians, the diagnosis they receive is based almost entirely upon post- mortem studies.

Research on donated organs has led to entirely new treatments for Alzheimer's disease and Motor Neurone Disease. These treatments were developed from the findings that cholinergic neurons are lost first and most in AD, work that was dependent on donated material...

Future developments in the understanding of neurological, neuropsychiatric and 'organic' psychiatric disorders will continue to be dependent on the use of donated organs"[(1)].

Summary

From the establishment of Ethics Committees, the Royal College of Psychiatrists has expected psychiatric research proposals to be submitted to LRECs.

In 1990 the College published guidelines concerned with research on patients with mental health disorders. These emphasised the importance of confidentiality and appropriate consent. Pre or post mortem consent for studies of the brain were not specifically mentioned.

In 1991 the "Red Book" drew attention to the guidelines issued by the College the previous year. The "Red Book" also required LREC approval for research on the recently dead in NHS premises.

In June 2000 the College guidelines, referring to archived samples, emphasised that LREC clearance was essential.

In April 2002 the College, responding to the Department of Health consultation on the use of human organs and tissues, emphasised that valid consent was mandatory.

The College has drawn attention to the important advances in the understanding and treatment of neurological and degenerative disorders which have resulted from post mortem research on the brain.

References

1. Royal College of Psychiatrists response to the Department of Health's draft interim statement on "Use of Human Organs Tissue", 2002.

SECTION 8

Approaches post mortems and organ retention

CHAPTER 42

Pathologists and post mortem reports

Introduction

One consistent feature of the many post mortem reports reviewed during this investigation has been the almost total absence of any record that a brain had been retained. This finding was consistent at all the locations where post mortem reports were available. Only a handful of reports mentioned brain retention, even when this had been for diagnosis.

This chapter describes why many pathologists, in their reports to Coroners, did not mention that the brain had been retained. It also records the views of morticians. The chapter is based on:

- findings made during this investigation;
- observations of pathologists, morticians and Coroners in many locations;
- guidance issued by the Royal College of Pathologists.

These sources identify a number of reasons that explain why brain retention was so rarely referred to in post mortem reports.

References to brain retention found in post mortem reports

Reports from the Manchester area

More than 120 post mortem reports from the Manchester area were reviewed during this investigation. These were all written between 1985 and 1995. In only two was brain retention mentioned. This finding surprised two pathologists at NMGH who had written some of the reports of post mortems at that mortuary. Their recollection was that they had usually referred to brain retention in their reports to the Coroner. The reports reviewed show otherwise.

Two pathologists at other hospitals agreed that they had not mentioned brain retention to the Coroner when the reason for retention was for research. In these cases, brain retention had no bearing on the cause of death. In the late 1980s organ retention was not a subject discussed among pathologists. The pathologists added that organ retention was so frequent at that time that no significance should be drawn from this omission.

Reports in other locations

Pathologists in other locations confirmed that they had not included organ retention in reports to the Coroner. Two Coroners who had later discovered this practice confirmed this. The pathologists all agreed there was nothing out of the ordinary about practice in Manchester. Practice there was no different from other parts of the country. Other Coroners reported that they had not known about brain retention and had expected the post mortem report to state whenever the brain, or other organ, was retained.

Why was brain, organ and tissue retention not mentioned by pathologists?

Various reasons were offered to explain why retention was so infrequently mentioned in reports to Coroners.

Avoidance of distress to relatives

The most common explanation offered was that pathologists did not wish to add to the distress of the relatives when this could be avoided. In some places it was reported to me that local understandings had developed with the Coroner so that the pathologist would allude to organ or tissue retention by including in the report "histology will follow" or "the results of more detailed investigations may become available", or words to similar effect. This would alert the Coroner that tissue, or an organ, had been retained and that further information from histological examination might become available later.

More than one pathologist reported that they had been told that "colleagues" had been given instructions by the Coroner not to include the retention of organs in post mortem reports. Two Coroners referred to this practice although they had not themselves given any such instructions. These recollections are "hearsay evidence" but in view of the consistency from unconnected sources they are included in this report. There is **nothing in writing** to confirm instructions of this kind were given by any Coroner.

Organ and tissue retention was not an issue among pathologists in the 1980s

Pathologists in Manchester and in other parts of the country were asked if organ retention was discussed by the specialty in the late 1980s. All replied that at that time organ and tissue retention was so much part of the post mortem room scene that it was not the subject of discussion within the specialty. Organ and tissue retention for research and teaching went unremarked and unquestioned.

The national collection of pituitaries

All pathologists and morticians were well aware of the national pituitary collection system, Chapter 5. Circular HC(77)29 issued by the Department of Health in 1977 was specifically intended to encourage removal of the pituitary glands when consent for a post mortem had been given by the relatives.

Pathologists remembered that the pituitary collection programme began as a research project. Pituitary collection had never been mentioned in post mortem reports. This had become part of post mortem routine. The fee paid for each pituitary added to the misunderstanding.

If it was acceptable to collect pituitaries for research but not mention this in post mortem reports, what was different about retaining brains for the same purpose?

Reasons why organ retention was regarded as "normal" during post mortems

Further reasons were advanced to explain why organ and tissue retention was considered a normal part of any post mortem.

Professional training in histopathology

Professor Lucas, during a meeting at the College of Pathologists, explained that post mortem procedures were learned by trainees observing how senior histopathologists undertook the examination. This was, in effect, training by apprenticeship. In the 1960s and 1970s senior members of the specialty had frequently retained organs and other specimens that "*were of interest*" for both teaching and research. Histopathologists in training had followed the practice of their seniors.

Organ retention was in the public interest and intended to improve knowledge and future patient care

In retaining organs and tissues primarily for diagnosis, pathologists had also been motivated by the public benefit that would result from histological or other examination of retained material for research and teaching purposes. The additional information gained would not only confirm diagnosis, but also enhance knowledge and thereby improve future health care.

In retaining organs for research, pathologists had intended to benefit patient care and serve the public interest by improving diagnostic accuracy. There were many research studies that could only be carried out on the organs of the dead.

Consent had been properly given for organ retention

Hospital post mortems

It was widely believed that the post mortem consent form signed by the relatives also indicated their agreement to the retention of organs and tissues. In the 1980s few consent forms made any specific reference to organ or tissue retention. A few forms asked a separate question about retention but most did not. In reality, many relatives did not realise that when they were asked to sign the post mortem consent form this would be regarded as consent for retention. Many relatives did not want to know any such details.

Coroners' post mortems

In the 1980s many pathologists believed that in a Coroner's case the consent of the relatives was not necessary for research. The Coroner had control of the body and could agree to organ retention. Whether the Coroner was in fact asked is a matter that has already been discussed.

In the 1980s, few NHS pathologists were aware that the Coroner could only consent to retention of organs that had a bearing on the cause of death, or as allowed in Coroners Rules 9 and 12, Chapter 5.

One pathologist wrote to me:

"For their part the pathologists believed that once a brain was retained for diagnosis it could be held after diagnosis was complete without informing the Coroner or the relatives. This belief was based on the fact that the brain had been originally held under the authority of the Coroner and was a belief reinforced in the training of the pathologists supported by precedence and established practice in other centres".

None of the pathologists seen during the investigation recalled that they had seen or been told about the Home Office 1989 letter which reminded Coroners that organs and tissues could only be retained with the agreement of the relatives.

The policy of carrying out a "full post mortem"

In the 1980s no distinction was made between hospital and Coroners' cases. Almost all would have been "full post mortems". Very few pathologists modified the post mortem procedure in a Coroner's case unless the Coroner had given specific instructions. This happened in some places, generally for reasons related to the religious beliefs of the deceased.

In pathology departments where a full post mortem was routine, samples of the brain would often be retained for histology. Everyone involved "knew". This applied both to hospital and Coroners' post mortems.

Pituitary collection had served to encourage the practice of a "full post mortem" as the brain had to be removed before the pituitary gland could be collected.

When brain retention was mentioned, why was this not noticed?

Although pathologists provided the Coroners with the cause of death before an inquest was resumed, the written post mortem report was by no means always available in time for the inquest. Due to the number of post mortem reports arriving after inquests, Coroners relied on their staff to bring to their attention any unexpected or unusual features that had not been reported in time for the inquest.

When a post mortem report did include a reference to brain retention (or to some other organ), it was not surprising that such rare references were not always noticed. When histology reports arrived weeks or in some cases months after the inquest, these were frequently simply filed.

Pathologists did not believe organ retention was in any way wrong

It is important to record that pathologists who retained organs and tissues did not consider the practice was wrong. This point was emphasised by Professor Lucas during the meeting at the Royal College of Pathologists:

"Pathologists did not consider they were doing anything controversial or wrong".

In the light of the comments made to me by other pathologists, it is clear that Professor Lucas' remark is an accurate reflection of what pathologists believed at that time. His observations were reinforced by many pathologists during this investigation.

Pathologists have been shocked and dismayed by the hostility the specialty has experienced since organ retention came to wide public notice. I am sure that pathologists genuinely believed that organ and tissue retention for research and teaching was in the public interest and would in due time result in better care for future generations.

Reservations of morticians about organ retention

Different views were held among the morticians. Some had no concerns about retention of organs in the late 1980s for the same reasons as pathologists. Other morticians had reservations about the scale of retentions in certain mortuaries, and the fact that the relatives were not told that organs had been removed.

One mortician in the Manchester area has, since 1990, kept a file with copies of all the consent forms for organ retention signed by relatives. He had noted and been concerned that the brain was the only organ for which the relatives were never asked to give consent.

Another mortician's reservations started when relatives viewing bodies after the post mortem asked about features on the body that had changed since the relatives had last seen the deceased shortly after death. The mortician knew the features in question were the result of organ retention or tissue removal about which the relatives had not been told. In one mortuary, the relatives had questioned why the ears of the deceased looked *"wrong"*. The reason, the mortician knew, was that the temporal bones had been removed for surgical training purposes.

When this mortician's reservations increased at the scale of retentions, he spoke to the Coroner knowing that in doing so an argument with the pathologists would follow. The Coroner put a stop to retentions from his cases but retentions from hospital post mortems continued.

In another location, a mortician became concerned when a femur was removed for research and replaced by part of a broom handle.

Summary

Historically, in the training of pathologists, organ and tissue retention was seen as an important part of the routine. There was nothing exceptional or unacceptable in keeping for histological study any organ or tissue that was of interest.

The national pituitary collection programme, encouraged by NHS Circular HS(77)28, misled pathologists and morticians to believe that removal of organs and tissues was permitted when the relatives had already consented to a post mortem. This policy inevitably led to a full post mortem so that the pituitary could be harvested.

The policy of a full post mortem did not distinguish between hospital and Coroners' post mortems. This would include examination of the brain and retention for fixation in appropriate cases.

Some Coroners left the decision to retain organs and tissues to the discretion of the pathologists.

Some Coroners discouraged specific references to organ retention in post mortem reports. Others preferred an oblique reference such as *"histology may be available later"*.

The retention of organs and tissues was considered to be "*in the public interest"*, but not a matter for routine inclusion in the post mortem report.

Organ and tissue retention were simply not an issue for pathologists in the late 1980s and early 1990s.

Some morticians were disturbed by the extent of organ retention, particularly when the results became noticeable to the relatives when viewing a body after post mortem.

A few morticians took these concerns to Coroners in the early 1990s. Where this happened the Coroners gave instructions that organ retention for research must stop. As morticians and pathologists work closely together, other morticians were reluctant to say anything to Coroners that would jeopardise their working relationships.

CHAPTER 43

The different purposes of Coroners' and hospital post mortems

Introduction

There are important differences between the purposes of Coroners' and hospital post mortem examinations. The majority of Coroners' post mortems are carried out to identify the cause of death, while hospital post mortems are intended to investigate the extent of disease(s) and to confirm (or revise) the cause of death that is already known. These different purposes indicate that the scope of a Coroner's post mortem can, and indeed should, be different from a hospital post mortem, particularly when the procedure is undertaken against the wishes of the relatives and/or the deceased.

This investigation has shown that the different purposes of Coroners' post mortems have been overlooked. The practice of a single standard post mortem has blurred the differences in many places.

This chapter describes these differences, and why they should influence the extent of Coroners' post mortems. Subsequent chapters address the attitudes of professional organisations, the public and religious faith groups to Coroners' post mortems where the requirements of the law properly take precedence over the objections of the relatives.

Historical perspective

The first examinations of human bodies after death were undertaken centuries ago and were for what would now be regarded as "research". The reason for examining bodies was to identify the internal structures, their relationships and functions. While the position of the major organs was known, many of their functions were not; for example, William Harvey in 1628 discovered that blood was circulated round the body by the heart.

Later, when the anatomy of the internal organs was known, dissections were undertaken for medical teaching purposes.

Investigation into the cause of death

The office of Coroner dates from the Middle Ages, when the role of the Coroner was to find out why a person had died. The post mortem examination was introduced much later as a better way of identifying the cause of sudden or unexplained death.

The Human Tissue Act, 1961

Before 1961, in some hospital deaths relatives had little choice about whether or not a post mortem examination was carried out. There were always some relatives who objected to post mortems for religious or other reasons.

The Human Tissue Act regularised the legal position. Since that date, the consent of relatives has been required for all hospital post mortems. (When a death occurs in hospital and the deceased has no known relatives, this responsibility falls to the hospital authorities.) The relatives can also place limits on the extent of the procedure.

The Human Tissue Act permitted the retention of organs and tissues, providing there was "*no objection*" from relatives. This wording, as Chapter 5 noted, is subtly but importantly different from "*with consent*", but it carries the implication that steps are required to see if the relatives have objections to organ retention.

How many relatives were actually asked if they had objections to tissue or organ retention during the period 1961 to 1995 will never be known. In those years it was generally assumed that, in consenting to the post mortem, the relatives also had no objection to retention of tissues or organs. The consent forms rarely referred to retention, Chapter 42. It appears from the recollections of relatives, and of those who spoke to them, that the question of retention was infrequently mentioned when relatives were asked to sign the post mortem consent form.

Until media publicity was given to organ and tissue retention it was unusual for the relatives to place restrictions on the extent of the examination, or on the retention of tissues.

The present position is very different. Many relatives are only prepared to agree to a hospital post mortem provided it does not include, for example, the opening of the skull or the retention of any organs or tissues.

Relatives should therefore always be asked about tissue and organ retention to ensure there are no objections.

The main differences between Coroners' and hospital post mortems

The two main differences between Coroners' and hospital post mortems are consent and prior knowledge of the cause of death.

Consent

For the relatives the main difference is that their consent is required for a hospital post mortem but they have no choice in the matter when the Coroner orders a post mortem. For relatives, particularly those with religious objections to post mortems, this difference is stark.

Prior knowledge of the cause of death

For the pathologist the main difference is that in most, but not all, Coroners' post mortems his task is to discover the cause of death. By contrast, in a hospital post mortem the cause will already be known. If this is not so the death should, by definition, have been referred to the Coroner.

For the Coroner identification of the cause of death is the foremost objective, and the decision to order a post mortem examination is for that sole purpose. However,

Coroners are not obliged to order a post mortem if there are alternative ways of identifying the cause of death.

The Coroner's responsibilities

Rule 36 of the Coroners Rules deals with *"matters to be ascertained at inquest":*

"The proceedings and evidence at an inquest shall be directly solely to ascertaining the following matters, namely:

a) *who the deceased was;*
b) *how, when and where the deceased came by his death;*
c) *the particulars for the time being required by the Registration Acts to be registered concerning the death".*

For deaths where there is no inquest the Coroner still needs to answer these questions, and (b) and (c) both relate to the cause of death.

It does not, however, follow that a post mortem examination is the only way to answer these questions. Nor does it follow that if an examination of the body is ordered there must be a "full post mortem" and that organs and tissues must be retained, though this may be necessary in some cases.

Deaths referred to Coroners

The majority of deaths referred to Coroners are sudden and expected deaths of unknown cause. In the minority, the cause will be known when deaths are reported for other reasons, for example, following an accident or a death during a surgical procedure. In such cases the cause of death is known but the Coroner still needs to satisfy Rule 36 on *"how the deceased came by his death".*

For deaths of unknown cause the Coroner needs to decide whether the cause can be satisfactorily established by reference to the deceased's existing medical condition(s).

In many such cases the probable cause of death becomes clear once the deceased's medical history is available. The Coroner can then decide whether this information is sufficient without resorting to a post mortem. Chapter 44 considers other means through which Coroners could answer the questions posed by Rule 36.

Thus for the Coroner and for relatives the important question is whether a post mortem examination is needed and if it is, the scope of the examination.

Objections by relatives to Coroners' post mortems

A coroner has the authority to order a post mortem examination in any death reported to him. The Coroner's right to insist on an examination is an essential legal safeguard.

As Chapter 42 indicates, however, many pathologists consider a "full post mortem" should be routinely undertaken. In deciding that a post mortem is necessary, against the wishes of the relatives, the Coroner will need to decide between a full post mortem or restricting the extent of the examination. Many Coroners have indicated their preference for respecting the objections of relatives, provided a limited post mortem satisfactorily identifies the cause of death.

Once the cause of death has been identified, the Coroner's purpose is satisfied and so is Rule 36. It is difficult to see how continuing to a full post mortem can be justified in these circumstances. "Routine procedure" and "medical curiosity" are insufficient to justify further disregard of the wishes of the relatives.

The same principle should apply to the retention of organs and tissues from a Coroner's post mortem. These should only be retained when they are relevant to the cause of death.

Chapter 45 illustrates the difficulties that post mortem examinations pose to some religious faith communities. The experience in coronial districts where relatives have been assured the examination will be limited to the minimum necessary has shown that this alone eases the objections of some relatives.

The hospital post mortem

The situation is different in a hospital post mortem. The purpose of the procedure is to examine the extent of the disease that led to death, to look for unexpected features, and to confirm the cause of death. In a proportion of cases the cause(s) will be revised as a result of the examination, but it is rare for a hospital post mortem to discover that death was not due to natural causes.

In a hospital post mortem it has been the practice since 1961 to carry out a full post mortem, including examination of the brain.

Pursuit of knowledge

As medical knowledge advanced, it was found that a better understanding of the direct and indirect causes of death could be learned from post mortem examinations. When deaths occurred in hospital, doctors increasingly wished to learn from post mortem examinations to confirm their diagnosis and to identify any other unrecognised factors that contributed to the cause of death. As a result, in many hospitals post mortem examinations were regularly requested. Before 1961 some hospitals even included consent to a post mortem as a condition of admission.

Many advances in medical knowledge and in the care of patients have come directly from the findings of post mortem examinations. The importance and value of the post mortem and its contribution to better patient care cannot be underestimated, Chapter 46.

Summary

There are different purposes for Coroners' and hospital post mortem examinations. These differences have become blurred by the policy of carrying out a "full post mortem" in all cases.

The distinction is particularly important when the relatives are opposed to the examination.

Coroners' post mortems are mostly undertaken to establish the cause of death, but once a cause has been found, there is no justification to extend the scope of the examination against the wishes of the relatives.

A more limited post mortem examination may ease the difficulties of some relatives who have religious or other objections to the examination.

In many Coroners' cases, organ retention is not necessary to establish the cause of death. Where retention is necessary, the extent should be limited.

The Human Tissue Act requires the consent of the relatives for a hospital post mortem and lack of objection to tissue and organ retention.

The cause of death will be known before a hospital post mortem. Otherwise the death would have been reported to the Coroner. The purpose is to confirm the cause and to find out if there were any other significant features of the death.

Hospital consent forms have in the past not referred to organ retention but consent for this was assumed when the relatives agreed to the post mortem.

The hospital post mortem was usually a full post mortem, but relatives can place restrictions on the extent of the examination.

Enquiries should always be made to ensure the relatives do not have objections to organ and tissue retention.

The importance of post mortem examinations in contributing to medical knowledge and to improvements in patient care cannot be underestimated.

CHAPTER 44

Legislation on the use of bodies, organs and tissues; Coroners' post mortems; procedures and alternatives

Introduction

This is the first of three chapters that address the fourth of my Terms of Reference. This chapter discusses the use of organs and tissues from hospital and Coroners' post mortems for research and teaching in the light of current legislation, and the findings made during this investigation. Alternatives to post mortems in some types of Coroners' case are considered.

The investigation of sudden, unexpected and violent deaths

There are three enduring reasons for the proper investigation of all deaths that occur suddenly after accidents or in unexpected and suspicious circumstances. These are:

- to discover the cause of death in sudden and unexpected deaths;
- to detect evidence of foul play;
- to identify avoidable factors and prevent the same circumstances recurring.

The responsibility to investigate such deaths and the powers to do so are now exercised by Coroners in the 136 districts in England. In practice, deaths are reported to Coroners by doctors, the police, the Registrars of Births and Deaths, and occasionally by relatives.

A legal framework for the investigation of unexpected deaths will always be necessary. At present, within each district the Coroner has the absolute right, subject only to intervention by the High Court, to decide whether a post mortem should be undertaken in any death reported to him.

Home Office review

In 2001 the Home Office set up a fundamental review of all aspects of the role of Coroners and coronial services. The Terms of Reference of the review are at Annex 7. Annex 7

As future arrangements for the investigation of deaths that are currently reported to Coroners and proposals for a medical auditor service are central to the work of the Coroner Services Review, these subjects are not discussed in this report. Some other subjects overlap with the review and these are noted accordingly where they occur in this chapter.

Background to retention of organs and tissues

Historically, the use of bodies and body parts for medical teaching and research was controversial because of the emphasis then given by Judeo-Christian religions on the importance of the body remaining intact.

Before the Anatomy Act of 1832 it was only lawful to dissect the bodies of criminals executed for murder, but not for other capital crimes. As a result, the "trade" of body snatching was developed to satisfy the requirements of medical schools to teach anatomy.

Rather than rob graves, Burke and Hare resorted to murder to provide bodies for the Edinburgh Medical School. The Anatomy Act was the direct result of their crimes. It became law after the execution of Burke, whose body was given to the Edinburgh Medical School for dissection.

The 1832 Act survived virtually unchanged until 1984 when it was replaced by the present Act.

There was in the 1832 Act an important principle that was carried forward into the Human Tissue Act 1961 and to the revision of the Anatomy Act in 1984, that **if the relatives objected** the body could not be used for the purposes permitted by the Act.

Anatomy Act 1832: objections by relatives

Section VII of the 1832 Anatomy Act permitted anatomical examination of those who had expressed this wish in life "*unless the surviving Husband or Wife, or any known Relative of the deceased Person, shall require the Body to be interred without such examination*". Put simply, any relative was given the legal right to object to the use of a body for anatomical dissection.

Appendix 47

The Human Tissue Act 1961

This Act was intended to regulate the retention of body parts from post mortems which had not previously been specifically regulated, provided the relatives had no objections.

In this context the Human Tissue Act, Clause 1(2), refers to the person in possession of the body "*having made such reasonable enquiry as may be practicable, he has no reason to believe -*

Appendix 2

(a) that the deceased had expressed an objection to his body being so dealt with after his death, and had not withdrawn it; or

(b) that the surviving spouse or any surviving relative of the deceased objects to the body being so dealt with."

Similar wording is contained in Section 4(3)(b) of the 1984 Anatomy Act.

Appendix 48

Both the Human Tissue Act and the Anatomy Act clearly intend that the views of the relatives should be sought. When the relatives object, the Acts are clear that these objections should prevail over the intended use of the body or organ or tissue.

Differences between the Anatomy Act and the Human Tissue Act

An important feature of the 1984 Anatomy Act was the introduction of regulations. These require detailed record keeping not only of all bodies and body parts held under the Act but also of the names and addresses of the relative or executor who has authorised the donation of the body and/or the retention of body parts.

The Human Tissue Act does not require any records to be kept.

Whereas the 1832 Anatomy Act included criminal penalties for non-compliance that have been maintained in the 1984 Anatomy Act, the Human Tissue Act does not include any penalties.

The "lack of objection" by the relatives was intended as an important safeguard. Had the Human Tissue Act required record keeping and included penalties for non-compliance it is unlikely that brain retention on the scale discovered during this investigation would have occurred.

Organ and tissue retention in hospital and Coroners' cases

For the reasons discussed in Chapter 43, the requirement of relatives' consent to a hospital post mortem has been ineffective in preventing organ and tissue retention without the knowledge of the relatives. Few relatives when asked to consent to a post mortem knew that organ and tissue retention might result from their agreement.

In a Coroner's post mortem, the Coroners Rules should have prevented retention of organs and tissues for teaching and research that had no bearing on the cause of death.

Coroners Act and Rules

As described in earlier chapters, the Coroners Rules derive their authority from the Coroners Act 1988, and Rule 9 states:

"*A person making a post-mortem examination shall make provisions, so far as possible, for the preservation of material which in his opinion bears upon the cause of death for such a period as the coroner thinks fit*".

To comply with the Human Tissue Act the relatives should have been asked if they had objections to further retention and to the use of organs or tissues for research or teaching, once the Coroner had no further need to retain the "*material*".

This rarely happened. Retention continued, as many pathologists were not given directions about disposal. Coroners report that they had left further retention to the discretion of the pathologists. Pathologists and Coroners had relied on "common sense" with the result that brains, other organs and tissues from Coroners' post mortems accumulated in pathology departments, Chapter 7.

It is no surprise that these accumulations of brains and other organs were later used for teaching or research, Chapter 34.

Had Rule 9 been observed, these accumulations would not have been available for research after the Coroner had no further need of the "*material*".

Alternatively, the relatives could have been asked whether they were content for the *"material"* to be donated for research or teaching. This is what now happens in an increasing number of places.

Consent forms for hospital post mortems

The inadequacies of hospital consent forms for post mortem have already been discussed. The forms used in the past did not give the relatives the information they needed to make an informed decision.

Many members of the public are also now much better informed of their rights.

For the future, the legal imperative for retention of body parts (including brains) after hospital post mortems is clear - **the relatives must give their consent.** The alternative phraseology, that the relatives "have no objection", does not satisfy the anxieties that relatives have expressed. Their trust in the present arrangements has been undermined.

The Department of Health is consulting on new forms that will rectify this deficiency and provide relatives with the information they need to make an informed choice on hospital post mortems and the retention of organs and tissues.

Refusals of hospital post mortems and threats to report deaths to Coroners

During the course of this investigation I was told by relatives of their experiences of pressure from doctors exerted on them to agree to a hospital post mortem. When these relatives refused they were told the death would be reported to the Coroner. In one case the relatives had already been given the death certificate, but had the presence of mind to speak immediately to the Coroner and explain what had transpired. When the death was later reported to him, the Coroner refused to order a post mortem.

While this incident is outside my Terms of Reference, the use of threats by doctors to report a death to the Coroner to force relatives to consent to a hospital post mortem is a form of duress and totally unacceptable.

Deaths reported to the Coroner and frequency of post mortems

The next sections of this chapter overlap to an extent with the Review of Coroner Services.

In England and Wales in 2001 over 200,000 deaths were reported to the Coroner. Post mortem examinations were undertaken in over 120,000 cases.

In England and Wales the overall Coroners' post mortem rate amounted to 23 per cent of all deaths, whereas in Scotland the post mortem rate on the instructions of the Procurator Fiscal was 15 per cent and in Northern Ireland nine per cent.

Are Coroners' post mortems always necessary?

The above differences in post mortem rates pose the question whether all Coroners' post mortems are really necessary. Several Coroners questioned the need for, and value of, post mortems in many of the deaths reported to them, as the examination added little information to that available from other sources. While all cases reported should be considered on their individual circumstances, Coroners identified the following categories of death where a post mortem may not be needed in every case.

Deaths in those with known life threatening disease.

A category of "natural" deaths currently reported to the Coroner are those where the deceased is known to have life threatening disease such as advanced cancer or severe heart disease. If the deceased had not seen a doctor in the last 14 days of his life, the doctor is not permitted to sign a death certificate. The 14 day time limit is arbitrary, but when the doctor knows that death was inevitable, the need for a Coroner's post mortem and the value of the examination is questionable.

Deaths from some types of accident

The circumstances of all deaths from accidents require investigation. Where injuries from an accident are incompatible with life, such as decapitation, the purpose and value of the post mortem examination can be difficult to justify.

The internal examination is of little help to the Coroner in determining how the deceased met his death. On the other hand, toxicology texts for alcohol and/or drugs may contribute vital information.

Extreme old age

The need for a post mortem examination in centenarians was questioned during the course of this investigation, but some Coroners consider a post mortem may still be necessary in extreme old age where there is no known pre-existing disease.

Alternatives to post mortem

There remain a substantial number of mainly sudden deaths reported to the Coroner that do not fall within the above categories. In these deaths, some means of identifying the cause is still required. During the investigation the following options were identified by Coroners and others.

Magnetic Resonance Imaging as an alternative to post mortem

While all sudden deaths require investigation, many will be due to natural causes such as a stroke or heart attack. A post mortem has hitherto been regarded as the only way to establish why the deceased died.

A preliminary trial carried out in Manchester compared the results of Magnetic Resonance Imaging (MRI) in cases of sudden death with the findings of conventional post mortems. This technique is already used extensively for imaging of the interior of the body for diagnostic purposes. Following that study, the Coroner for Central Manchester will now accept a cause of death identified through MRI when the findings are clear-cut. Where no cause of death can be found on the MRI scan, a post mortem examination will follow.

Other Coroners have been willing to accept a cause of death identified by this technique. However, MRI is successful in only a proportion of cases. The use of the technique does not guarantee that a post mortem will be avoided. All Coroners who have accepted a cause of death based on MRI emphasise that there must be certainty that the cause of death has been established.

MRI has been used by the Jewish faith community in Manchester and by others who, for reasons discussed in the next chapter, object in principle to interference with the body after death. Coroners who will accept MRI all emphasise that the option of this technique is open to all relatives who will meet the costs in order to avoid a post mortem examination, and is not confined to particular faith groups.

The potential of MRI as an alternative to post mortem requires further evaluation. The costs are substantial and current availability is very limited.

A limited post mortem

Many relatives do not understand why it is necessary to conduct a full post mortem when an obvious cause can be found from a limited examination. In practice, the main objection is to the opening of the skull to examine the brain when the cause of death has been identified in the chest or abdomen. The relatives argue that the post mortem examination should end once a cause of death has been found.

Coroners who contributed to this investigation generally agreed with this argument. Some had given instructions that the skull should not be opened without their consent when a cause of death had been found in the chest or abdomen.

The concept of a limited post mortem could be extended further.

Toxicology

Coroners often referred to toxicology as "an under-used resource". The findings from specific tests for drugs and other toxic substances are reported by Coroners to be more informative than post mortem examination in some cases.

The importance of toxicology as an adjunct but not an alternative to post mortem has been emphasised in the First Report of the Shipman Inquiry.

A different approach to the investigation of sudden death

Several Coroners expressed concern at the number of post mortem examinations which did not add significantly to the information already known about the patient's medical condition before death. There were often cases where no doctor was willing to sign the death certificate as the deceased had not recently been seen.

A Coroner who is concerned about the proportion of post mortems that yield little additional information to what is already known about the medical condition of the deceased but which cause much distress to the relatives, commented to me that:

- a careful description of the scene and circumstances of a death,
- a meticulous external examination of the body, and
- toxicology testing as appropriate

could provide a sufficient basis to establish that the cause of death was not "unnatural" .

These are matters that are under consideration by the Review of Coroners Services and the Shipman Inquiry, but such an approach would only be relevant to deaths of those known to have pre-existing life threatening diseases.

Deaths in suspicious circumstances

It must be emphasised that deaths with any unusual or suspicious features will always require a post mortem, as will some other categories of death reported to Coroners, for example those due to industrial diseases.

Retention of organs and tissues after a Coroner's post mortem

In all post mortems undertaken for the Coroner there will be some where the pathologist is unable to determine the cause of death from the naked eye findings and histological examination will be necessary. The pathologist must be able to retain organs and tissues, including the brain, in these cases.

When organs or tissues are retained it is essential that the relatives are told what has been retained and why retention is necessary. With this information the relatives can decide whether:

- to delay the funeral so that the organs and tissues can be returned to the body before burial or cremation;
- to dispose of the retained organ or tissue separately when the Coroner's investigations are complete;
- to donate the retained parts to the hospital or other institution for medical teaching or research.

Under Rule 9, the retention of "*material*" remains in force until the Coroner decides further retention is not required. Retention can be extended provided the relatives have no objections, but to comply with the Human Tissue Act they must be asked.

There is an important exception where criminal and/or civil actions may follow. The Crown Prosecution Service has provided guidance on circumstances when retention may be justified in criminal cases. The legal considerations when civil proceedings may follow are beyond the scope of this investigation.

An alternative to brain retention in Coroners' cases

For the reasons described in Chapter 7, it is normally impossible to carry out histological examination of the brain in less than four to six weeks while the brain is "fixed". In other parts of the world, notably New Zealand, the use of microwaves has been attempted to expedite fixation to allow the brain to be reunited with the body within 48 hours of the post mortem examination.

The acceptability of this technique has not been explored among those who object to organ retention. There is, however, a substantial practical objection, as many neuropathologists describe the resulting histological examination as "unsatisfactory".

Organ transplantation

The possibility of organ transplantation when the deceased carried an organ donor card adds a further urgent dimension to the removal of major organs for life-saving procedures to benefit others. In natural deaths that are not reported to the Coroner, the relatives, where they are readily contactable, can give consent to organ removal for transplantation.

Many deaths where organ donation might follow need to be reported to the Coroner. In these circumstances organ removal for transplantation is at the Coroner's discretion, provided the relatives also agree. During this investigation, Coroners who mentioned transplantation stated that they would normally agree to organ removal for transplantation provided this did not impede their pathologist's ability to determine the cause of death.

Audit of Coroners' post mortems

The review of Coroner services is considering how these services should in future be subject to audit and quality assurance.

This investigation has shown that there are no current checks on the standard of Coroners' post mortems and no independent quality assessment of other aspects of the service. These findings reinforce the provisional conclusions of the Coroner Services Review that audit and quality assurance should be built into any new arrangements.

Responsibility for Coroners' post mortems carried out in NHS mortuaries

One crucial finding from this investigation is the uncertainty over who is responsible for the conduct of staff involved in post mortems undertaken for Coroners in NHS hospital mortuaries. While the pathologist undertakes the post mortem on the instructions of the Coroner, the other staff are NHS employees.

In the incident in the Medico Legal Centre at Sheffield, reported in Chapter 36, the City Council investigated what had happened as the Council were responsible for the premises and mortuary staff involved but not for the pathologist.

There is no similar clarity of responsibility where Coroners' post mortems are carried out in NHS hospital mortuaries. In an NHS mortuary the body of the deceased will be under the jurisdiction of the Coroner, but the mortuary staff will be employees of the NHS and the Coroner will pay the pathologist.

While there may be a fee paid to the NHS Trust for each post mortem (or an annual contract between the Coroner and the NHS Trust for use of the mortuary), the practical consequences cause confusion.

Many Coroners reported that they did not regard themselves as responsible for the actions of NHS employed staff when the latter were assisting the pathologist with a Coroner's post mortem, while Trusts considered the Coroner was responsible for bodies that were under his control.

Coroners who were legally rather than medically qualified stated they could not be held responsible for the actions of NHS mortuary staff or supervise what happened in the mortuary to ensure that organs and tissues were not inappropriately removed.

Put simply, the issue is *"who should police the mortuary"* to check that organs and tissues are not retained after Coroners' post mortems, except when retention is authorised by the Coroner and/or with the consent of the relatives?

The responsibility for the conduct of Coroners' post mortems in NHS mortuaries is further confused when examinations of hospital and Coroners' cases are undertaken at the same time or in random order.

<u>Summary</u>

The Home Office has established a fundamental Review of Coroner Services.

Post mortem examinations will always be required to identify the cause of death when this is unknown. This responsibility rests with the Coroner.

Hospital post mortems can only proceed with the consent of the relatives, but the Human Tissue Act requires that organs and tissues are only retained when the relatives have no objection.

It must never be assumed that the relatives have no objections. Some inquires must be made on this point.

In a Coroner's case, Rule 9 of the Coroners Rules authorises retention of "*material*" where this is relevant to the cause of death.

When the Coroner decides the "*material*" is no longer needed, organs and tissues can only be further retained so long as the relatives have no objection. There is exception when criminal proceedings may follow.

The continued retention of organs and tissues for civil proceedings requires clarification.

A large proportion of Coroners' post mortems are carried out where the circumstances of the death may not need a "routine" post mortem. Alternatives to post mortem examination should be considered in such cases.

For other unexplained deaths, the potential of Magnetic Resonance Imaging requires further evaluation.

The use of a "limited post mortem" should be explored where there are personal or religious objections to post mortem.

Retention of the brain for further examination presents particular difficulty as fixation normally takes four to six weeks.

Toxicology is significantly under-used, and its potential value as an adjunct or alternative to a post mortem in certain cases should be explored.

A quality assurance system for Coroners' post mortems should be introduced.

Where the relatives object to a Coroner's post mortem, a full post mortem cannot be justified where a more limited procedure identifies the cause of death.

It is not clear who is responsible for the misconduct of NHS mortuary staff employed in NHS mortuaries during post mortems carried out for the Coroner.

CHAPTER 45

Views of relatives and religious faiths on post mortems and organ retention

Introduction

This is the second of three chapters that address the fourth of my Terms of Reference. The lack of objection of relatives to organ and tissue retention is a central issue for the future and for research that involves organs and tissues from post mortems.

While public attitudes may have changed and many people have no concerns about post mortems or the retention of organs, there are faith communities whose fundamental objections to both have not altered. The chapter considers how best these objections can be recognised and what measures are available to meet, in part, the religious requirements of these faiths.

Historical Christian objections

In the 18th and early 19th centuries, such was the demand by anatomists for cadavers to dissect that grave robbing became common. At that time Christian theology laid emphasis on the importance of the resurrection of the body. Relatives who could afford to, fortified graves to prevent robbers jeopardising the bodily resurrection of the deceased.

The legislation of the late 18th century permitted the dissection of the bodies of criminals executed for murder but not of those executed for other crimes. Murderers were considered beyond redemption.

Attitudes to post mortem examination in the last 40 years

Attitudes of the Christian denominations to dissection have changed since those times, but even in the 1960s and 1970s very few members of the public knew what a post mortem examination involved, indeed few wanted to know. Relatives did not ask what was involved.

Thirty years ago the public were much more inclined to accept what doctors advised without question or challenge. When a hospital post mortem was suggested the relatives were expected to agree. The doctor's opinion that a post mortem was needed was trusted. Indeed, there was surprise and often an argument when the relatives refused to give consent.

As earlier chapters have shown, organ retention was virtually unknown except to pathologists, morticians and the health professionals. These matters were not appropriate for discussion with relatives. If questions were asked bland replies were often given "to avoid distress". The deficiencies of consent forms have been discussed already.

These attitudes underlay the omission of references to organ retention in post mortem reports to Coroners.

When a Coroner ordered a post mortem the only route open to relatives to prevent the examination was an application to the High Court for an injunction. Such applications were exceptionally rare. The High Court remains the route available for relatives to make their case that a post mortem should not take place.

Changing attitudes

In the 1980s and 90s attitudes began to change. Patients and relatives were less deferential to doctors and more willing to question the doctors' views. When a person died, many relatives wanted to know why a hospital post mortem was necessary. If they did not consider the reasons were sound, a growing number of requests were refused. These refusals have been reflected in the steady decline in the number of hospital post mortems that began long before the recent publicity given to the scale of organ retention.

As public awareness grew, the fall in the number of hospital post mortems increased, but it was the report from the inquiry into the Royal Liverpool Children's Hospital, published in January 2001, which placed post mortems and organ retention under intense media scrutiny.

Nevertheless, in today's secular society many people have no objections to post mortem and to organ retention; indeed they consider that post mortem research should be encouraged to improve patient care and treatment in future.

Objections to post mortems

Many of those who reject post mortems and organ retention do so for religious reasons. Unlike others in the community, the faith groups have always known what was involved. Their objections are longstanding and deeply held, unlike the changing attitudes of secular society. The faith groups have vigorously expressed to Coroners their objections to post mortems.

Organ and tissue retention in Coroners' cases

As public attitudes have changed so has the practice of organ and tissue retention in Coroners' post mortems. While some relatives still prefer not to be told the details, the majority now want to know whether organs and tissues have been retained and why, and what will happen to these organs and tissues when the Coroner no longer needs them.

Many Coroners have responded to concerns by introducing forms that are completed by the pathologist at the end of every post mortem. The forms record what tissues have been retained and, equally important, the relatives' instructions regarding their eventual disposal. Annex 113 is an example of the form now in use in one coronial district. There are similar forms used in many other districts.

Annex 113

Positions of faith communities

The Hindu, Jewish and Muslim faith communities are prominent among those who reject post mortems and organ retention. These practices are incompatible with their religious laws and beliefs. The requirements of the faith communities were explored through meetings with senior representatives of the Hindu, Jewish, and Muslim faiths.

The Registrars of the London Beth Din and the Manchester Beth Din, the Sadhus of the Shri Swaminarayan Mandir (Hindu Temple) in Neasden, and the Muslim Burial Council of Leicestershire each provided comprehensive descriptions of the reasons why their respective faiths reject post mortems and organ retention. The faith communities believe, on the basis of their religious laws and centuries old principles, that:

there should be no assault of any kind on the body of any deceased person.

To the faith communities, interference with the body between death and burial or cremation breaks religious law. It is the duty of the relatives to prevent a post mortem if this can lawfully be done. For some faiths, any interference with the body after death will prejudice the future of the deceased in their next life.

These faith communities are not alone in their rejection of post mortems. Objections are still held by some Christian denominations.

There are others whose objections have no religious basis but who believe the human body after death has a special status. A post mortem is an affront to that special status and does not respect the dignity of the deceased.

Whilst a description of the faith communities' reasons for their objections to post mortems and organ retention go beyond the scope of this report, the objections of the communities are very sincere and deeply held. In a multicultural society these objections must be recognised and respected wherever possible.

All the faith communities accept that in this country legal requirements will dictate that a Coroner's post mortem examination is a legal necessity in cases such as murder, suicide or other suspicious circumstances. The faith communities are greatly concerned that post mortems are too readily undertaken when there are no such compelling reasons, for example when the deceased was already ill with a known terminal disease.

There are similar concerns when organs are retained on the instructions of the Coroner and these are not returned to the bodies from which they have been taken. Such retention prevents disposal of the whole body in accordance with the religious observance of the deceased.

It is the more important in a multicultural society that the sincerely held beliefs of minorities, including the faith communities, are acknowledged and respected.

The use of Magnetic Resonance Imaging as a non-invasive method of determining the cause of death has been welcomed by leaders of some faith communities as a way of ensuring that both the sensitivities of religion and the demands of the law can be harmonised where this technique avoids a post mortem in some cases, but by no means all.

<u>What can be done to recognise these objections?</u>

1. Discussion with the relatives about the reasons for a post mortem

The principle must be frankness about the reasons for the examination.

One consistent complaint during this investigation has been the lack of information provided to the relatives about the post mortem. Some relatives were not informed there would be a post mortem, others were told that a post mortem was "routine", or words to that effect. None was told that the Coroners Rules allow them to request a representative to attend the post mortem.

The relatives and the faith communities want to know why a post mortem is necessary, not that it is "routine". Time spent explaining the reasons may not lessen their objections but will help to avoid misunderstandings.

It will not be possible to contact relatives before the post mortem in every case, but when this is not practicable, the relatives should be informed as soon as possible. (An exception may be deaths under investigation by the police where a relative is in custody.)

The simple expedient of explaining to relatives why the post mortem is necessary, and when and where it will take place will avoid the commonly voiced complaint that "*we were not told what was happening and why.*"

2. Why organs or tissues are retained

There must be openness about the retention of organs and tissues and why this is necessary.

The cases in this report show how damaging the discovery of a retained organ can be, particularly when this comes to light after the funeral or cremation. The consequence has been that some relatives and faith communities no longer trust the information they have been given.

There is no easy way to re-establish trust, but there are measures that can be taken to increase the confidence of relatives and to demonstrate to those with religious objections that their concerns have been recognised.

3. Measures to assist those who have objections to post mortems and organ retention

The presence of a medically qualified representative at the post mortem, as provided for by Rule 7(2)a of the Coroners Rules, could provide reassurance that no organs or tissues have been covertly retained. This could prevent a recurrence of the disbelief that has been voiced by relatives whose trust has been undermined.

Where for valid diagnostic reasons an organ has to be retained, the relatives should be given time to decide what should happen to the retained organ when this is no longer needed for the Coroner's purposes.

The retention of "slides and blocks" may be more acceptable than whole organ retention, though not the complete solution.

Practical measures

Coroners have introduced a number of procedures to demonstrate to the faith communities that their religious concerns and observances have not been forgotten. Extra organisation and effort is required to modify procedures to meet the needs of the faith groups.

Reducing delays

For those relatives whose religious beliefs require burial or cremation on the day of death, rapid completion of the post mortem and of any investigation should take place as soon as possible.

During my investigation, districts have been visited where strenuous efforts are made by all involved to expedite the post mortem examination and release the body for burial or cremation. The speed with which post mortems have been undertaken in some districts has indicated to the faith communities that their concerns have been recognised by the release of the body at the earliest opportunity.

There will be a minority of cases where early release of the body is not possible. The faith communities have recognised that, in such cases, the law and the principles of justice must prevail over their religious requirements.

Observance of rituals

For some faith communities, the body of the deceased should not be left unattended and/or special prayers should be said over the body during the period between death and burial or cremation.

Where these rituals do not interfere with the investigation of the cause of death, the opportunity to follow religious observances will reduce distress.

In some districts, when bodies have been removed to public mortuaries, rooms are provided where relatives and religious representatives may sit with the body and follow the observances of their faith.

Some rituals such as the washing of the body cannot, however, be carried out until after the post mortem examination, as any interference with the body could remove vital evidence before it has been examined by the pathologist.

While the washing of the body may, for these reasons, have to be delayed until after the post mortem, there are mortuaries where rooms are provided for these rituals.

Limiting the extent of the examination in a Coroner's post mortem

The scope of a coroner's post mortem was discussed in Chapter 43. The case for limiting the extent of the examination is particularly relevant in post mortems when the Coroner knows that there are religious objections to the examination. Once the cause of death has been identified, to continue with a full post mortem is an unacceptable denial of the wishes and rights of the relatives and an unjustified assault on the body of the deceased.

The fact that the examination was authorised by the Coroner does not justify extending the procedure, for example, to open the skull, if the cause of death has been found in the chest or abdomen.

The need for "consent" is the cornerstone of modern medical practice, and should also be required for carrying out a more extensive post mortem than is required to determine the cause of death for the Coroner's purposes.

Faith communities that require disposal through cremation

The Hindu faith requires cremation of the body but the preferred method of cremation in the open is not available in this country. However, many crematoria make special arrangements for the relatives to participate in the disposal in a manner that is as close to the traditional practice as English law permits.

While discussion of methods of body disposal are beyond my terms of reference, the requirements of the Hindu faith illustrate that in a multicultural society the procedures of post mortems and retention of organs should be modified as far as possible, to take account of the religious beliefs of the faith communities.

Disposal of retained organs

There is one particular problem which results from past covert organ retention. Among the retained organs held in NHS hospitals, Universities and other locations are some removed from those whose religion demands that any retained organ should be reunited with the body or, if this is not possible, interred in a burial ground of the deceased's faith.

A number of retained brains were identified during the course of this investigation that come into this category. There will be other retained organs taken from deceased persons of the faith communities in places I have not visited.

Where a retained organ can be identified as belonging to a member of a faith community, the guiding principle should be that the opportunity is given for the relatives and/or the religious authorities of the relevant faith community to be consulted about what should happen to the retained organ.

For some faith communities organs retained in these circumstances present a doctrinal dilemma. The principle is that the relatives and/or the religious authorities must have the opportunity to decide how to dispose of the retained organ in keeping with the religious beliefs of the deceased.

Summary

There are long standing and deeply held objections to both post mortems and organ retention. These are founded in religious belief in the sanctity of the human body.

Public attitudes to post mortems and to organ retention began to change in the last two decades, but did not become the focus of public attention until the scale and circumstances of organ retention at the Royal Liverpool Children's Hospital became known.

The lack of openness about organ and tissue retention has caused distrust even among relatives who have no objections in principle to retention, when this took place without their knowledge.

Certain faith communities, Hindu, Jewish and Muslim, have always rejected post mortems for religious reasons. There are also some Christian communities and individuals who believe post mortems violate the body.

In a multicultural society it is important to acknowledge the strongly held objections of the faith communities, and make adjustments to procedures to accommodate religious observances where these do not interfere with the proper investigation of the death.

In all Coroners' cases, the relatives should be given an explanation of why a post mortem is necessary and, if organ retention is required, why this too is necessary in determining the cause of death.

There are practical ways in which a Coroner's post mortem can be adjusted. For example, the post mortem can be expedited so that burial or cremation takes place as soon as possible when religious belief requires this.

Organs should be retained only on the specific instructions of the Coroner where, for evidential reasons, there is no alternative, but with the knowledge of the relatives.

The relatives should be consulted regarding their wishes for eventual disposal of any organ retained.

Once the Coroner's need to retain an organ has ended, the relatives' instructions for disposal should be carried out.

SECTION 9

The importance of post mortem research to the future of Health Care

CHAPTER 46

The benefits of post mortem research: clinical and ethical aspects of the retention of organs and tissues

Introduction

This is the last of three chapters that address the fourth of my Terms of Reference. The chapter draws attention to the great advances in knowledge and improvements in the care of patients in succeeding generations that have resulted from post mortem research on the brain. These benefits have only been possible through post mortem research.

The chapter also considers the ethical and clinical basis on which research on the brain should continue in the light of my findings on retention of organs from Coroners' post mortems.

Post mortem research on the brain is essential for future improvements in prevention and treatment of neuropsychiatric diseases and to improvements in patient care. There is no alternative to post mortem study for continued progress in the understanding of disease processes that affect the brain. The importance of this field of research cannot be over-emphasised.

The benefits of research on the dead

Historically, the study of diseased organs and tissues after death has led to greater understanding of the processes that led to death. The findings from post mortems have advanced medical knowledge and the care of patients in ways that could not have been achieved by research on surgical specimens obtained during life.

There is abundant evidence in the medical literature that shows how much succeeding generations have benefited from the findings made from post mortems on the bodies of previous generations.

Research on the brain

In almost all organs disease processes can be studied through removal of small quantities of tissue at the post mortem. The brain is an exception to this general rule as it is the organ of the body least amenable to detailed study during a post mortem examination. The reasons for this were described in Chapter 7. If histological examination of the brain, or part of it, is necessary there will be a delay of four to six weeks while the brain is fixed. There is no satisfactory alternative method to expedite histological examination.

The clinical need and value of research on post mortem brains

In discussion with neurologists, psychiatrists, neuropathologists and many others during this investigation, I have been provided with specific examples of beneficial results from research on post mortem brains. Many studies have revealed mechanisms and processes in the brain that led directly to improvements in the range and effectiveness of treatments for conditions that had not previously been treatable, for example in Parkinson's disease.

Post mortem studies have also led to practical preventative strategies. The head protection that is now worn in amateur boxing bouts is designed to avoid brain damage from repeated blows to the head. These measures, and the limits set on the number of rounds in amateur and professional fights, are the direct result of research undertaken by Professor Corsellis. His research conclusively linked the resulting brain damage to their previous boxing careers, Chapter 33.

The recent death of a professional football player, renowned for his ability to head the ball into the goal when footballs were considerably heavier than they are today, illustrates that brain damage in sport from repeated minor head injuries was not confined to boxing.

It would be possible to draw up a very long list of research to illustrate how new knowledge and improvements in prevention, treatment and patient care are the direct result of research. Construction of such a list goes beyond my Terms of Reference. However, during the course of this investigation I have received illustrative examples from experts who have long experience in these specialised research fields. These will be found at Annex 114, and I am indebted to those who have provided these contributions. This annex can only include a few examples from an enormous research literature.

Annex 114

The value of brain research

This report has focused on what went wrong with post mortem research on the brain in some places. However, there have been many post mortem studies in which the organs were retained with the full knowledge and consent of the relatives. It is essential that the benefits to future generations from such research are recognised.

The observations and correspondence from eminent consultants in neurology, psychiatry and neuropathology and the papers they have provided prove, if any such proof was needed, that brain research in this country has been original, clinically valuable and of worldwide significance.

Brain archives

Another element in the success of brain research in this country has been the availability of brain collections and archives. These collections have been crucial to the success of brain research. To give one important example, without brain collections and archives it would not have been possible for variant CJD to have been recognised as a new disease in 1996.

There will inevitably be other situations where research on brain collections and archives will be the only way to find out if an apparently new disease is indeed new, or the re-emergence in a modified form of a disease that has been previously described.

Without brain collections and archives, research in neuropathology and neuropsychiatry will be seriously jeopardised. Brain archives and the information these contain must be recognised as essential research tools to improve the care of patients. The potential of DNA research on the brain has yet to be explored, and for this brain archives will be essential.

Histological research on retained brain tissues

One particular benefit of archived brain tissues is the opportunity these provide for further research into the histological features of neuropsychiatric disorders. At the Queen's Medical Centre, Nottingham, research of this kind is described as "diagnostic review", Chapter 28. This research has a number of important purposes based on brain histology:

- advancement of knowledge;
- improvement of diagnostic accuracy;
- quality control and medical audit;
- continuing medical education and training.

Advancement of knowledge

Knowledge of neuropsychiatric disease has made major advances through research on histological diagnoses. New disorders, such as variant CJD, have been identified. In future, similar opportunities will undoubtedly occur.

Improvement of diagnostic accuracy

Through review of histology of the brains of patients with Alzheimer's disease, a different condition of dementia with Lewy bodies was identified. This discovery has resulted in changes in the drug treatment of patients with this condition to prevent drug-related deaths.

In the context of particular patients, re-appraisal of brain histology can benefit families when a second related individual becomes afflicted by a similar disease and the original diagnosis of the first relative is called into question.

Quality control and medical audit

Histological review is an important method of quality control in histopathological practice and thereby in the identification and avoidance of misdiagnoses.

Continuing education and training

Continuing medical education and the promotion of good medical practice can both benefit from regular histological self audit. This enables histopathologists to maintain and enhance their individual standards of practice and to compare the quality of their diagnoses with their peers.

Consented research on the brain

It is a challenging task to ask relatives for consent to brain retention, and the sensitivity required in making such requests should not be under-estimated. However, experience since the 1970s shows that relatives are willing to agree when the purpose of the research is properly explained to them.

One of the earliest studies in this country by Dr Bird at Cambridge benefited from the enthusiastic support from relatives of patients with Huntington's disease. Many relatives of patients with this progressive incurable disease were active supporters of Dr Bird's research. They spread information to other relatives and encouraged the donation of brains, Chapter 26.

Since 1982 the Cerebral Function Unit in Manchester has collected brains of patients with progressive dementias with the full consent of relatives, Chapter 8.

Other large prospective studies, for example CFAS, OPTIMA and HOPE, have adopted similar procedures, Chapters 26 and 30. In these investigations the relatives are fully informed about the purposes of the research before they are asked about brain retention towards the end of the life of the patient. Their written consent is recorded, but a further check is made after the patient's death to confirm that the relatives have not changed their mind.

The relatives' support for the research is often indicated by the fact that they are the first to contact the research team after the patient has died.

While the difficulties of obtaining consent must not be under estimated, many investigations have been successfully carried out since the 1970s with the full knowledge and agreement of the relatives.

There must be no recourse in future to collection of brains from Coroners' cases without the knowledge of the relatives.

"Control" brains

Many research teams report that it is much more difficult to collect brains from normal individuals as "controls" for their research. In some places brains of "controls" have been collected from hospital post mortems with consent. Prospective studies such as CFAS and brain banks for specific conditions such as Parkinson's disease, encourage relatives to donate their own brains as "controls" and in this the teams have experienced some success.

While the collection of "control" brains certainly presents greater difficulties, the principle must be the same as the collection of brains from patients with neuropsychiatric disease. **Consent of the relatives is an absolute requirement.**

Past unlawful practices

After the Human Tissue Act of 1961, the previous practice of collecting tissues and organs without the knowledge and consent of the relatives continued to be widespread and with little regard for legal and ethical considerations.

Retention of organs and tissues was part of the post mortem room culture of the time. Organ and tissue retention was not the subject of comment or discussion. No one thought use of organs and tissues was in any way wrong. The research was intended for "the public good". Good intentions do not, however, justify disregard of ethical principles or ignorance of the law.

There must in future be no resort to collection of brains, or of other organs, from Coroners' cases just because these are easy to obtain without the knowledge of the relatives.

Ethics committee approval

In the 1970s and 1980s, with the increase of the role and influence of Ethics Committees, there was a growing awareness in some places that research on the dead might also require the consent of the relatives. This recognition started with research that documented the patient's condition in life and investigated the brain after death.

In the 1980s, the "in life" dimension of research resulted in some teams routinely submitting applications that included research on post mortem brains for Ethics Committee approval.

The 1991 NHS guidance made it clear that all research *"on the recently dead in NHS hospitals"* needed Ethics Committee approval. Appendix 12

The joint team in Manchester continued collecting brains from Coroners' cases until 1996, without the knowledge of the relatives or of any Ethics Committee. In other places the practice of collecting brains from Coroners' cases continued even later, only to end with publication of the report of the Royal Liverpool Children's Inquiry.

For the future, Ethics Committees have an important responsibility to see that consent of the relatives is integral to the methodology of all studies that use organs and tissues, irrespective of whether these are obtained from hospital or Coroners' post mortems.

Research funding bodies

In the past, organisations that fund post mortem research relied on statements by the applicants that ethics approval had been obtained. For the future, research funding organisations should insist on seeing the terms of approval by the relevant Ethics Committee.

The risk to future research potential

This country has been one of the leaders in the international effort to carry out post mortem research in neuropsychiatric conditions. Several research teams working in different parts of the country have made major international contributions.

This country's research potential has been jeopardised by covert brain retention which relatives believe has betrayed their trust as well as disregarding the Human Tissue Act. Public confidence and trust in medical science has been undermined and with it the willingness of relatives to agree to post mortem research.

The rest of this chapter sets out ways in which public trust and confidence can be restored. This is in everyone's interest.

Restoration of trust

Introduction

With openness and integrity the following measures will provide further reassurance and the basis on which confidence can be rebuilt.

Consent by the relatives

The first and essential requirement is that the relatives must always be asked for their consent for the collection and use of post mortem brains in research, including the retention of "control" brains.

Strict adherence to the principle of consent must be the key priority.

In other spheres of medical practice the patient's consent (or, for research involving children, their parents' agreement) must be obtained before any research can be ethically undertaken. The same principle must be applied to post mortem research, except that the consent will be obtained from the relatives after death in addition to any consent given in life by the deceased.

Relatives must also be asked if retention is to be for research, teaching or training purposes.

Consent forms

All hospital consent forms for post mortem examinations must include separate entries for consent for the examination and consent for retention of the brain and for other organs and tissues.

If the relatives ask for additional information about retention they must be told what is involved. If they wish, the relatives can place restrictions on what is retained and the purposes for which it is used.

Referral to an Ethics Committee

All research on brains and brain tissues from post mortems must be submitted to a properly constituted Ethics Committee. The Committee must be given all the relevant information. As part of its evaluation, the Ethics Committee must be able to check how consent will be obtained; this is particularly relevant to collection of "controls". The methods through which brains are obtained must be transparent and open to validation.

Checks by research funding bodies

When an application for research funds is received, the funding organisation should check what arrangements have been made to obtain consent from the relatives and the terms of the ethical approval obtained.

Checks on consent in mortuaries

A system should be established in each mortuary so that a named individual has responsibility for checking that consent has been given by the relatives before any organ or tissue is retained for research at the end of the post mortem.

Record keeping

Proper records must be maintained of all organs and tissues retained whether retention is for diagnosis, research or teaching purposes. Retention must be recorded in the post mortem report. This applies equally to hospital and Coroners' cases.

A named person in each NHS Trust should be responsible for ensuring the accuracy and completeness of all records of retained organs and tissues, and that these are kept up to date.

Reports

Regular reports on the progress of each research project using retained organs and tissues must be made to the Ethics Committee, the responsible NHS Trust and the organisation(s) funding the research.

Brains retained from Coroner's post mortems for diagnosis

When the brain is retained for diagnosis, the relatives must be informed and asked about what is to happen once the Coroner no longer needs the brain for his purposes.

In practice the choice for the relatives is limited to:

- return of the brain to the relatives for burial or cremation;
- disposal by the hospital on behalf of the relatives;
- donation of the brain for research or teaching, including diagnostic review.

The relatives' choice must be unfettered. There will be many who prefer the second or third of the above options; for others, the return of the brain for burial is of paramount importance for religious reasons.

Research on other organs and tissues

The same measures should apply to retention of other organs and tissues. There are indications that given these conditions, relatives will consent to research on brains if the purpose of the research is fully explained to them. In one centre, consent is now obtained in the many cases where specialist teams have been set up to provide relatives with as full an explanation as they want about the purpose of research.

Provided the conditions are scrupulously observed there should be minimal risk of brains, or other organs, being collected for research unethically or unlawfully.

Summary

Research on post mortem brains has led to many important advances in knowledge and to the improvement of treatment and care for patients with neuropsychiatric diseases.

The value of post mortem research on the brain cannot be underestimated.

Brain collections and archives are essential to the future of neuropathology and neuropsychiatric research. The collections provide the only means by which new diseases can be distinguished from old diseases with new features.

Consent from relatives has been obtained in the past and is vital for the future. It is essential that the reasons for research are explained to them.

There must be no return to the collection of brains or other organs from Coroners' post mortems as a convenient and easy source of specimens for research.

Public trust and confidence has been undermined by retention of brains, organs and tissues from post mortems without the knowledge of the relatives.

A named person in each NHS Trust should be responsible for ensuring the accuracy and completeness of all records of retained organs and tissues.

Research undertaken "in the public interest" cannot justify or excuse disregard of the Human Tissue Act.

Ethics Committees and research funding organisations are well placed to review the arrangements proposed for obtaining the consent of relatives.

The benefits of neuropsychiatry research, in which this country has made a very substantial contribution to international knowledge, have been put at risk.

The foremost priority must now be the restoration of public trust that all retention of organs and tissues will in future be with consent. A series of measures are proposed to achieve the restoration of confidence.

SECTION 10

What has already changed and further changes that are needed

CHAPTER 47

Changes to procedures of Coroners' post mortems to prevent unauthorised brain retention

Introduction

Chapter 24 described the circumstances in Manchester through which the joint programme obtained brains from Coroners' cases without the knowledge of the relatives. Subsequent chapters have shown that the use of brains from Coroners' cases for research was commonplace in other locations.

This chapter considers how procedures have already changed to prevent the unauthorised research use of brains from Coroners' cases. The previous chapter suggested some measures that would reduce the possibility of brains being used for research or teaching without the knowledge and agreement of relatives. This chapter sets out other measures intended to prevent the recurrence of organ retention without the knowledge and consent of the relatives.

While the chapter focuses on retained brains, the measures described also apply to other organs and tissues retained from Coroners' cases for diagnosis.

The priority for the future

The restoration of confidence and trust must be the immediate and top priority. The principle is that the relatives must be fully informed, unless they decline the information offered. All discussions with the relatives about hospital and Coroners' post mortems should be characterised by "transparency and openness".

In all circumstances where the Human Tissue Act applies, objections expressed by the relatives must be respected. Their agreement to organ retention for research or teaching must never be assumed.

Brain retention in Coroners' cases

There were a number of reasons why brains were used for research without the relatives' knowledge and agreement.

- Post mortem reports concealed brain retention

  Brain retention was hidden by the omission of any reference in post mortem reports to the Coroner. This was intended to avoid distress, but that good intention has left many relatives feeling deceived and betrayed.

- Ignorance of the Human Tissue Act

  It is surprising that so many pathologists and morticians stated during this investigation that they were unaware of the limitations imposed by the Human Tissue Act and that relatives had the right to object to the use of brains for research or teaching.

- Misunderstanding of Coroners Rules 9 and 12

  The misunderstanding of these Coroners Rules was perhaps the principal reason why brain retention for research occurred so frequently. Pathologists who had discretion from Coroners to retain the organs and tissues that they considered necessary for diagnosis believed that they also had the Coroner's authority to retain brains for research.

  Some, but by no means all, researchers also believed that brains could be lawfully obtained from Coroners' cases without the knowledge or agreement of the relatives.

- Proper use of Rules 9 and 12

  These Rules give the Coroner authority to retain "*material*". The Coroner must clearly be asked before any research is conducted under these Rules. This is what happened before the research studies at the Clinical Research Centre and at St George's Hospital began, as described in Chapter 32.

- Coroners' verbal consent for brain retention for research

  During the course of this investigation, several pathologists have referred to verbal consent given by Coroners to brain retention for research. It has been impossible to confirm these accounts due to the passage of time and the deaths of those involved. There is nothing in writing to confirm or refute these recollections.

  However, such has been the frequency of these recollections that it seems probable that in the 1980s some Coroners did indicate to their pathologists that brains could be retained for research.

- Misuse of brains after the Coroner's purposes had been completed

  Research in many locations has been carried out on brains of Coroners' cases originally retained for diagnosis. The need to ask the relatives about further use of brains was not recognised. Some pathologists and researchers were ignorant of the Human Tissue Act. Others failed to appreciate that it applied to them.

  Brains from Coroners' post mortems were an easy source of research material and relatives were not asked if they had objections to this use.

The current position

Hospital post mortems

Public attitudes to post mortems have changed significantly since 1985-1996, the years mainly covered in this report. The decrease in the number of hospital post mortems shows that relatives are now much less willing to agree to a hospital post mortem.

The reports of the Royal Liverpool Children's HospitalInquiry, the Bristol Royal Infirmary Inquiry and the work of the Retained Organs Commission have alerted the public to the issues of organ and tissue retention. When the relatives do consent to a hospital post mortem, permission to retain organs and tissues is more often refused.

The publicity given to retained organs has reminded pathologists, morticians, researchers and all others involved of their legal and ethical obligations and of the need for the relatives to be consulted about the use of retained organs for research.

Coroners' post mortems

Many Coroners have given instructions to pathologists that nothing must be retained without their knowledge.

Some Coroners will no longer authorise a full post mortem and/or the opening of the skull without their agreement on a case by case basis.

Special forms have been introduced to record what organs, tissues and other specimens have been retained and pathologists are required to complete these at the end of each post mortem. These forms list all organs and tissues that have been retained and why retention was needed. An example of a form in use in one district is Annex 113
at Annex 113.

Pathologists are now unlikely to omit reference to retained organs and tissues from post mortem reports.

For their part, relatives are better informed and ask well-directed questions of the Coroner's Officer before a post mortem takes place.

In many districts Coroner's Officers have been instructed routinely to make enquiries of the relatives before the post mortem examination to ascertain their views on organ and tissue retention. The relatives' instructions for disposal are included in the forms used in some districts.

There are, however, some relatives who prefer not to know the details about a Coroner's post mortem examination. If that is their wish relatives are entitled "not to know". It would be wrong to force details on relatives who do not wish to be informed, but the fact that they have declined information should be recorded.

Possible changes to the law

The Department of Health has issued a consultation document entitled *"Human Bodies; Human Choices"*. This document asked for opinions on possible changes in the law.

Until the Human Tissue Act and/or the Coroners Rules are amended, every effort must be made to re-establish the confidence and trust of relatives within the existing legal and ethical framework. The wishes of the relatives must be respected whenever the law requires "consent" or "lack of objection".

Unless this principle is followed trust will not be re-established and anxieties will remain that Coroners' post mortems are being used as a covert way of obtaining organs and tissues for research. It was the covert retention of brains from Coroners' post mortems that led to this investigation.

Ethics Committees

Ethics Committees have an important responsibility to ensure that, in future, research on post mortem brains is only undertaken when consent has been properly obtained. In the past, Ethics Committees were not fully involved or informed.

- The retention of organs for research

In the late 1980s when research involved patients in life and further study of their brain after death, it was clear that Ethics Committee approval was required. There was less clarity about the role of Ethics Committees in research that began after the death of the patient but required access to the patient's medical records.

- Disclosure of all relevant details to Ethics Committees

Researchers have always been expected to disclose all relevant factors to Ethics Committees. The collection of brains and other organs from Coroners' cases was widespread in the 1970s and continued in some locations into the mid 1990s. Without knowing all the relevant details it is axiomatic that Ethics Committees can be misled.

It is my opinion that some Ethics Committees were misled, and that some of the studies investigated in this report would not have been permitted to use brains from Coroners' cases without the knowledge of the relatives if the LRECs had known about this practice.

The current position

In 1991 the guidance on the responsibilities of Ethics Committees was clarified. This required that any research on the *"recently dead in NHS premises"* should be submitted to an Ethics Committee.

For reasons unconnected to post mortem research studies, Ethics Committees have become more aware of the need for the consent of relatives where the mental capacity of the patient is impaired.

Ethics and organisations that host research

In the late 1980s, universities and other institutions that hosted research funded from other sources left the researchers to decide whether to obtain ethical clearance and did not enquire about the need for such clearance.

The current position

Universities and other institutions have now set up their own Ethics Committees. These committees require all researchers to notify them of applications made to Ethics

Committees and of ethical approvals received from LRECs or other Ethics Committees. For example, Manchester University Ethics Committee placed this requirement on all staff of the University for research begun since 1994.

Research funding organisations

Organisations that fund post mortem research should ensure that any research they support has the appropriate consents. Under former arrangements this did not happen routinely.

- In the 1970s and 1980s not all research funding organisations required applicants to submit evidence that an Ethics Committee had approved their projects. The decision whether to seek Ethics Committee approval was left to the applicants. In 1983 the Medical Research Council's conditions for project grants included under a heading *"Human Subjects": "Local ethical committee approval is required for research that includes clinical trials and/or involves human subjects (whether patients or normal) and appropriate evidence of such approval must be* Annex 110 *incorporated in the application".* These requirements were later strengthened, Chapter 38.

- Other research funding organisations made similar requirements for applicants.

- Despite the guidance, two research teams examined in this study did not in the mid-1980s observe the MRC's guidelines and policies.

The current position

In 1995 the Medical Research Council's Guidelines on MRC-funded brain banks and brain research emphasised that any studies involving the recently dead should comply with the guidance and be referred to Ethics Committees.

The latest MRC requirements were published in April 2001 in *"Human Tissue and Biological Samples for Use in Research"*[1]. This emphasises:

> *"Informed consent is required from the donor (or the next of kin, if the donor has died) whenever a new sample is taken wholly or partly for use in research";*
>
> *"All research using samples of human biological material must be approved by an appropriately constituted Research Ethics Committee".*

The guidance also has a section that addresses the use for research of old samples:

> *"Researchers should satisfy themselves that the samples were not obtained in an unethical or improper way and that there was valid consent to the taking".*

Action to ensure guidance is observed

These statements of principle are welcome, but without back-up are not enough.

To make certain that researchers observe the MRC's guidance, the Council and other organisations that provide funds for post mortem research should put in place their own procedures to ensure the guidance is followed. Otherwise, a repetition of the 1980s incidents in which researchers failed to follow the MRC's stated policies could be repeated.

Research funding bodies should not delegate this responsibility. Provided the MRC's principles are scrupulously observed, research on the brain will only be undertaken with the knowledge and agreement of the relatives.

<u>Access to medical records</u>

In the 1980s there was no specific NHS guidance on access to the records of dead patients, but in 1983 the General Medical Council issued guidance to doctors on *"Professional Conduct and Discipline"*: Appendix 13

> *"the death of the patient does not absolve the doctor from the obligation to maintain secrecy*" and "*information may also be disclosed if necessary for the purpose of a medical research project which has been approved by a recognised ethical committee"*.

This guidance was sent to all registered medical practitioners, but it was still widely believed that access to medical records for research on the dead did not require any specific clearance.

<u>The current position</u>

Since the 1980s there have been major changes in the arrangements for access to patient data.

The General Medical Council has updated its guidance to doctors in *"Good practice in research. The role and responsibility of doctors"*[2].

The Caldicott Report of December 1997, which was distributed under HSC(98)089, recommended the appointment of Caldicott guardians and has set out new requirements for access to personalised data on NHS patients.

The Medical Research Council in its "Ethics Series" has issued *"Personal Information in Medical Research"*.

These documents provide the basis on which Ethics Committees review the acceptability of any research protocol that involves access to medical and/or personal information about deceased persons.

For the future, the Department of Health is consulting on a code of practice for the NHS on confidentiality matters.

Guidance from the Royal College of Pathologists

In the 1980s and 1990s the difference between a Coroner's and hospital post mortem became blurred.

Chapter 40 described the policy of a full post mortem examination that was recommended by the Royal College of Pathologists in the guidance issued in 1993 in the College's *"Guidelines for Post Mortem Reports"*:

> *"that a single standard should be applicable to all post mortem examinations, whether funded by the NHS, Coroner or Procurator Fiscal".* Appendix 29

The current position

The College published revised guidelines in March 2000. Further advice has subsequently been issued in *"Guidelines on Autopsy Practice"* and further guidance is in preparation. Appendix 46 Appendix 49

Public awareness of post mortem practice and consent forms

In the late 1980s the public were very largely unaware of what a post mortem entailed. Many relatives did not ask or wish to know the details.

The current position

In the aftermath of the publicity about organ retention, the public are much better informed about the nature of a post mortem examination. This awareness provides a further safeguard against unauthorised use of retained organs.

Consent forms

In 2002 the Department of Health circulated for consultation a paper with five different consent forms for post mortem examinations.

Before the Department's consultation document had been issued, many NHS Trusts had already amended their consent forms so that the relatives who consented to a post mortem are now separately asked for their consent to organ or tissue retention. For those relatives who prefer not to know the details of a post mortem examination, one of the Department of Health consultation consent forms was designed for that purpose.

Neuropsychiatric research

In the 1980s some studies were undertaken with the knowledge of the relatives when these investigations began before the death of the patient. Others, as this report has demonstrated, were conducted without the knowledge of the relatives.

During this investigation no current study has come to light in which the relatives are not consulted when a brain is obtained for research purposes.

In view of the events of the past two years, it would be remarkable if any research teams today are unaware of the need to obtain the agreement of relatives for post mortem studies involving the brain.

Unresolved matters

There remain a number of subjects on which action is still required. This, the last section of the report, addresses these problem areas.

1. Who is responsible for staff in an NHS mortuary when a Coroner's post mortem is carried out?

- Public mortuaries were and are still the responsibility of the local authority and, with the exception of the pathologist who is appointed by the Coroner on a case by case basis, all the staff of the mortuary are employees of the local authority.

- The position was and remains confused where a NHS hospital mortuary also serves as the public mortuary. The pathologist is accountable to the Coroner on a case by case basis, but it is far from clear whether the Coroner or the NHS management are responsible for any irregularities that occur in the mortuary when a post mortem is carried out on a Coroner's case.

- Coroners, particularly those who are legally qualified, have stated to me that they do not consider they are or can be responsible for the actions of NHS employed staff in NHS premises when irregularities occur.

- Where hospital mortuaries doubled as community mortuaries, the hospital managers did not regard the Coroner's post mortems as coming within their responsibility.

This confusion over who is responsible for staff involved in Coroners' post mortems carried out in NHS premises remains unresolved. This question has been discussed with Coroners, pathologists, hospital managers and morticians. No one was clear where the responsibility lies. Whatever the legal position may be, none of those directly involved knew who was accountable.

I recommend that this confusion be resolved quickly.

2. Training in forensic histopathology

- The discipline of forensic pathology has fallen between the responsibilities of the Department of Health and the Home Office. While hospital histopathology is clearly an NHS discipline, forensic pathology is not regarded as a Department of Health responsibility but a matter for the police and the Home Office.

- The large majority of Coroners' post mortems are sudden and unexplained deaths with no suspicious circumstances. Most of these post mortems are undertaken by an NHS pathologist at the request of the Coroner. The NHS does not pay for these duties and the NHS does not provide training for Coroners' post mortems.

- Training opportunities in forensic pathology have reduced as the uncertain position of forensic pathology has continued since the 1980s.

- The Home Office maintains a list of forensic pathologists who are usually called upon to undertake post mortems in criminal cases. Most Home Office pathologists undertake their duties as independent contractors.

While responsibility for forensic pathology and training for this discipline is beyond my Terms of Reference, I feel obliged to draw attention to the unsatisfactory position of the specialty, which has continued for far too long.

3. Quality assurance in Coroners' post mortems

- The NHS has developed a quality assurance programme in pathology.

- There is no quality assurance system of any kind for Coroners' post mortems.

- This is a subject outside my Terms of Reference on which the Coroners services review is currently consulting.

In the light of my findings, the importance of a quality assurance system for Coroners' post mortems is clearly required.

References

1 "Human tissue and biological samples for use in research: Operational and Ethical Guidelines": MRC Ethics Series, April 2001.
2 General Medical Council: "Good practice in research: the role and responsibility of doctors", 2002.

SUMMARY

Preamble

The Summary should not be read in isolation, but in the context of relevant chapters of the report as a whole.

Introduction

This report was instigated by the discovery by Mrs Elaine Isaacs in April 2000 that the brain of her late husband, Mr Cyril Isaacs, had been removed during the post mortem examination carried out at Prestwich mortuary on 27 February 1987.

Mr Isaacs' brain was removed without the knowledge or consent of Mrs Isaacs and in clear breach of the requirements of the Human Tissue Act, 1961.

Mr Isaacs' brain and many others were retained as part of an arrangement that had started in 1985 when the Coroner for the North Manchester district, Mr North, had agreed to a proposal that his office staff should identify, from among the deaths reported to the Coroner, those where the brain might be suitable for research at Manchester University. Mrs Joyce Langan, the senior member of the Coroner's office staff, had ascertained that Mr North had agreed to the proposal before any brains were retained for research.

This research programme was jointly undertaken by staff of the Departments of Psychiatry and Physiology. The initial team comprised Dr Bill Deakin, now Professor Deakin, in the Department of Psychiatry, and Dr Alan Cross and Dr Paul Slater in the Department of Physiology. For the avoidance of doubt, the programme organised by Dr Deakin, Dr Cross and Dr Slater is referred to as the "Joint Programme" to distinguish it from other research programmes in Manchester University which were in progress at the same time.

It is important to note that there was in Manchester a separate research programme in the Cerebral Function Unit (CFU), which is part of the Department of Neurology, that also collected brains from the same mortuaries as the joint programme. The CFU's research programme had the full support and knowledge of the relatives and approval from the Ethics Committees who had been provided with comprehensive details of the research. The Cerebral Function Unit's research continued during the same time period as the joint programme.

The existence of more than one programme created confusion in some mortuaries.

Discovery of the retention of Mr Isaacs' brain

When Mrs Isaacs discovered her late husband's brain had been retained, without her knowledge, she was dismayed and incensed as the religious beliefs of her husband and family, as Orthodox Jews, required burial of her husband's body in a complete state. At the time of her husband's death, Mrs Isaacs had drawn attention to the requirements of her husband's faith and her own objections to any post mortem examination of her husband's body. The objections of the family had been recognised to the extent that the time of the post mortem had been rescheduled to enable Mr Isaacs' funeral to take place on the day after his death.

Mrs Isaacs had been reassured that contact would be made with her husband's general practitioner, which she assumed would avoid a post mortem because of her husband's treatment for mental disorders in the weeks prior to his death. The possibility that any part of her husband's body would be retained at the post mortem did not enter her mind.

When she discovered the truth, Mrs Isaacs immediately began investigating the circumstances and drew attention to what had happened to her Member of Parliament, Mr Ivan Lewis MP, who in turn raised the matter with Mr Alan Milburn, Secretary of State for Health.

Mr Milburn requested the Chief Medical Officer, Professor Sir Liam Donaldson, to meet Mrs Isaacs. Following a meeting on 4 May 2001 between Sir Liam, Mrs Isaacs, her son, Dr Austin Isaacs, Mr Lewis and officials of the Department of Health and the Home Office, Mr Milburn decided that an independent investigation should be undertaken. It was against this background that I was asked to undertake an investigation with the following Terms of Reference:

"H.M. Inspector of Anatomy has been asked to carry out an independent investigation with the following Terms of Reference:

1. To investigate and document the procedures and circumstances which led to the removal and retention of organs of the late Cyril Mark Isaacs during the autopsy performed at Prestwich Mortuary on 27 February 1987;
2. To investigate what subsequently happened to the organs removed and retained;
3. To review whether similar removals of organs occurred at other public mortuaries after deaths outside hospitals;
4. To examine these events in the light of clinical and ethical policies, relevant legislation, religious beliefs, and the expectations and rights of relatives;
5. To report conclusions and recommendations to the Secretary of State for Health."

The initial phase of the investigation

From my early enquiries in Manchester University, Prestwich Hospital and the Coroner's Office for the North Manchester coronial district, it became clear that the retention of Mr Isaacs' brain was not an isolated incident, but part of a larger system for the collection of brains for the joint programme. The brain books of the joint programme show that a total of at least 311 brains were obtained between November 1985 and April 1997. There is evidence in the brain books that other brains were collected in addition to those identified as part of the joint programme.

Of the brains collected, the large majority (230) were obtained from Coroners' cases. Most of these cases were sudden deaths in the community and a minority, deaths in hospital reported to the Coroner.

Approximately 25 per cent of all the brains collected were from hospital in-patient deaths without the involvement of the Coroner.

For in-patient deaths in both categories, there was no evidence, from the limited number of case records available, that consent had been obtained from the relatives. The collection of brains from patients who died in the long-stay wards of mental hospitals was encouraged. The brains of patients with mental handicap, as it was then described, were also included in the programme.

Why were brains collected?

The joint team planned to investigate the neurochemistry of the brains of those suffering from various disorders, including Alzheimer's disease and schizophrenia. Newly developed techniques were used to compare the results of investigations of abnormal brains with those of people who had died with no neurological or psychiatric diseases. It was the comparison with "normal" brains that necessitated the collection of "normal" brains as controls.

Brains from Coroners' cases

The large majority of the "normal" brains were obtained from post mortems carried out for Coroners, while the brains of patients with diseases were collected both from Coroners' post mortems and from hospital post mortems on patients from mental hospitals.

Sources of brains

Prestwich hospital mortuary

The arrangements for obtaining brains from Prestwich mortuary were made through Dr Deakin's contacts with the consultant psychiatrists at Prestwich hospital and after Dr Slater's discussions with the North Manchester Coroner's office in Rochdale.

In the initial two years, 1985-1987, the large majority of the brains (44 of 58) were collected from Prestwich mortuary and identified for the joint programme through the arrangements with the North Manchester district Coroner's office in Rochdale. Mrs Joyce Langan, who was then the senior member of the Coroner's office staff, believed these arrangements had the Coroner's approval.

The identification of brains through the North Manchester Coroner's office began in November 1985 after a number of telephone calls had been received in the Coroner's office. Mrs Langan's clear recollection is that she had not identified any cases for the joint programme until Mr North had indicated his agreement. Later, on an unrecorded date but probably in 1986, when Dr Slater was in Rochdale to collect a brain from the public mortuary, he visited the Coroner's office. Mr North was not there at the time, so Dr Slater left a letter which Mrs Langan placed on Mr North's desk.

In May 1987 the joint programme ceased receiving brains from all the mortuaries that had been involved in providing brains prior to that date. No further brains were received by the joint programme for the next ten months. This temporary ending of brain referrals occurred seven weeks after the inquest into Mr Isaacs' death and after Mrs Isaacs had written three letters to Mr North to question the verdict of suicide. This may have been pure coincidence, but none of those involved at the time has been able to give a convincing explanation that the two events were not related.

Both Dr Slater and Professor Deakin have stated that they were unaware that Mrs Isaacs had begun correspondence with the Coroner in 1987.

Only nine further brains were collected between August 1988 and September 1989 when post mortems at Prestwich mortuary ceased.

Bury, Oldham and Rochdale mortuaries

The arrangement for identification of suitable cases through the North Manchester Coroner's office was not confined to Prestwich mortuary. After the interval when no brains were collected in 1987/88, the arrangement involving the North Manchester district Coroner's office resumed and was extended to identify suitable cases from Coroner's post mortems at mortuaries in Bury, Oldham and Rochdale. The arrangement to identify cases from these mortuaries continued until Mrs Langan retired in 1996.

North Manchester General Hospital (NMGH) mortuary

At NMGH a different arrangement was in place to identify brains for the joint programme. The collection of brains from NMGH mortuary followed Dr Deakin's approach to consultants, psychiatrists and pathologists at the hospital and a letter from Dr Deakin to Mr Peter Leatherbarrow, the mortician at the hospital, following approval of an application to the Ethics Committee responsible for NMGH, dated 17 July 1986. This application does not mention Coroner's cases.

Mr Leatherbarrow was uneasy and took the letter to the Senior Consultant Pathologist, Dr Glyn Brown, who was aware of the Ethics Committee clearance and reassured Mr Leatherbarrow that the supply of brains to the joint programme was in order.

Only three brains were collected from NMGH before collection was suspended in May 1987. When collection resumed in 1988, the NMGH mortuary was the main source of brains for the programme and over the next four years provided more than 130 brains, two-thirds of which were from Coroner's cases.

The system depended on the mortician, Mr Leatherbarrow, identifying cases where the brain might be suitable for the joint programme.

North Manchester General Hospital is in the jurisdiction of the Central Manchester Coroner, Mr Leonard Gorodkin. The Coroner and his office were unaware of these arrangements as the post mortem reports submitted to them did not refer to brain retention.

Warrington General Hospital mortuary

The third largest source of brains was the mortuary of Warrington General Hospital. While in terms of numbers this mortuary provided only 23 brains, these included 15 Coroner's cases. Many of these, and the eight hospital cases, were from patients in Winwick, a nearby mental hospital.

The arrangement to collect brains of patients who died in Winwick Hospital, Warrington, was made following Dr Deakin's approach to consultant psychiatrists at the hospital. The basis on which brains were obtained in this coronial district is less clear. In 1989 a newly appointed Coroner's Officer questioned the retention of brains for research. He was reassured by a member of the Coroner's office staff that retention was in order.

Other mortuaries

Small numbers of brains were obtained from four other mortuaries. These, with two exceptions, were all from hospital post mortems.

Proposed enlargement of the programme

In March 1995 an attempt was made to enlarge the programme and a draft letter prepared for local pathologists. The draft letter refers to discussions with local Coroners about access to tissue from Coroners' cases in terms that suggested the contact with Coroners was a new initiative. This disregards the fact that, by 1995, more than two-thirds of all the brains collected for the programme had been obtained from Coroners' cases.

Following advice from local pathologists that Coroners' cases would require consent of the relatives, a meeting was set up with Mr Gorodkin.

Ethics Committee clearance

Brain collection for the joint programme started in November 1985, before any Ethics Committee had considered the research proposals of the programme. On 15 January 1986 the Salford Ethics Committee, which had the responsibility for considering research at Prestwich Hospital, was the first Ethics Committee to consider an application from the joint programme.

The application referred only to the collection of brains from in-patients for which the relatives had given ante mortem consent, and the importance of relating post mortem findings to the patient's mental health condition in life was emphasised.

The North Manchester Ethics Committee (NMEC) considered a different application in July 1986. While the application to the Salford Ethics Committee did not mention the collection of "control" brains, the application to the NMEC did mention this. However, the application to the NMEC did not mention that the majority of the brains already collected had come from Coroners' cases or that it was intended to continue this arrangement.

The application to the NMEC and to the other Ethics Committees stated *"We will need to look at the deceased patient's notes at some stage after collecting each patient's brain"*. For the brains of "control" cases, this would require access to the patient's medical records.

When the joint team needed to obtain information about Coroners' cases where no in-patient notes were available, the team sent a letter to the deceased's general practitioner. This letter is notable for two features. First, the letter states:

"These studies have Ethical Committee approval".

However, the Salford EC and the NMEC had not been informed that the "controls" would be mainly Coroners' cases and that approaches would be made to general practitioners of Coroners' cases. The Salford EC was never informed of the collection of brains from Coroner's cases or from other deaths in the community.

The second misleading feature of the letter refers to *"brain samples"* when in fact the whole brain had been retained in most cases. The letter left general practitioners with the impression that the studies met the existing Ethical Committee guidelines.

Apart from the protocol dated 17 July 1986 and a single letter, there are no papers available about the consideration given by the South Manchester Ethics Committee (SMEC). The surviving letter, dated 21 November 1986, suggests that consideration by the SMEC took place after consideration by the Salford and North Manchester Ethics Committees. The unsigned letter asks the South Manchester Ethics Committee Secretary for comments on a draft letter to GPs. The draft letter is not attached. However, Professor Deakin states that the draft letter was approved by the SMEC.

No papers are available to indicate what response was given by the South Manchester Ethics Committee regarding the draft intended for GPs. There is no indication that similar letters were sent to the NMEC. The Salford Ethics Committee certainly did not receive a similar letter as this would have been recorded in the minutes where no reference to it can be found.

The General Medical Council in its Guidance issued to all practitioners in August 1983 had advised that the fact of death did not absolve the general practitioner from keeping medical and personal information confidential, but that information may be disclosed for a medical research project *"which has been approved by a recognised Ethical Committee"*.

The reference to Ethics Committee approval in the joint team's letter, which at best is economical with the truth, would have led some general practitioners to disclose information about their deceased patient in circumstances that no Ethics Committee had been asked to consider.

Between 1989 and 1991 further Ethics Committees were approached with the protocol that had been sent to the NMEC in 1986. No additional information was provided. The Committees were reassured that the application had approval from the Ethics Committees of Salford, North and South Manchester. By the time these Committees were approached, the research team would have been aware that two-thirds of the brains they had collected had been obtained from Coroners' cases. There was no mention of this in the protocol.

In 1991 the Department of Health issued new guidance to Ethics Committees which required them to consider all research in NHS hospitals on the recently dead. No action was taken by the joint research team to inform the various Ethics Committees of changes to their protocols following the 1991 circular, or to keep the Committees informed of the progress of their studies. Had reports been made, the Committees should have been informed of the dependence of the research programme on brains obtained from Coroners' cases.

Why were brains collected without the knowledge of relatives?

At the mortuaries at Prestwich, Rochdale, Oldham and Bury the pathologists and morticians believed they were following the Coroner's instructions as the Coroner's office staff had initiated the process and informed the joint programme of the availability of each brain. The Coroner's Officers in this district were also aware that the instruction had originated from the Coroner's office. The staff did not question the collection of brains, authorised by the Coroner.

The morticians at Prestwich, Bury, Rochdale and NMGH were well aware that in hospital cases the consent of the relatives was required. In Coroners' post mortems, however, the morticians believed that consent of the relatives was not needed, as the Coroner's authority was all that was required. At the mortuary at NMGH the pathologists and the mortician had been further reassured by the documentation provided by the joint research team which indicated the research had been approved by the Ethics Committee.

These mortuaries had since 1982 been collecting brains with consent from the relatives for the research programme of the Cerebral Function Unit. The CFU research had Ethics Committee approval, as it involved assessment of the patients in life and study of the brain after death if the relatives agreed.

Not all the CFU patients had a post mortem examination and for those that did not, the morticians were asked to remove the brain without the supervision of a pathologist. The morticians meticulously checked each patient's notes to ensure a consent form had been completed before they removed the brain.

Fees to morticians

Morticians in the 1980s were accustomed to receiving fees. These had been paid since the 1960s for the National Pituitary Collection Programme. They also received fees from pathologists for each Coroner's post mortem with which they assisted. Fees to morticians had previously been paid for brains supplied to the Anatomy Department of Manchester University.

From the start of the joint programme, morticians were offered a fee for each brain collected. Dr Deakin wrote to Mr Leatherbarrow at NMGH in 1986 suggesting up to two brains per week might be provided: *"We can arrange payment of £10 per brain before tax, which is deducted at source"*.

Although the offer of a fee is not in itself remarkable, the level set was interpreted by at least one mortician (at another hospital) as an inducement to encourage provision of a regular supply of brains.

It is notable that no fee was paid for brains collected for the Cerebral Function Unit research programme, although the removal of brains involved the mortician in additional work. On occasion, morticians were asked to attend the mortuary in the middle of the night to remove brains for the CFU programme.

The morticians' employers were unaware of the fee arrangements which, in one instance, paid the mortician over £400 in a period of 12 months.

<u>How did Prestwich mortuary become involved?</u>

From the early 1970s, Dr Bird in the Cambridge brain bank was actively collecting brains of patients with Huntington's disease. For this pioneering programme, Dr Bird had the enthusiastic support of the relatives of patients with this progressive, incurable disease. Through these relatives, pathologists throughout the country became aware of the programme, and Dr Bird was offered brains, with consent, from many parts of the country.

In 1972 Dr Rockley, a Consultant Psychiatrist at Prestwich Hospital, who had heard about this research, wrote to Dr Bird. Following from this contact, in April 1973 the first brain from a patient with Huntington's disease was referred by the pathologist at Prestwich Hospital to the Cambridge brain bank.

Over the next 13 years the brains of 28 patients were referred from Prestwich mortuary to the Cambridge brain bank. The first referrals were brains of patients with Huntington's disease that were sent, with consent and the full support of relatives. Later, brains of patients with schizophrenia were also referred by pathologists. In patients whose deaths had been reported to the Coroner, the referral of the brain was made by the pathologist without reference to the North Manchester Coroner's office.

By 1985 the pattern of referral by pathologists between Prestwich mortuary and the Cambridge brain bank was well established and only brains that matched the specification set out in protocols distributed by the Cambridge brain bank were referred to the bank. No "normal" brains were referred from Prestwich mortuary to the Cambridge brain bank.

The case notes of the last case referred from Prestwich mortuary to the Cambridge brain bank include a note giving the telephone number of the North Manchester Coroner's office and Mrs Langan's name as the contact point for further details, but the staff of the Coroner's office were not involved in the referral to Cambridge.

Dr Deakin, Dr Cross and Dr Slater visited Prestwich Hospital and mortuary in 1985. Dr Deakin suggests the date was either 19 or 22 April, although this date is unconfirmed. The team travelled in Dr Deakin's Vauxhall car. The visit was to meet the consultant psychiatrists at the hospital and explain the research programme to them. The team also visited the mortuary. They did not meet Dr Farrand, the pathologist who undertook most of the Coroner's post mortems at Prestwich in the late 1980s, but did see the mortician Mr Walkden. The visit is remembered by others at Prestwich Hospital.

How did the Coroner's office become involved?

I have been unable to discover when in 1985 the first contact was made between the joint research team and the North Manchester Coroner's office in Rochdale. There are no extant documents. The Coroner's office has been searched but no trace of any letters or other written evidence of the arrangement has been found.

It is clear, however, from the recollections of Dr Slater and Mrs Langan that there were a series of telephone calls between them initiated by Dr Slater.

Both Mrs Langan and Dr Slater remember these calls but not the dates. During these telephone calls Dr Slater asked Mrs Langan about the possibility of brains being obtained for the joint programme, with the agreement of the Coroner. Dr Slater did not speak to the Coroner.

Mrs Langan's recollection is that the calls were made before any Coroner's cases were identified to the research programme. Mrs Langan remembers that the phone calls were followed some time later by a visit from Dr Slater to the Coroner's office in Rochdale. Mr North was not in the office. Mrs Langan remembers that Dr Slater left a letter, which she had typed for Dr Slater, for Mr North's consideration.

The date of Dr Slater's visit remains uncertain but is remembered by other members of the office staff.

Mrs Langan states that, in keeping with the procedures in the Coroner's office at the time, she and other members of the Coroner's office staff would have taken no action without the agreement of the Coroner. She assures me that no cases were identified to the joint programme until Mr North had indicated that he agreed to the proposals Dr Slater had made in his telephone calls.

Dr Slater's recollections of the telephone calls and of details of his visit to the Coroner's office are less definite. Dr Slater remembers he left a letter for Mr North after his visit to the Coroner's office, but states that he never received a reply. Dr Slater is certain his visit was not in 1985 but later, perhaps as late as 1988. Dr Slater is clear that brains had already been identified by the Coroner's office before his visit to the office in Rochdale. The entries in the first of the brain books serve to confirm this.

In the absence of any contemporaneous data, I cannot be sure when the arrangement began or of the date of Dr Slater's visit to the Coroner's office. The available information suggests this was probably in 1986.

What is clear is that from the start of the joint programme on 1 November 1985 there was a steady flow of referrals to the programme from the Coroner's office.

The Coroners

Mr Bryan North – North Manchester (1978-1994)

None of the post mortem reports submitted to Mr North makes any reference to retention of the brain. However, the fact that brains were being retained was well known by all members of his office staff.

Mr North assures me that he did not know. He has provided me with copies of letters he wrote before and after Mr Isaacs' brain was retained in 1987. These letters spell out in clear terms the requirements of the law and state that the consent of the relatives must be obtained if the brain is to be retained for research purposes.

I find it hard to believe that Mr North was completely unaware of the activities of his staff over a ten-year period from 1985-1994.

Mr North resigned as Coroner in June 1994 on the grounds of ill health and his deputy, Mr Barrie Williams, filled the post on an interim basis until formally appointed in 1995.

Mr Leonard Gorodkin – Central Manchester (from 1978)

Although the largest number of brains was obtained for the programme from Coroner's cases in NMGH, I am satisfied that Mr Gorodkin and his staff were completely unaware of what was happening. Mr Gorodkin had made his position on organ retention clear to his pathologists and staff for many years. Mr Gorodkin has only authorised the retention of any organ for examination in order to establish the cause of death. If any organ is required for any other purpose, there would have to be consent of the next of kin.

I have examined more than 50 of the 100 Coroner's cases from NMGH submitted to Mr Gorodkin and, with a single exception, there was no mention that brains had been retained for research purposes. In view of the number of post mortem reports received, Mr Gorodkin relied on his office staff to scrutinise these and alert him to unexpected particulars.

The first occasion Mr Gorodkin could have become aware of the joint programme was during the meeting held at Professor Deakin's request on 26 June 1995.

The late Mr Hibbert – Cheshire (1988-1992)

Mr Hibbert's office staff were aware that brains were collected for research at Manchester University. When questioned by the new Coroner's Officer in 1989, they had reassured him that the brain could be retained. There is nothing to suggest Mr Hibbert was aware that brains were going to Manchester University for unconsented research. I have examined all the post mortem reports provided by the Coroner's office of the cases from Warrington General Hospital. None includes any reference to retention of the brain.

Mr Barrie Williams – North Manchester (from 1995)

After Mr Williams was appointed Coroner, the identification of suitable cases to the joint programme was a well established routine in the office, but by 1995 the number of brains identified in the Coroner's office was small compared with earlier years. Mr Williams assures me that he was totally unaware of the long-standing arrangements. Nothing was said to me by any of his staff to the contrary.

Pathologists

Examination of the post mortem reports provided for the Coroners in Manchester, North Manchester and Cheshire districts showed that, with two exceptions, these contained no mention of retention of the brains. This finding came initially as a surprise to me, as the removal of a major organ for research or for diagnostic purposes would appear to be a significant feature of the examination.

Discussion with Dr Farrand, who had carried out the post mortem on Mr Isaacs, and with other pathologists in the Manchester area, indicated that this omission did not surprise them. The removal of brains and other organs was so frequent in the 1980s that it was not a matter of comment or discussion among pathologists at the time.

There are a number of explanations for this lack of reference to organ retention.

First, before the Human Tissue Act in 1961, pathologists had been used to removing organs at post mortems that appeared to be of interest for research or teaching purposes. This practice had continued during the 1960s, little influenced by the Human Tissue Act.

Second, pathologists carrying out post mortems were trained by their seniors and followed their example and the practices of earlier years set by their seniors.

Third, some pathologists were reportedly asked by Coroners not to distress relatives by referring in their post mortem reports specifically to the retention of organs. There is nothing in writing to confirm that such instructions were given, but avoidance of distress of the relatives was so frequently mentioned that I am satisfied some Coroners did ask pathologists to refrain from mentioning organ and tissue retention in their post mortem reports.

Fourth, it is noteworthy that Schedule 10 of the Coroners Rules, which sets out the format for the post mortem examination report, refers obliquely to organ or tissue retention. The schedule does not require a list of organs and tissues that have been retained.

The Guidelines for Post Mortem Reports, issued by the Royal College of Pathologists in August 1993, recommend that the post mortem report should indicate whether material has been taken for histology and what other material has been saved. The College's 1993 Guidelines were based on best practice during previous years.

While brain retention was not overtly reported to the Coroners in and near Manchester, the practice was no different from that in other parts of the country.

Brains were very widely retained after Coroners' post mortems both for diagnosis and for use in research without any reference to retention being made in the post mortem reports sent to Coroners.

Morticians and Coroner's Officers

The morticians who put aside brains from Coroners' cases for the joint programme in North Manchester were under the impression that the instructions had come from the Coroner. At least one of the morticians became concerned that the relatives were in ignorance, but believed the Coroner's authority was sufficient.

For similar reasons, the Coroner's Officers in the North Manchester district were misled. However, a newly appointed Coroner's Officer in the Cheshire district questioned the retention of a brain on the first occasion he became aware of the system. The Coroner's Officer was wrongly reassured.

In the Central Manchester district the position of the mortician, Mr Leatherbarrow, has already been described. The Coroner's Officers and staff of Mr Gorodkin's office were unaware of the large number of brains that were being collected for research.

NHS authorities

All the mortuaries that provided brains for the programmes were in NHS hospitals with the exception of the Rochdale public mortuary. Hospital cases were referred to Rochdale mortuary as no post mortems were carried out at Birch Hill Hospital during the period in question.

The NHS authorities were unaware of the collection of brains for research from Coroners' cases, including those of deaths among inpatients that had been reported to the Coroner for other reasons.

What happened to the brains collected in the joint programme?

Most of the brains collected were used for the joint research programme. During the research procedures, the brain substance and structure were lost, so that at the end of the procedure there was no residue for disposal.

Some brains that were collected were not used in the research programme, as investigations of the deceased's medical history showed that they had not suffered from the neuropsychiatric disease for which their brain had been obtained, or, in the case of "controls", that the medical history was unavailable or indicated some previous mental illness. Brains unsuitable for use in the research programme and brain tissues not used for research were disposed of by incineration as clinical waste.

A small number of brains unsuitable for study in the joint programme were transferred to research teams in other locations. On three occasions samples of brain were provided for research carried out with pharmaceutical companies.

In no cases were the brains returned to the family for burial.

What happened to Mr Isaacs' brain?

This investigation started with the retention of Mr Isaacs' brain; it is therefore important to record my findings of what happened in his particular case.

The brain books of the joint programme indicate that Mr Isaacs' brain was not used for research as Dr Rosenberg, Mr Isaacs' general practitioner, did not provide any information about Mr Isaacs' previous health.

Two members of the research team recalled that a number of brains were disposed of in approximately 1993. Their conclusion was that Mr Isaacs' brain had been disposed of at that date. There is, however, no written evidence of this.

It was important to ensure that Mr Isaacs' brain had not been transferred for research, either to another research team in Manchester or to teams in other parts of the country that had received a small number of brains collected by the joint programme.

The records of other brain collections in Manchester were checked. There is no record in any of these to suggest Mr Isaacs' brain was transferred.

There are also references in the joint programme brain books to seven other locations or individuals who might have received Mr Isaacs' brain. These were all visited and their records checked. There is no record of Mr Isaacs' brain being transferred elsewhere.

Other research records in Manchester University were examined to see if any other organs of Mr Isaacs had been retained. Nothing was found in any of these checks to suggest that any of Mr Isaacs' other organs were transferred elsewhere. This point confirms the recollections of Dr Farrand, the pathologist, and Mr Walkden, the mortician, who were present at the post mortem examination.

My conclusion is that Mr Isaacs' brain was disposed of after it was decided that it could not be used in the research programme. None of his other organs was retained for research.

The wider scope of the investigation

In the next phase it was necessary to investigate whether brains had been collected in other locations for research without the knowledge of the relatives. The Census of retained organs carried out by the Chief Medical Officer in 2000 had shown that brain retention was widespread in the years 1970-1999.

In view of the large number of NHS hospitals that had reported collections of brains during the Census, it was decided to focus the investigation on the universities and NHS Trusts that had had some contact with the joint programme in Manchester, as indicated by entries in the brain books. Within the time scale of the investigation, it was simply not possible to visit every location that had reported a collection of retained brains in the CMO's Census.

Different types of brain collections and brain archives

The wider phase of the investigation showed there are three types of collection that include brains from Coroners' cases, unknown to the relatives.

Brains specifically collected for research

These collections are few in number and are distinguished from the other collections by the fact that the brains were obtained solely for research. There was no prior intention to carry out any diagnostic procedure or to inform the Coroner of the results of the research investigations. Many of the brains obtained from the joint programme in Manchester were in this category, as were some of the brains collected by the brain bank in Cambridge.

Brains initially collected for diagnostic purposes, but later used for research

These collections include by far the largest number of brains held in the centres that I have investigated. The brains were referred for histological examination from hospital and Coroners' post mortems. Once the histological examination had been concluded the brains were set aside, but at a later date were used in research studies. Some of these studies had a direct relevance to the disease or condition from which the deceased had suffered, but this was not necessarily always so.

A diagnostic report would have been made available to the referring doctor in the case of a hospital post mortem, or to the Coroner as appropriate, but the results of the research investigation would not be sent to the referring doctor or to the Coroner.

Accumulations of brains

The third type of brain collection are those where brains initially referred for diagnosis are set aside once the diagnostic process is completed. Over time, more and more brains have accumulated without any research or other use being intended.

Some accumulations have occurred simply because neither the Coroner nor the pathologists gave instructions regarding disposal of these brains.

In practice, many brain collections include brains from the latter two categories. However, the important difference between the first category and the other two is that the sole reason for retaining the brain was for research (or, in some locations, for teaching use).

Did research on brains take place elsewhere without the knowledge of the relatives?

As a direct result of the findings in Manchester, it was necessary to follow up the brains transferred from Prestwich mortuary to the Cambridge brain bank to see if there was a link to the North Manchester Coroner's office. I am satisfied that the Coroner's office was not involved in the referral of brains to Cambridge.

Other brain collections that had a direct link to the joint team were at the Clinical Research Centre at Northwick Park (now closed), Oxford, St George's Hospital in London and the Corsellis collection, now held at the West London NHS Mental Health Trust.

During the investigation I was approached by relatives who believed that organs had been retained during Coroners' post mortems in other locations, including Nottingham and London.

A series of visits demonstrated that research on brains retained in the first two categories described above was frequently undertaken, but the circumstances of these studies varied widely.

The responses to the questionnaires from centres that held brain collections and archives but which I have not visited, show that the retention of brains from Coroners' cases was very widespread. In only four locations were any attempts made to obtain consent from the relatives, and these were sporadic.

The Cambridge brain bank

This brain bank was one of the first in the world to be set up, and started as a result of the interest of Dr E D Bird in researching the brains of patients with Huntington's disease. This programme, which began in 1970, had the enthusiastic support of the relatives who encouraged other relatives to contact Dr Bird whenever the death of a patient with Huntington's disease occurred.

Dr Bird's programme took place within a research unit supported by the Medical Research Council (MRC). The programme evolved so that in 1985 the MRC awarded a major programme grant for the banking of brains and brain tissues. The brain bank was expected to supply other researchers with suitable samples.

In 1987 the main purpose of the Cambridge brain bank changed after Cambridge was one of the centres chosen to carry through a large scale prospective study of ageing, including the dementias of old age. Before this study began, a research nurse had been appointed by the brain bank for a local epidemiological study of dementia which had also been funded by the MRC. One of the main tasks of the research nurse was to make contact with the relatives during a patient's illness and, when a patient died, to request consent for study of the brain.

The current research programme of the Cambridge brain bank takes place with the full knowledge and consent of the relatives.

This, however, has not always been the case. From the late 1970s, many brains were collected from Coroner's post mortems carried out at the mortuary at Addenbrooke's Hospital without the knowledge of the relatives. A simple system was in use to identify brains that would be of interest to the brain bank, either as index or "control" cases.

The senior technician in the brain bank would visit the mortuary early each morning to review the list of post mortems for the day. The technician would then report to the person in charge of the brain bank who, in turn, would ask the pathologist to retain the brain of any case of interest to the brain bank, provided it was not required for diagnostic purposes. Later in the day the brain would be taken to the brain bank.

The brains were identified from Coroner's cases and from hospital post mortems. In the latter case, consent forms had been signed by the relatives.

The late David Webb

The system for identifying brains that would be of interest to the Cambridge brain bank is illustrated by the case of the late David Webb. This has many similarities to the retention of the brain of Mr Isaacs in Manchester. In January 1988 Mr Webb, who had suffered from depression, was found dead in his car which was filled with exhaust fumes. His body was taken to the mortuary at Addenbrooke's Hospital where a post mortem was carried out two days later on the instructions of the Coroner for South and West Cambridgeshire.

Mr Webb's widow, who was aware that organ retention from Addenbrooke's mortuary was not uncommon, emphasised to the police officer, who was acting as Coroner's Officer, Mr Webb's personal convictions which should have precluded any retention of his organs for research.

It was not until 12 years later, as a result of the problems of organ retention revealed by the report of the investigation into the Royal Liverpool Children's Hospital, that Dr Webb, Mr Webb's widow, discovered that her husband's brain had been retained by the Cambridge brain bank for an investigation of the brains of victims of suicide. Although Mr Webb's brain, and the brains of 42 other suicide victims, had been collected by the brain bank, this research was never undertaken as funding was not obtained.

The Addenbrooke's Hospital mortuary serves not only the hospital but also the coronial districts in and around Cambridge. At the time of Mr Webb's death, Mr John Smith was the Coroner for South and West Cambridgeshire, but not the City of Cambridge. Mr Smith and his staff were unaware of the organ retention practices that were current in Addenbrooke's mortuary in the late 1980s.

In 1988 the Coroner for the City of Cambridge was Mr Sterndale Burrows, who had an office in the mortuary at Addenbrooke's Hospital.

When Mr John Smith was appointed Coroner for Cambridge City in 1991 following the death of Mr Sterndale Burrows, he became aware that organ retention had been common practice in the Addenbrooke's hospital mortuary.

Mr Smith gave instructions that no organs were to be retained from Coroner's cases without his knowledge and then only for diagnostic purposes, unless the consent of the relatives was obtained.

It is notable that Professor Gresham, the Professor of Pathology at Cambridge, and the late Mr Arthur Turner, the Chief Mortician at Addenbrooke's, were joint authors of a book on post mortem procedures that recommended the retention of organs for research and teaching purposes.

The retention of organs at Addenbrooke's Hospital mortuary in the 1980s and earlier years was not confined to brains, although these represent the largest number of organs retained.

Research conducted under Coroners Rules 9 and 12

Investigations at the Clinical Research Centre, Northwick Park, and at St George's Hospital, London, showed that a number of Coroners in the London area had been approached by research teams at these locations who had asked for the Coroners' agreement to the collection of brains or brain samples under Coroners Rules 9 and/or 12.

These rules provide that the Coroner may authorise retention of tissues and organs (referred to as *"material"*) where an investigation may provide evidence that is directly relevant to the cause of death.

The first of these studies was undertaken at the Clinical Research Centre with the agreement of Dr D R (Bob) Chambers, Coroner for St Pancras, later the Inner North London District. This research study involved the collection of brains of those who had committed suicide. The brains were studied and compared with the brains of patients with neuropsychiatric diseases, including Alzheimer's disease and schizophrenia. These brains were obtained with the consent of the relatives of patients who had died in Shenley Hospital, a long-stay mental hospital in Hertfordshire.

Similar studies of the brains of suicides under Coroners Rules 9 and 12 were carried out at St George's Hospital, beginning in 1984. For these investigations the collection of brain samples was authorised by a number of Coroners in South and West London and adjacent districts. In one investigation some of the Coroners also authorised the collection of brain samples from "controls" matched by gender and age who had died of unrelated disease.

Research on brains initially referred for diagnostic purposes

Investigation of the brain collections held at the Radcliffe Infirmary, Oxford, at the Queen's Medical Centre, Nottingham, and in other places showed that all brains in these collections had been obtained for diagnosis and that those of interest for research had been retained after the diagnostic procedures were complete. These brains had later been used in research studies and, at Nottingham, also held for "diagnostic review".

In this context the term "diagnostic review" was used at Nottingham to describe the re-examination of categories of brain specimens to see if the existing diagnostic criteria could be further redefined to identify previously unrecognised sub-categories within the larger diagnostic group. For example, Alzheimer's disease was considered as a single diagnosis; it is now sub-categorised to include different types of dementia that have the same clinical picture but different histological findings.

Diagnostic review is an important procedure for the advancement of the knowledge of neuropsychiatric disease. Similarly, brain collections such as those at Oxford, Cambridge, Edinburgh, Nottingham and elsewhere have been used to discover if a condition such as variant CJD is a new disorder or one that has been observed in the past. Studies of this kind can only be carried out by reference to brain collections and archives.

Knowledge of the relatives

Many of the investigations referred to in the preceding paragraphs involve the study of brains or brain samples from Coroners' post mortems without the knowledge of the relatives. In those locations where research was carried out under Coroners Rules 9 and 12, the Coroners were aware of the studies and had authorised the investigations. In other locations there is no documentary confirmation that the Coroners were informed but, for the reasons mentioned, it is improbable that the Coroners would have been aware of every case where a brain was retained because the post mortem reports were almost always silent.

Questionnaire to NHS Trusts that were not visited as part of this investigation

The total number of retained brains reported to the Chief Medical Officer's Census in 2000 was 28,107. These brains had been obtained between 1970 and 1999. These returns included separate totals (i) for hospital and Coroners' cases, and (ii) for brain archives. The data for the 6,491 brains held in archives did not distinguish between hospital and Coroners' cases. Many Trusts reported holding no brains from Coroners' cases.

There were, however, more than 20 Trusts that in 2000 reported holding an archive or a collection that included more than 50 brains from Coroners' cases collected between 1970 and 1999. In 1999, the last year covered by the Chief Medical Officer's Census, a total of 650 brains from Coroners' cases had been retained.

A questionnaire requesting further details of the consent arrangements when brains had been collected was sent to the Trusts which had reported holding large numbers of brains from Coroners' cases. (Trusts were not asked to recount the brains in their collections.) The questionnaire was not sent to Trusts that had already been visited during this investigation.

The responses from 17 NHS Trusts in England which I have not visited show that the practice of using brains from Coroners' cases in research was very widespread. These Trusts between them hold 25 brain collections, including nine categorised as archives. The brains held in these collections and archives were mainly obtained between 1970 and 1999. In some places research and/or teaching use of brains from Coroners' cases continued throughout the 1990s, in some only ending when publicity was given to unconsented organ retention.

In total the responses from the Trusts show that more than 14,600 brains from Coroners' cases are held in the collections which reported to the Chief Medical Officer's 2000 Census, and that a further 8,000 brains are held in archives. The number of Coroners' cases within the archived collections is unknown. These figures relate to brains held in collections and do not include those from Coroners' cases which have been disposed of after the diagnostic procedures for which the brains had been retained had been completed.

The responses to the questionnaires show that the large majorities of the brains from Coroners' cases were retained for diagnostic reasons and used for research after diagnosis was complete. The collection of brains solely for research was reported by seven Trusts. These responses confirm that the collection of brains for research purposes was not confined to the joint programme in Manchester and to the Cambridge brain bank.

The extent to which Coroners were aware of the retention of brains varied from one location to the next. Only one of the Trusts in responding to the questionnaire reported that the Coroner had given written authorisation for the collection and use of brains in research. This excludes studies that were specifically carried out under Coroners Rules 9 and 12.

Frequently, the responses stated that the Coroners had given verbal agreement. As these centres have not been investigated and many of the Coroners have passed on, it is impossible to determine how far the pathologists simply assumed that they had the agreement of the Coroner for their actions.

Teaching use of retained brains

I was informed of an investigation carried out by Sheffield City Council in 1987 when it was discovered that brains from the public mortuary were being provided for teaching use in the Anatomy Department of Sheffield University. This incident was fully investigated at the time and reported in the national media. It is, however, relevant to this investigation as other medical schools had obtained brains for teaching purposes from public mortuaries up to and including the late 1980s.

Following this discovery, my predecessor as HM Inspector of Anatomy, the late Dr Paul Mason, wrote in February 1987 to all anatomy departments to ensure that the collection of brains for teaching use took place only with the knowledge and agreement of the relatives.

Concern about the transmission of diseases such as CJD has, since the early 1990s, precluded the collection of brains for medical education purposes, even in situations where the relatives have given their consent.

The position of organisations and other bodies regarding organ retention from Coroners' post mortems

Ethics Committees

The position of Ethics Committees in the Manchester area has been described already. In other locations, Ethics Committees were generally consulted when research involving retention of organs was undertaken in an investigation that first studied the patient in life and later the brain after death.

Until 1991 most Ethics Committees appear not to have taken a close interest in research that was exclusively undertaken post mortem. In that year a new circular from the Department of Health placed on Ethics Committees the responsibility to consider *"research on the recently dead"*.

Nevertheless, prior to 1991, whenever Ethics Committees were informed that "controls" were to be studied, the Committees would have expected to be fully informed about the circumstances in which the "controls" were obtained.

Apart from the joint research programme at Manchester, the brain bank at Cambridge is the only other programme visited during this investigation that systematically collected brains for research unrelated to the cause of the death and without the knowledge of the relatives. There is no evidence that this method of collection of brains was ever submitted for approval to the Cambridge Ethics Committee.

The responses to the questionnaire suggest that this practice occurred in nine other locations where brains from Coroners' cases were collected as "controls".

Research funding organisations

Several organisations funded post mortem research on the brain in the 1980s and 1990s.

The North West Regional Health Authority

The North West Regional Health Authority (NWRHA) was the first to finance the research undertaken by the joint programme. The applications made to the NWRHA were, like the applications submitted to Ethics Committees in the Manchester area, silent on the question of Coroners' post mortems. For the second and third applications to the NWRHA this was relevant, as the main source of brains collected for the programme between 1985 and 1988 had been from Coroners' post mortems.

Two of the applications to the NWRHA mention "controls", but not Coroners' post mortems.

The Mental Health Foundation

An application to the Mental Health Foundation for a grant to start in September 1988 refers to obtaining brains from the Lancashire area "*via the Rochdale Coroner*". This is the first reference in any application to the involvement of the North Manchester Coroner's office in Rochdale.

The Medical Research Council

The Medical Research Council (MRC) is foremost among those organisations that funded research on the brain. The first reference to MRC support for brain banking identified in this investigation was the grant awarded in 1950 to support the collection of brains by Dr Corsellis at Runwell Hospital.

In subsequent decades, the MRC had two separate roles; the first as a funder of research projects and programmes, including the Cambridge brain bank which began in 1970 within an MRC-funded unit; the second as the Government's leading institution for the financing of medical research.

As a research funding organisation, the MRC provided programme grant support for the Cambridge brain bank in 1985, and funded several other brain banking programmes in subsequent years. Separately, the Council has financed many research projects submitted through its competitive grants system. Among these were three project grants awarded to the joint programme in Manchester in 1988 and 1989.

In considering grant applications in the late 1980s, the Council relied on the research applicant to submit his research for Ethics Committee approval. The MRC did not separately evaluate the ethics of the projects. However, the MRC's Terms and Conditions for Project Grants and the Council's grant application forms became progressively more stringent in the information requested about ethics approval during the 1980s.

In its wider role, the MRC was in 1962/3 the first organisation in the UK to formulate guidelines for consideration of the ethics of research on patients. From these guidelines, and the report of the Royal of College of Physicians in 1966, the whole Ethics Committee structures have developed.

As part of its responsibilities for developing medical research, the MRC has, from time to time, organised reviews of research fields to identify which new research initiatives and developments would have the best prospect of success.

In this context, in 1974 the MRC organised a review of brain banking. This review was chaired by the late Professor Corsellis. The review meeting included many of the Council's scientific staff who were themselves undertaking research on the brain. At that meeting, and at later meetings about the collection of pituitaries, the Council were made aware, through comments recorded in the notes of the meetings, that Coroners' post mortems were being used as a source of post mortem material. At one meeting in December 1977 the legal position of such use was questioned, and the DHSS was consulted. The DHSS in turn contacted the Home Office, but the eventual reply, if any, given by the DHSS to the MRC is not available.

The Council did not, however, directly question the use of Coroners' post mortems as a source of research material in the 1980s when awarding grants for post mortem research.

The Wellcome Trust

The Wellcome Trust also funded post mortem research. Like the MRC, the Trust expected the researchers to submit their applications to Ethics Committees whenever this was appropriate. The Trust did not itself consider the ethical aspects of research involving post mortem examinations.

The Royal College of Pathologists

Although the College had encouraged pathologists to conduct "full" post mortems in the late 1980s, it was not until 1991 that the College, jointly with the Royal College of Physicians and the Royal College of Surgeons, issued formal guidance in a report entitled "*The Autopsy and Audit*".

In 1993 the Royal College of Pathologists issued their own document on *"Guidelines for Post Mortem Reports"*. This emphasised:

"a single standard should be applicable to all post mortem examinations, whether funded by an NHS Coroner or Procurator Fiscal".

The guidelines supported the *"desirability of retention of tissues for histological examination in most cases"* and encouraged the comprehensive reporting of all findings.

There was no reference to the different purpose of a Coroner's post mortem from a hospital post mortem undertaken with the consent of the relatives and, in the context of organ retention, no mention of the need to check that the relatives did not object.

The importance of audit was re-emphasised.

The College, responding to the growing awareness of the distress caused by the retention of organs and tissues and the public's reluctance to agree to hospital post mortems, a trend which had started in the 1960s, issued new guidance in March 2000 entitled *"Guidelines for the Retention of Tissues and Organs at Post Mortem Examination"*. This report was published before the Redfern Report on the problems of organ retention at the Royal Liverpool Children's Hospital.

In the guidelines issued in 2000 the College emphasise the legal and ethical principles that must apply to all retention of tissues:

- retention of tissue must be lawful;
- reasons for retention of tissue must be defensible, open and justifiable in law and in clinical practice;
- unless the post mortem is directed by law, the procedures must be sufficiently flexible to reflect the wishes of relatives, while maintaining standards of diagnostic accuracy.

The guidelines state it is unlawful for a pathologist to perform a post mortem examination, or to retain any tissue, without proper authorisation. It is emphasised that the retention of organs and tissues from a Coroner's post mortem, other than for investigation of the death, must be in accordance with the Human Tissue Act.

These guidelines from the College rightly reflect the importance and need for consent by the relatives for tissue retention. There are, however, a number of pathologists who believe that a full post mortem should be carried out in every Coroner's case, even though this is not necessary in all cases to achieve the Coroner's purpose, which is solely to establish the cause of death. This position is based on the knowledge that many abnormalities that may have a bearing on the cause of death are discovered only after a full post mortem examination.

The Royal College of Psychiatrists

The Royal College of Psychiatrists has emphasised the importance of approval of research by Ethics Committees from the start of the Ethics Committee approval system. Ethical clearance is particularly important in research on patients with psychiatric conditions where the capacity of the individual to consent may be reduced.

In the 1991 guidance from the Department of Health to Ethics Committees, the advice given by the Royal College regarding research on mentally disordered people was commended as a source of additional guidance for mental health research.

While the Royal College of Psychiatrists has not issued guidance specifically on post mortem research on the brain, the College would expect any research studies that investigated the patient's mental health in life and studied the brain after death to be approved by an Ethics Committee.

In June 2000 the Royal College recommended that the approval of any research using records or archive samples must be sought from the appropriate Ethics Committee.

The General Medical Council

The General Medical Council's series of guidance documents on *"Professional Conduct and Discipline: Fitness to Practise"* have, since 1980, included recommendations that affect the conduct of doctors carrying out research on post mortem material.

In August 1980 the Council's guidance emphasised the importance of maintaining confidentiality:

"It is a doctor's duty strictly to observe the rule of professional secrecy by refraining from disclosing voluntarily to a third party information which he has learned directly or indirectly in his professional relationship with the patient. The death of the patient does not absolve the doctor from the obligation to maintain secrecy".

When the guidance was revised in August 1983, further emphasis was given that the death of the patient did not absolve the doctor from the obligation to maintain secrecy.

However:

"Information may be disclosed if necessary for a medical research project which has been approved by a recognised Ethical Committee".

The guidance on research and on maintaining professional confidentiality has been further developed in later documents issued by the Council, in particular on the principles for obtaining valid consent. The latest guidance refers specifically to the involvement of Research Ethics Committees in considering studies where participants are unable to give consent for the use of data identifiable to them.

Why did research on organs and tissues obtained from Coroners' post mortems continue unchecked for so long?

There is no one single reason that accounts for the extensive and prolonged use of organs and tissues from Coroners' post mortems in research.

A major misunderstanding of the Human Tissue Act and the Coroners Rules was the fundamental reason. Pathologists, morticians, researchers and others believed that the Coroner's consent was all that was required for the retention of any organs and tissues for research or teaching. The fact that Coroners could only consent to the retention of "material" relevant to the cause of death was widely unknown or disregarded.

While organs and tissues were retained in the erroneous belief that the Coroner had authority to permit retention without reference to the relatives, this justification could not be invoked in districts where the Coroner was unaware of the retention and had never even been asked. The examples in this report show that some Coroners were unaware that organ retention was taking place.

The apprenticeship training of pathologists was identified during a meeting at the Royal College as having a major influence on the practice of pathologists in the 1970s and 1980s. Pathologists had been trained by their seniors to carry out a full post mortem examination and it was common practice to retain organs and tissues that were of interest for research or for teaching.

Pathologists were also motivated by benefits to the "public good" resulting from research on post mortem tissues. The purpose of carrying out a full post mortem and of retaining tissue was better to identify the cause of death and to improve the quality of care for future generations. Pathologists did not consider their practice was in any way wrong or unacceptable to relatives.

The circumstances of organ retention in the North Manchester coronial district appear exceptional in that the Coroner's office staff were directly involved in identifying cases where the retained brain might be suitable for the joint research programme.

Pathologists, morticians and the Coroner's Officers (who were then serving police officers) in the North Manchester district were all misled to believe that the retention of brains for research was lawful if it was with the authority of the Coroner.

Was the Coroner for North Manchester district aware of organ retention from cases reported to him?

There is a conflict of evidence on whether Mr North was aware of the retention of organs of cases reported to him. Mr North's letters to pathologists who asked about access to retained organs for research clearly state the correct legal position. However, if Mr North was aware that brains were being retained on the instructions of his staff, he did nothing to stop the practice. I find it hard to believe Mr North did not know.

One practical reason that hid organ retention from relatives was the omission of any mention of organ and tissue retention from reports submitted to the Coroner. Indeed, the relevant appendix to the Coroners Rules refers only obliquely to tissue retention.

Where have these procedures led?

The report of the investigation at the Royal Liverpool Children's Hospital brought into the public domain the extent of the practice of organ retention after hospital post mortems on children. The Census of retained organs carried out by the Chief Medical Officer in 2000 indicated that a very large number of organs and tissues from adults and children had been retained from both Coroners' and hospital post mortems in the years 1970-1998, and that organ retention was continuing on a large scale during 1999.

The public's confidence in the medical profession to seek consent has been seriously undermined by these findings. The hospital post mortem rate, which was already falling, has reduced further and there is a very great reluctance among many of the population to agree to any form of organ or tissue retention.

These events have unsurprisingly had a very dramatic effect on reducing the availability of organs and tissues on post mortem research. Past undisclosed organ retention has put at risk the excellent work of many research teams who have scrupulously observed all the ethical and legal requirements and have routinely obtained consent from the relatives before any organ retention took place.

Researchers in this country have been among the leaders of the international research effort to discover new knowledge from post mortem studies of the brain and, from the knowledge gained, to improve future patient care and prevent neuropsychiatric disease and premature deaths.

There are many people who wish to help future generations through the study of their organs and tissues after death. However, it will be a disaster if this report leads to a further reduction in the availability of organs and tissues for post mortem studies when the lawful requirements, ethical approval and consent of the relatives have all been obtained.

Action already taken

Following the publicity already given to organ retention in Coroners' cases, many Coroners have given instructions to their Officers and to their office staff that relatives must be given a proper explanation about the reasons for a post mortem examination. If there are objections, arrangements have been made in some districts for further discussion before the examination goes ahead.

Some Coroners have given instructions that no organs and tissues are to be retained except with their consent and then only for diagnostic reasons. Consent for retention unrelated to the cause of death may only take place after reference to the Coroner and then only when the relatives have confirmed their agreement.

Coroners have introduced forms to be completed after every post mortem to record what, if any, tissues have been held back and the relatives' instructions regarding eventual disposal.

Objections to post mortems

The above measures will provide some reassurance to those who have no objections in principle to post mortems and organ retention. However, there are, in our multicultural society, faith groups who on account of their religious beliefs cannot accept post mortems and, particularly, organ retention. For these groups, which include the Hindu, Jewish and Moslem faith communities, the need for a post mortem is incompatible with their beliefs.

There are also some Christian denominations and individuals who have religious objections. Others of no religious persuasion sincerely believe that the post mortem examination is an affront to the respect and dignity that should be accorded to the human body after death.

For all these groups, post mortems and organ retention create grave difficulties when the examination is carried out on the instructions of the Coroner, as they have no choice in the matter.

While these faith communities and individuals recognise that their beliefs cannot be accommodated within the requirements of the law, their views are sincerely held and it is important that their religious requirements and observances are acknowledged, provided that these do not impede the Coroner's investigations.

Where there are no suspicious circumstances there are other ways than post mortem to investigate a sudden death. These methods need further exploration. The technique of Magnetic Resonance Imaging (MRI) has been accepted by some Coroners as an alternative to a post mortem when the MRI technique provides a definitive cause of death. The MRI technique requires further evaluation.

Alternative systems for death certification are being considered by the Fundamental Review of Coroner Services; the alternative procedures for death certification which the review is considering go beyond the scope of this investigation.

For the faith communities, limited post mortems are more acceptable than full post mortems, and post mortems without organ and tissue retention are preferable as the body can then be buried or cremated whole.

For some faith communities, burial or cremation on the day of death is of the greatest importance and arrangements have been made in many places for the Coroner's procedures to be expedited to permit the observance of this religious requirement.

There are other religious rituals and observances, for example the saying of prayers over the deceased, which can be facilitated in deaths reported to the Coroner and which in some districts have been permitted and found not to impede the Coroner's investigations.

Inevitably there will be a minority of deaths reported to the Coroner where the nature of the death and/or a criminal investigation will not permit religious observances.

The way forward

The investigation of events that followed Mr Isaacs' death has shown that the retention of his brain for research was not an isolated incident. Research on organs, particularly brains, retained after Coroners' post mortems was widespread during the 1980s and 1990s as well as in earlier years.

The relatives were almost always unaware that organs and tissues had been retained. The discovery of organ retention has caused much distress, particularly among the faith communities where post mortems and organ retention conflict with religious observance.

While for others in our multicultural population a post mortem examination is the acceptable way of identifying the cause of death, the problems of covert and unconsented organ retention have undermined public confidence. Much of this research was, however, intended for the public good and carried out on organs that were initially obtained for sound diagnostic reasons.

Since the publicity given to organ retention in the Redfern Report and others, a number of important safeguards have been introduced. If these are strictly observed, it should be impossible for organs and tissues from Coroners' and hospital post mortems to be retained for use in research or teaching without the knowledge and consent of the relatives.

The restoration of public confidence must be the first and urgent priority. Confidence must be re-established that post mortems in general, and Coroners' post mortems in particular, will not be used as a source of organs and tissues for research and teaching without proper consent.

In 2001 over 200,000 sudden deaths were reported to Coroners in England and Wales. These included a minority of unnatural deaths and deaths in suspicious circumstances. The large majority were, however, due to natural causes. Nevertheless, some investigation into the cause of all these deaths is essential though a post mortem examination will not be necessary in every case. The system for investigating deaths reported to the Coroner must be freed from any suspicion of covert organ retention.

A further urgent reason for restoration of public confidence in the post mortem procedures are the many improvements in patient care that have resulted from knowledge gained from post mortem research. If the benefits from post mortem research are to continue, all pathologists, others involved in post mortems and research teams must be scrupulous in observing all the legal and ethical requirements.

The recommendations in this report are intended primarily to assist in the restoration of public confidence. They will also facilitate the continuation of research on post mortem organs and tissues, but only with the full knowledge and consent of the relatives.

Annexes

Appendices

Acronyms

Acronym	Chapter	Description
CFAS	26, 30, 38, 46	Cognitive Function and Ageing Study
CFU	C, 8, 9, 12, 13, 16, 23, S	Cerebral Function Unit
CJD	5, 7, 28, 46, S	Creutzfeldt Jacob Disease
COMBAT	26	Charitable organisation that provided support for people with Huntington's Disease and their families
CRC	9, 10, 32, 38	Clinical Research Centre
LREC	UQ, 6, 12, 14, 24, 30, 38, 39, 41, 47, An	Local Research Ethics Committee
MRC	UQ, 5, 7, 9, 11, 25, 26, 31, 32, 38, 47, S, Ap	Medical Research Council
MRI	C, 9, 44, S	Magnetic Resonance Imaging
NCEPOD	40	National Confidential Enquiry into Perioperative Deaths
NCPU	7, 26, 38	Neurochemical Pharmacology Unit
NMEC	13, S	North Manchester Ethics Committee
NMGH	C, 9, 10, 13, 16, 21, 22, 23, 24, 25, 42, S	North Manchester General Hospital
NWRHA	UQ, 9, 10, 11, 14, 23, 25, S, Ap	North Western Regional Health Authority
OPTIMA	30, 46	Oxford Project to Investigate Memory and Ageing
QMC	28, 29	Queen's Medical Centre, Nottingham
SEC	12, 14, 18	Salford Ethics Committee
SHSA	37	Special Hospitals Service Authority
SMEC	13, 18, S	South Manchester Ethics Committee

Notes

An: List of Annexes
Ap: List of Appendices
C: Conclusions
S: Summary
UQ: Unanswered Questions

Glossary of Terms

Alzheimer's Disease

A progressive form of dementia occurring usually in late middle age. It is associated with diffuse degeneration disease of the brain.

Autopsy

Examination of a body after death in order to determine the cause of death or presence of disease processes. (Also referred to as post mortem examination or necropsy).

Community or Public Mortuary

A mortuary owned by the local authority with facilities for the storage and preservation of material and for the conduct of post mortems on persons who have died in the community.

Controls (as applied to pathology)

Specimens of organs or tissues obtained from individuals who are not affected by the disease process that is being investigated. These "normal" control organs or tissues can be compared with those obtained from those individuals possibly affected by the disease process that is being investigated.

Coroner

An independent judicial officer acting on behalf of the Crown to investigate the cause and circumstances of violent or unnatural deaths, or sudden deaths of an unknown cause. Coroners must be legally and/or medically qualified, although most are now drawn from the legal profession.

Coroner's Officer

A Coroner's Officer is either a serving police officer permanently seconded to the Coroner's office to undertake the day-to-day routine of investigation of deaths reported to the Coroner, or a civilian appointed for the same purpose. The Coroner's Officer's duties may entail the Officer compiling a report in respect of each sudden death. She/he may compile the report her/himself or collate reports provided by uniformed police officers and other witnesses. Increasingly the position of Coroner's Officer has been made a civilian rather than a police appointment.

Coroner's Post Mortem

Post mortem examination carried out on the instructions of the Coroner. The consent of the next of kin is not required for a Coroner's post mortem. The purpose of a Coroner's post mortem examination is to provide the Coroner with information relevant to determining the cause of death. The Coroner is not required to order a post mortem examination in every case reported to him where information obtained from other sources provides satisfactory evidence to establish the cause of death.

Coroners Rules 1984

The Rules set out in secondary legislation the procedures that Coroners should observe in the exercise of their duties. The present Rules, enacted by Parliament, became operative on 1 July 1984. The Rules set out procedures to be followed in arranging post mortem examinations, burial orders, inquests, records to be kept and documents and forms to be used.

Coroner's Staff

The administrative office staff employed by the local authority to assist the Coroner in carrying out his duties.

Dementia

A disorder of brain function, usually chronic and progressive, that is the result of brain disease but may follow severe head injuries. Dementia is characterised by memory loss, particularly short-term loss, changes in personality, inability to attend to personal care, confusion and disorientation.

Down's Syndrome

A congenital disorder that is the single most frequent cause of mental retardation. It is the result of the affected person usually having 47 chromosomes rather than the usual 46. Down's Syndrome is characterised by learning difficulties of varying severity and sometimes physical abnormalities.

Ethics Committee (EC)

A committee set up to advise NHS bodies (or other organisation) on the ethical acceptability of research proposals involving human subjects or human material. Ethics Committees provide independent advice and members of the committees include in their membership both lay and professional members who bring together a broad range of experience and expertise to reconcile scientific and medical aspects of research with the interests and welfare of research subjects.

Histology

The study of the internal structure of cells and tissues by means of special staining techniques combined with light and electron microscopy.

Hospital Mortuary

A mortuary on a hospital site with facilities for the storage of bodies of those who have died in the hospital and usually for the conduct of post mortems.

Huntington's Disease

A progressive hereditary disease characterised by involuntary movements and dementia. The genetic defect has now been identified and genetic screening is available for those at risk.

Inquest

A public hearing called by the Coroner in specific circumstances to ascertain the identity of the deceased and to establish how, when and where the death occurred. The proceedings are inquisitorial by nature. An inquest is appropriate when the person:

(a) died a violent or unnatural death; or
(b) died a sudden death of which the cause is unknown; or
(c) died in prison or in such a place or in such circumstances as to require an inquest under any other Act.

Jewish Burial Board

A co-operative organisation within a Jewish community that makes arrangements for funerals and pays burial costs and fees for its members.

Magnetic Resonance Imaging (MRI)

A non-invasive method of imaging the body and organs within it. The technique has been used in some locations with the agreement of the Coroner to identify the cause of death as an alternative to post mortem. However, the technique is applicable for this purpose in a minority of cases of sudden death and requires further evaluation.

Mortuary Technician

An employee of the hospital or local authority who is responsible for the operation of the mortuary in respect of the reception and storage of bodies. Where a post mortem is undertaken, the technician assists and is directed by the pathologist during the examination.

Neuropathology

A study of diseases affecting the nervous system by microscopic examination of tissue samples to identify diseases and injuries to the brain and spinal cord.

Organ

A part of the body that forms a structural unit and/or is responsible for a particular function (or functions). Organs may be composed of more than one tissue and may be large, for example the liver, or very small, for example the pituitary.

Parkinson's Disease

A disorder predominantly of middle aged and elderly people characterised by tremor, rigidity, mask-like facial immobility and a poverty of spontaneous movement. The first and most prominent symptom is tremor, which often initially affects one limb and then spreads progressively to affect other limbs.

Schizophrenia

A mental disorder (or group of disorders) of variable severity characterised by a disintegration of the process of thinking, of contact with reality, and of emotional responsiveness and usually extensive withdrawal of an individual's interest in other people and their outside world. Delusions and hallucinations (especially hearing voices) are frequent features, and a patient with this disorder often feels that their thoughts, sensations, and actions are controlled by, or shared with, others.

Tissue

A collection of cells specialised to perform a particular function. The cells may be of the same type (e.g. in nervous tissue) or of different types (e.g. in connective tissue). Aggregations of tissue constitute organs.

Tissue Blocks

Tissue blocks are small samples taken from organs which are then stabilised by a process called "fixation" so that wafer thin slices may later be cut for examination on glass slides under the microscope.

Toxicology

The study of poisonous materials and their effects upon living organisms. Toxicological investigations may form part of a post mortem examination to discover if drugs, or other chemical substances, were implicated or caused death.